NEUROPEPTIDE INFLUENCES ON THE BRAIN AND BEHAVIOR

Advances in Biochemical Psychopharmacology
Volume 17

Advances in Biochemical Psychopharmacology

Series Editors:

Erminio Costa, M.D.

Chief, Laboratory of Preclinical Pharmacology
National Institute of Mental Health
Washington, D.C.

Paul Greengard, Ph.D.

Professor of Pharmacology
Yale University School of Medicine
New Haven, Connecticut

Neuropeptide Influences on the Brain and Behavior

Advances in Biochemical Psychopharmacology
Volume 17

Edited by

Lyle H. Miller, Ph.D.

Department of Psychiatry
Temple University School of Medicine
Philadelphia, Pennsylvania

Curt A. Sandman, Ph.D.

Department of Psychology
The Ohio State University
Columbus, Ohio

Abba J. Kastin, M.D.

Endocrinology Section
Veterans Administration Hospital and
Department of Medicine
Tulane University
New Orleans, Louisiana

Raven Press ■ New York

Raven Press, 1140 Avenue of the Americas, New York, New York 10036

Made in the United States of America

Library of Congress Cataloging in Publication Data.

Miller, Lyle.
    Neuropeptide influences on the brain and behavior.

    Includes index.
    1. Neuropsychology. 2. Peptide hormones.
3. Neuroendocrinology. I. Sandman, Curt A., joint
author. II. Kastin, Abba J., joint author. III. Title.
(DNLM: 1. Neurochemistry. 2. Peptides—Pharmaco-
dynamics. 3. Hormones—Pharmacodynamics. 4. Brain—
Drug effects. 5. Behavior—Drug effects. WL104
M684n)
QP360.M52   612'.822   76-5663
ISBN 0-89004-130-X

Preface

In the last thirty years there has been a phenomenal increase in knowledge of hormonal influences on behavior. The early studies dealing with the involvement of the pituitary-adrenal axis in stress reactions have, for example, stimulated investigation into the direct effects of ACTH and its fractions on the central nervous system and behavior. Research in the United States and abroad has widened the neuropeptide field to include MSH and its fractions, vasopressin, and a host of other polypeptide hormones. Extensive, multidisciplinary research programs throughout the world bring additional factual information regarding the behavioral significance of the neuropeptides to our constant attention.

While the data base has proliferated at a constantly accelerating pace, its theoretical integration has lagged. Behavioral research on the neuropeptides has reached the point where it seems that an investigator has the choice of repeating similar studies with minor modifications or of developing new paradigms which may, or may not, be productive. It is time for reflection on the theoretical implications the neuropeptides hold for the more traditional views of brain-behavior relationships. It is time for the development of some sort of theoretical overview that will aid in the development of new paradigms and lead to additional insights into the nature of neuropeptide influences on the central nervous system and behavior.

The papers in this volume provide comprehensive overviews of ongoing peptide research, as well as syntheses of the existing neuropeptide data against the background of the literature in relevant brain-behavior areas, including attention, learning, memory, emotion, pharmacology, neural substrates, psychophysiology, electrophysiology, and biochemistry.

Lyle H. Miller
Curt A. Sandman
Abba J. Kastin

Acknowledgments

We wish to thank Betty Flowers, Julie Lore, Darlene Miller, Martha Rudrauff, Nancy Thode, and Patti Watson for their invaluable assistance at the conference and for their contributions to the preparation of the manuscripts. We gratefully acknowledge the financial support of Organon, N.V., the Veterans Administration, Abbott Laboratories, Hoffman-La Roche, and MacNeil Laboratories.

Contents

Contributors

Michael S. Beattie, M.A.
Laboratory of Comparative and Physio-
  logical Psychology
The Ohio State University
1314 Kinnear Road
Columbus, Ohio 43212

Sanford I. Cohen, M.D.
Division of Psychiatry
Boston University School of Medicine
720 Harrison Avenue
Boston, Massachusetts 02118

David de Wied, M.D.
Rudolf Magnus Institute for
  Pharmacology
State University Utrecht
Padualaan 8 Utrecht, The Netherlands

Elemér Endröczi, M.D., D.Sc.
Central Research Division and Institute
  of Experimental and Clinical
  Laboratory Investigations
Postgraduate Medical School,
  P.O.B. 112
1389 Budapest, Szabolcs u. 35 Hungary

Paul Garrud, M.D., D. Phil.
Department of Experimental
  Psychology
Oxford University
South Parks Road
Oxford OX1 3UD England

W.H. Gispen, Ph.D.
Division of Molecular Neurobiology
Institute of Molecular Biology
State University Utrecht
Padualaan 8 Utrecht, The Netherlands

Paul E. Gold, Ph.D.
Department of Psychology
University of Virginia
Charlottesville, Virginia 22901

Jeffrey A. Gray, Ph.D.
Department of Experimental
  Psychology
South Parks Road
Oxford, England OX1 3UD England

Henk M. Greven, M.D.
Department of Pharmacology
Organon International, N.V.
Oss, The Netherlands

John W. Hennessy, Ph.D.
Stanford University School of Medicine
  Department of Psychiatry and
  Behavioral Sciences
Stanford, California 94305
Presently: Irish Foundation for Human
  Development
Psychomatic Unit, Garden Hill
Dublin 8 Ireland

Paula L. Hoffman, Ph.D.
Department of Physiology and
  Biophysics
University of Illinois at the Medical
  Center
901 South Wolcott Street
Chicago, Illinois 60612

Abba J. Kastin, M.D.
Endocrinology Section of the Medical
  Service
Veterans Administration Hospital and
  Department of Medicine
Tulane University School of Medicine
New Orleans, Louisiana 70146

Gregory A. Kimble, Ph.D.
Department of Psychology
University of Colorado
Boulder, Colorado 80309

Seymour Levine, Ph.D.
Department of Psychiatry and
  Behavioral Sciences
Stanford University School of Medicine
Stanford, California 94305

James L.McGaugh, Ph.D.
Department of Psychobiology
University of California
Irvine, California 92717

Donald R. Meyer, Ph.D.
Department of Psychology
The Ohio State University
202 Kinnear Road
Columbus, Ohio 43212

Lyle II. Miller, Ph.D.
Department of Psychiatry
Temple University School of Medicine
Philadelphia, Pennsylvania 19140

Allan F. Mirsky, Ph.D.
Department of Psychiatry (Neuropsy-
chology) and Neurology
Boston University School of Medicine
80 East Concord Street
Boston, Massachusetts 02118

Merle M. Orren, Ph.D.
Department of Psychiatry (Neuropsy-
chology)
Boston University School of Medicine
80 East Concord Street
Boston, Massachusetts 02118

Nicholas P. Plotnikoff, Ph.D.
360 West Sheridan Place
Lake Bluff, Illinois 60044

Karl H. Pribram, M.D.
Departments of Psychology and of
Psychiatry and Behavioral Science
Stanford University
Stanford, California 94305

M.E.A. Reith, Ph.D.
Division of Molecular Neurobiology
Institute of Molecular Biology
State University Utrecht
Padualaan 8 Utrecht, The Netherlands

Henk Rigter, Ph.D.
Department of Pharmacology
Organon International, N.V.
Oss, The Netherlands

Curt A. Sandman, Ph.D.
Department of Psychology
The Ohio State University
Columbus, Ohio 43210

P. Schotman, Ph.D.
Division of Molecular Neurobiology
Institute of Molecular Biology
State University Utrecht
Padualaan 8 Utrecht, The Netherlands

Charles Shagass, M.D.
Department of Psychiatry, Temple
University, and Eastern Pennsylvania
Psychiatric Institute
3300 Henry Avenue
Philadelphia, Pennsylvania 19129

William P. Smotherman, Ph.D.
Department of Psychiatry and
Behavioral Science
Stanford University School of Medicine
Stanford, California 94305

Henk van Riezen, M.D.
Department of Pharmacology
Organon International, N.V.
Oss, The Netherlands

Roderich Walter, Ph.D.
Department of Physiology and
Biophysics
University of Illinois at the Medical
Center
901 South Wolcott Street
Chicago, Illinois 60612

V.M.Wiegant, Ph.D.
Division of Molecular Neurobiology
Institute of Molecular Biology
State University Utrecht
Padualaan 8 Utrecht, The Netherlands

H. Zwiers, Ph.D.
Division of Molecular Neurobiology
Institute of Molecular Biology
State University Utrecht
Padualaan 8 Utrecht, The Netherlands

Neuropeptide Influences on the Brain and Behavior, edited by L.H. Miller, C.A. Sandman, and A.J. Kastin. Raven Press, New York © 1977.

Introduction: Perspectives on the Behavioral Effects of the Neuropeptides

*Curt A. Sandman, **Lyle H. Miller, and †Abba J. Kastin

*Department of Psychology, Ohio State University, Columbus, Ohio 43210; **Department of Psychiatry, Temple University, Philadelphia, Pennsylvania 19129; †Department of Medicine, Veterans Administration Hospital, and Tulane University, New Orleans, Louisiana 70140

NEUROPEPTIDE INFLUENCES

Early Conceptions

Exciting challenges to classically held beliefs regarding the functioning of the endocrine and central nervous systems have been accumulating. Historically the pituitary-adrenal axis has been implicated in the stress response of most animals (24). This response was thought to be mediated only by target organs far removed from the brain. Thus the actions of pituitary hormones were thought to be due to their peripheral actions and were considered to be slow-acting and primarily passive. However, Selye's (24) analysis of the pituitary-adrenal axis significantly changed earlier conceptions of the endocrine system since he speculated that the endocrine system could play a central role in the organism's response to the external environment.

Parallel and often overlooked developments were occurring with respect to the relationship between brain chemistry and behavior. The early experiments of Thompson and McConnell (26) and then the plethora of replications and extensions indicated that amino acids may influence behavior. This line of development culminated with the discovery by Ungar (27) of a polypeptide with 10 amino acids (scotophobin) which appeared to mediate the aversive response to darkness in rats. This dramatic report of polypeptide effects on behavior is still a subject of scientific debate. Nevertheless it moved the study of peptides into a new domain in which the central nervous system effects of peptide

1

chains (neuropeptides) became a focus of investigation.

The early work of Mirsky et al. (11) and of Miller and his colleagues (9, 10) anticipated the advances of Ungar. These investigators were among the first to discuss the central nervous system effects of the polypeptide ACTH and relate the effects to psychological processes. Their early conception that the ACTH molecule influenced behavior by increasing fear was challenged by the later report of de Wied and Bohus (4). In a major break from the historical precedent of assuming that ACTH was related only to stress, de Wied and Bohus (4) proposed that ACTH, MSH, and their smaller fragments improved memory. However, work in our laboratories (17, 18, 19, 23) has strongly suggested that improved attention (which might influence short-term memory processes) is a more parsimonious explanation of the spectrum of findings that have been reported for ACTH, MSH, and their fragments. The interpretation of these data are probably not terribly important. What is important is that data from several laboratories using different approaches and techniques all concluded that polypeptides influenced the brain and thus legitimized the field of the neuropeptides.

Challenge to Classical Conceptions

One of the most significant outcomes of neuropeptide research has been the challenge presented to classical views of brain functioning evident in physiological psychology. Traditionally physiological psychology has proceeded as if discrete behaviors were exclusively located in specific structures of the brain. This conception and its attendent methods (mostly surgical interventions) have produced a static view of brain-behavior relationships. The assumption that the functioning of an organ can be determined best by removing it and examining the residual deficit is indeed tenuous. Nevertheless the methods predominate and their clinical applications (lobotomies, etc.) have left an ugly scar.

The alternative conception implicit in research with the neuropeptides is that behavior and its physiological substrate are a process. Behavior is infinitely complex and an approach which ascribes function solely to brain structures cannot accommodate even the artificial and induced behaviors of laboratory rats. Research with neuropeptides indicates that behavioral changes can be mediated by polypeptide chains. This mediation can be determined as a partial function of the conformation and structure of the molecule, as a partial function of its size or molecular weight, and as a partial function of the quantity which is present.

These neuropeptide chains are in a constant state of
flux and replacement and can be quickly degraded or
cleaved by enzyme actions. The organism can produce or
release the peptides when necessary, and the quantity
or sequence of amino acids produced or released appears
to vary with situational or environmental requirements
(21). Thus the neuropeptides present a dynamic system
that allows the organism to adapt flexibly to its environment. It may be that a neuropeptide analysis of
behavior, one that can relate an infinite series of
permutations of amino acids to the infinite complexity
of behavior, will replace the classical but static
structure-function analysis of behavior. Several of
the assumptions required of this speculation have received dramatic support from laboratory analyses of
behavior.

One major assumption is that behavior should vary as
a function of treatment with specific peptides. There
are countless examples of the behavioral consequences
of treatment with peptides contained in this volume
and elsewhere (22). However a more telling and radical
statement of this assumption would be that behavioral
deficits are reversible.

Reversibility of behavioral deficit. If one can assume
that functions such as memory and attention relate to
processes in the brain and not structures, then deficits in functioning, of any kind, should be reversible.
At least two examples of dramatic reversibility of
functioning have been reported as a result of neuropeptide intervention. Rigter and his colleagues (15, 16)
have demonstrated that memory impairment in rats produced by electroconvulsive shock (ECS) or by CO_2 can be
reversed if the animals are pretreated with fragments
of MSH or ACTH. Thus, the authors argue, the deficit
of retrieval of information usually observed after ECS
or treatment with CO_2 and often ascribed to structural
impairment, can be reversed by a neuropeptide.

Sandman et al. (20) have reported that patients
suffering "chronic" intellectual deficits (mentally
retarded) and who evidenced massive impairment of attention showed dramatic improvement in intellectual
functioning after treatment with fragments of MSH or
ACTH. The attentional deficits in these subjects,
generally thought to be permanent and intractable were
ameliorated by treatment with a neuropeptide. These
data pose serious problems for viewpoints which advo-
cate that abilities or functions reside exclusively in
discrete areas of the brain. Only a more fluid conception of brain functioning can accommodate these findings. We believe that function must be construed part-
ly as a result of neurochemical events in the brain
and that the neuropeptides must be given a prominent

role in the determination and understanding of behavior.

Specificity of neuropeptide activity. A second major assumption of this position is that the behavioral or physiological influences of peptides are specific and not diffuse. Evidence for the specificity of action of neuropeptide chains derives from several sources. The work of Ungar, discussed earlier, illustrates the relationship of a specific chain of amino acids to avoidance of the dark. This certainly is a prime example of the specificity of peptide action. Recent studies by Beckwith et al. (1) and Dunn et al. (5) indicate that administration of MSH, ACTH, or their fragments result in different physiological and behavioral patterns. Moreover, the report of Plotnikoff and Kastin (13) indicate that different psychopharmacological profiles exist for several of the neuropeptides.

Among the most impressive evidence regarding the specificity of action of peptides comes from the work of Renaud et al. (14). These investigators have observed that hypothalamic peptides have differential effects on single cells of the brain. This research indicates that TRH, LHRH, and somatostatin exert direct effects on the brain in specific ways suggesting that a general activational interpretation of peptide influences is untenable. A further implication of this work is that the peptide substances serve a neurotransmitter or neuromodulatory function in the brain (14).

In an elegant group of studies Gispen et al. (6) have demonstrated that the family of enkephalins and endorphins exert behavioral influences which appear to be related to their structure or conformation. For instance grooming behavior in rats was elicited by LPH 61-91 but smaller fragments (i.e., LPH 61-76; 61-69, etc.) were not potent elicitors of this behavior. It also appeared that LPH 65-69 was completely inactive in this procedure. Others (2, 7, 12, 28) have indicated differential influences of these related peptides in tests of analgesia. Relatively minor structural modifications of these peptides (e.g., replacing an amino acid with another amino acid or substituting a D-isomer for the naturally occurring *l* form) can result in major behavioral and physiological changes (28). Thus, as Walker et al. (28) have suggested, the conformation of the peptides is as critical in determining its type or duration of action as the size or the dosage of the molecule.

It is apparent that several specific actions of several discrete peptide chains have been elucidated. It appears that a major focus of the recent research effort has been directed at the description of

specific actions of neuropeptide molecules. The optimistic forecast is that more behavioral and physiological actions will be related to the structure or conformation of the neuropeptides.

LIMITATIONS

Pharmacology or Psychology

There are always many limitations in a new field,
but neuropeptide research suffers from unique methodological problems. A few of the difficulties are the
result of a highly interdisciplinary field in which
some groups view behavior as a bioassay for peptide
effects while others view behavior as indicative of a
psychological process. The result is that factors
important to one group, such as testing a variety of
behaviors, may be a source of error to another group,
who instead wish to discover a single consistent behavioral test with which to develop parametric pharmacological principles. Nevertheless the goal of re-
searchers now is to elucidate the behavioral effects of
peptides. Before this goal can be realized all groups
will have to address the methodological issues raised
by pharmacological and behavioral research strategies.

Pharmacological or Physiological

One major criticism of the research concerning the
effects of neuropeptides is that they represent pharmacological rather than physiological phenomena. While
it is true that relatively large quantities of neuropeptides are introduced into the organism in behavioral
studies, it is impossible to determine if a systemic
injection of 10 µg or 30 mg is detected by the brain
as larger quantities than 1 pg released by the pituitary. Since the toxicity of the neuropeptides appears
to be nonexistent it is difficult to separate pharmacological from physiological states. However there are
data which suggest that physiological influences of the
neuropeptides are similar to the effects observed by
administering peptides to the organism. Sandman et al.
(21) have indicated that the endogenous release of MSH
and ACTH occur during behavioral conditions which are
conceptually consistent with the behaviors influenced
by systemic injections of these peptides. In another
example of this phenomenon Bohus et al. (3) have demonstrated that rats with hereditary diabetes insipidus
(a deficiency in antidiuretic hormone, ADH) extinguish
an avoidance response faster than normal rats. Injection of ADH to normal rats prolongs extinction of this
behavior. At the present stage of research concern
with the issue of "physiological or pharmacological"

is premature. Although a complement of both approaches should exist, the initial focus must necessarily be to describe as many effects as possible.

PROSPECTS

Clinical Utility

One of the great promises provided by the neuropeptides is their potential as clinically useful compounds. Molecules such as vasopressin or the fragments of ACTH or MSH which selectively influence attention or memory would appear to be of considerable clinical importance. The endorphins with opiate-like activity also must be considered among the most prominent of clinically useful substances. Although there are several studies of the influence of peptides with normal human populations only a handful of studies of patient populations have been reported.

The earliest study by Kastin et al. (8) indicated that infusions of MSH could induce menstrual bleeding in amenorrheic women. Additionally they reported slowing of the EEG and increases in anxiety. More recently, Sandman et al. (20) have indicated that intellectual deficits of a population of mentally retarded subjects were ameliorated by treatment with the 4-10 fragment of MSH/ACTH. Further, Strand et al. (25) demonstrated that a pathological decline in amplitude of evoked muscle action potentials was arrested by infusion of ACTH 4-10. Thus even though few clinical studies have been conducted, those which have convincingly indicate that the neuropeptides offer tremendous promise as clinically useful agents.

Enzymatic Degradation

Future research will probably focus upon relating smaller and smaller sequences of amino acids to behavior. Concomitant with this focus will be an examination of the enzymatic degradation of the endogenous substances. As smaller sequences are shown to have adaptive value the biological significance of these molecules will need to be discerned.

Self-Regulation

An exciting probable focus of attention will be the examination of the relationship of amino acid chains contained within a single larger molecule. It is conceivable that feedback or self-regulatory functions are contained within larger prohormones. The fact that β-lipotropin contains fragments of MSH, and ACTH, and the endorphins, and that these substances all have be-

havioral actions suggests that the concept of regulation should be examined with the LPH molecule.

CONCLUSION

Interest in the actions of neuropeptides on behavior
is of relatively recent origin and in the process of
rapid evolution. Only recently have investigators begun to realize the potential of neuropeptide research
for gaining an understanding of the brain and behavior.
While it has been the goal of physiological psychology
to elucidate the structural basis of behavior, future
research with the neuropeptides may confirm our belief
that behavior is a function of process rather than
structure. There appears to be an attractive parallel
between the actions of amino acids in determining physical structure and the role of neuropeptides in influencing behavior. It may be that specific neuropeptide
molecules are uniquely coded for discrete arrays of behavior.

REFERENCES

1. Beckwith, B. E., Sandman, C. A., and Kastin, A. J. (1976):
   Influence of three short-chain peptides (α-MSH, MSH/ACTH 4-10,
   MIF-I) on diamensional attention. *Pharmacol. Biochem. Behav.*
   (Suppl.), 5:11-16.
2. Bloom, F., Segal, D., Ling, N., and Guillemin, O. (1976):
   Endorphins: Profound behavioral effects in rats suggest new
   etiological factors in mental illness. *Science,* 194:630-632.
3. Bohus, B., van Wimersma Griedanus, Tj., and de Wied, D. (1975):
   Behavioral and endocrine responses of rats with hereditary
   hypothalamic diabetes insipidus (Brattleboro Strain). *Physiol.
   Behav.,* 14:609-615.
4. de Wied, D. and Bohus, B. (1966): Long-term and short-term
   effects on retention of a conditioned avoidance response in
   rats by treatment with long acting pitressin and α-MSH. *Nature,* 212:1484-1488.
5. Dunn, A. J., Iuvone, P. M., and Rees, H. D. (1976): Neurochemical responses of mice to ACTH and lysine vasopressin.
   Pharmacol. Biochem. Behav. (Suppl.), 5:139-145.
6. Gispen, W. H., Rieth, M. E. A., Schotman, P., Wiegant, V. M.,
   Zwiers, H., and de Wied, D. (1977): CNA and ACTH-like peptides: Neurochemical response and interaction with opiates.
   (This volume.)
7. Jacquet, Y. F. and Marks, N. (1976): The C-fragment of β-
   lipotropin: An endogenous neuroleptic or antipsychotogen?
   Science, 194:632-635.
8. Kastin, A. J., Kullander, S., Borglin, N. E., Dahlberg, B.,
   Dyster-Aas, K., Krakau, C. E. T., Inguar, D. H., Miller, M. C.,
   Bowers, C. Y. and Schally, A. V. (1968): Extrapigmentary ef-
   fects of melanocyte-stimulating hormone in amenorrhoeic women.
   Lancet, 1:1007-1010.

9. Miller, R. E. and Caul, W. F.   (1973):   Effect of adrenocorticotrophic hormone on appetitive discrimination learning in the
rat. *Physiol. Behav.*, 10:141-143.

10. Miller, R. E. and Ogawa, N.   (1962):   The effect of adrenocorticotrophic hormone (ACTH) on avoidance conditioning in the
adrenalectomized rat. *J. Comp. Physiol. Psychol.*, 55:211-213.

11. Mirsky, A., Miller, R., and Stein, M.   (1953):   Relation of
adrenocortical activity and adaptive behavior. *Psychosom.
Med.*, 15:574-588.

12. Pert, C. B., Pert, A., Chang, J. K., and Fong, B. T. W.
(1976):   [D-Ala^2]-met enkephalinamide: A potent, long-lasting
synthetic pentapeptide analgesic. *Science*, 194:330-332.

13. Plotnikoff, N. P. and Kastin, A. J.   (1977):   Neuropharmacological review of hypothalamic releasing factors. *(This volume.)*

14. Renaud, L. P., Martin, J. B., and Brazeau, P.   (1976):   Hypothalamic releasing factors: Physiological evidence for a regulatory action on central neurons and pathways for their distribution in brain. *Pharmacol. Biochem. Behav.* (Suppl.), 5:171-
178.

15. Rigter, H., Janssens-Elbertse, R. and van Riezen, H.   (1976):
Reversal of amnesia by an orally active ACTH 4-9 analog (Org
2766). *Pharmacol. Biochem. Behav.*, 5:53-58.

16. Rigter, H. and van Riezen, H.   (1975):   Anti-amnesic effect
of ACTH 4-10: Its independence of the nature of the amnesic
agent and the behavioral test. *Physiol. Behav.*, 14:563-566.

17. Sandman, C. A., Alexander, W. D., and Kastin, A. J.   (1973):
Neuroendocrine influences on visual discrimination and reversal learning in the albino and hooded rat. *Physiol. Behav.*,
11:613-617.

18. Sandman, C. A., George, J., McCanne, T. R., Nolan, J. D.,
Kaswan, J., and Kastin, A. J.   (1977):   MSH/ACTH 4-10 influ-
ences behavioral and physiological measures of attention. *J.
Clin. Endoc. Metab.*, (in press).

19. Sandman, C. A., George, J. M., Nolan, J. D., van Riezen, H.,
and Kastin, A. J.   (1975):   Enhancement of attention in man
with ACTH/MSH 4-10. *Physiol. Behav.*, 15:427-431.

20. Sandman, C. A., George, J., Walker, B. B., and Nolan, J. D.
(1976):   Neuropeptide MSH/ACTH 4-10 enhances attention in the
mentally retarded. *Pharmacol. Biochem. Behav.* (Suppl.), 5:23-
28.

21. Sandman, C. A., Kastin, A. J., Schally, A. V., Kendall, J. W.,
and Miller, L. H.   (1973):   Neuroendocrine responses to physical and psychological stress. *J. Comp. Physiol. Psychol.*,
84:386-390.

22. Sandman, C. A., Miller, L. H., and Kastin, A. J.   (1976):   The
neuropeptides: Pharmacology, physiological substrates and behavioral effects. *Pharmacol. Biochem. Behav.* (Suppl.), 5:1-3.

23. Sandman, C. A., Miller, L. H., Kastin, A. J., and Schally, A.
V.   (1972):   Neuroendocrine influence on attention and memory.
J. Comp. Physiol. Psychol., 80:54-58.

24. Selye, H.   (1956):   *The Stress of Life.*   McGraw-Hill, New York.

25. Strand, F. L., Cayer, A., Gonzalez, E., Stoboy, H.   (1976):
    Peptide enhancement of neuromuscular function: animal and
    clinical studies. *Pharmacol. Biochem. Behav.* (Suppl.), 5:179–
    188.
26. Thompson, R. and McConnell, J. V.   (1955): Classical condi-
    tioning in the planarian, *Dugesia Dorotocephlia*. *J. Comp.
    Physiol. Psychol.*, 48:65–68.
27. Ungar, G.   (1973): The problem of molecular coding of neural
    information. *Naturwissenshaften*, 60:307–312.
28. Walker, J. M., Berntson, G. B., Sandman, C. A., Coy, D.,
    Schally, A. V., and Kastin, A. J.   (1977): An analog of en-
    kephalin having prolonged opiate-like effects *in vivo*. *Sci-
    ence*, 196:85–87.

Neuropeptide Influences on the Brain and Behavior, edited by L.H. Miller, C.A. Sandman, and A.J. Kastin. Raven Press, New York © 1977.

Critical Appraisal of Peptide Pharmacology

Henk van Riezen, Henk Rigter, and Henk M. Greven

Department of Pharmacology, Organon International B.V., Oss, The Netherlands

INTRODUCTION

Pharmacology investigates the effects of chemical substances on living organisms for the purpose of predicting their possible therapeutic effects, and for understanding their mechanisms of action. Proper interpretation of the actions of a compound must be based on a thorough knowledge of the physiological functions involved and their regulation. Therapeutic predictions must be based on knowledge of the etiology and natural course of diseases and how they affect physiological processes.

When a valid animal model for a human disease exists, it is possible to search for a possible cure by testing a large number of new substances in this model. Peptide research, however, follows another approach. After having identified peptide hormones, the pharmacologist wants to know their exact function and possible therapeutic usefulness. Thus, he begins with profiling, using a wide variety of test models and a wide range of doses to find out which effects are consistently found at the lowest doses and characterize the substance. On the basis of this profile and his knowledge of the functions affected, he tries to determine the site and mechanism of interaction between the substance and the organism and to predict its possible applications in human therapeutics.

In this chapter we will discuss, first, some of the problems which specifically face a peptide pharmacologist; second, the possible physiological role of peptides in behavior; third, their site of action; and, fourth, the specificity of peptide effects.

PROBLEMS OF PEPTIDE PHARMACOLOGY

Once resorbed or injected, more stable chemical substances have ample time to reach their target organs and interact with their receptors. Their metabolism is slow in comparison to the processes of distribution and pharmacological activity. The magnitude of their effects usually parallels their free plasma concentration curve. Substances affecting the brain may have difficulty entering brain tissue, their effects may appear later and may not relate simply to plasma concentration.

Metabolism

Peptides are less stable. The enzymes of living organisms metabolize them very effectively and quickly. For example, Redding and Kastin (41) reported that the half-life of MSH is 1.5 min. Witter, Verhoef, and de Nijs (8, 63, 66) found that the half-life of ACTH 4-10 is less than one and a half min, while a behaviorally more potent ACTH 4-9 analogue had a half-life of 5 to 10 min, after i.v. administration to rats. This ACTH 4-9 analogue (Org 2766) was designed to be maximally resistant to enzymatic breakdown (28). It is behaviorally active in rats in doses a thousand times lower than the active doses of ACTH or ACTH 4-10 itself (46). The preliminary results of a study of its penetration into the brain are presented in Table 1. It can be seen that 5 min after intravenous administration approximately two thousandths of the administered dose is present in the whole brain of a rat. The content in

TABLE 1. *Recovery of intact peptide in µg per total brain (1.5 g) of rats and in part of the administered dose (40 µg/rat) with different routes and at different times after administration*

Route of administration	Min after administration	Total in brain (µg)	Part of dose
i.v.	5	$66.8 \cdot 10^{-4}$	$175 \cdot 10^{-6}$
	15	$39.6 \cdot 10^{-4}$	$99 \cdot 10^{-6}$
	30	$18.0 \cdot 10^{-4}$	$45 \cdot 10^{-6}$
s.c.	10	$11.8 \cdot 10^{-4}$	$27 \cdot 10^{-6}$
	30	$6.0 \cdot 10^{-4}$	$15 \cdot 10^{-6}$
	60	$3.6 \cdot 10^{-4}$	$9 \cdot 10^{-6}$
per os	30	$10.8 \cdot 10^{-5}$	$4 \cdot 10^{-6}$
	60	$11.2 \cdot 10^{-5}$	$4 \cdot 10^{-6}$
	120	$8.4 \cdot 10^{-5}$	$3 \cdot 10^{-6}$

*Based on data from Verhoef and Witter, ref. 63.

the brain, 120 min after oral administration of 40 µg, is three millionths of the original dose. As demonstrated by Rigter (46), rats show improvement of retrieval of a passive avoidance response after administration of a similar dose.

The fact that peripheral metabolism seriously interferes with studies of receptor-structure activity relationships has been demonstrated by the results of the Chapel Hill group (65). They obtained completely different relationships in their barbiturate antagonism experiments depending upon whether the peptides were administered centrally or peripherally. The effects of peripheral metabolism are even more obvious in the work on the peptide agonists of the morphine receptor.

Here, the blood-brain barrier prevents access of the most potent peptide to the receptor and only by local application could the tentative agonist, the C-terminal fragment of lipotropin, be shown to be 200 times more active than the smaller fragments (5,18).

Dose Response Relations

It is clear that peptides must be extremely active in order for behavioral effects to be seen after peripheral administration. It is not surprising that the conditions for showing such effects are not always favorable and that it is sometimes difficult to reproduce specific peptide effects. For that reason it is important to investigate a wide dose range and to control the experimental conditions rigidly. With careful experimentation, dose-response relationships can be found, as was demonstrated, for example, by Rigter for the effect of ACTH 4-10 on conditioned taste aversion (45) and for effects of Org 2766 on amnesia (46). de Wied has shown dose-response relations for the extinction of pole jump conditioning (9, 10) and retention of passive avoidance (1) for, among others, ACTH fragments, T.R.H., and vasopressin.

Often dose-response relationships are not widely explored. Most of our own work with ACTH-like peptides showed that supra-maximum doses usually have the same effect as the maximum dose. The danger of giving a very high dose, to insure a demonstrable effect, is clearly demonstrated by the findings of McGaugh et al. (34), who showed that while "low" doses of ACTH facilitated consolidation, a "high" dose blocked consolidation of memory for a passive avoidance of drinking.

Gold found the same with ACTH 4-10 (23, 24). Bennett reported similar findings for consolidation of footshock avoidance (19), and Plotnikoff and Kastin reported it for MSH effects on footshock induced aggression (39).

Specificity

Using a single test system, it is often found that several different types of peptides have similar behavioral effects. This nonspecificity of tests for CNS activities of drugs is not restricted to the field of peptide pharmacology. It is a general problem (3). Its relevance for peptides has been demonstrated by Plotnikoff (39). This is not at all surprising. An animal in a test situation is extremely restricted in its behavioral repertoire. Therefore, compounds with similar effects do not have to have similar sites or mechanisms of action. It is good practice for pharmacologists not to generalize from one test, not to assume that similar acting peptides react with the same receptor, until it is demonstrated that, without changing the dose ratio, they behave similarly in a wide range of tests. MSH, ACTH 4-10, and Org 2766 delay extinction of pole jump conditioning, and also delay extinction of appetitive responding (9, 28, 49). Rigter (46) showed that they antagonize amnesia in exactly the same way. These peptides also delay the extinction of conditioned taste aversion (45). From all available data it is clear that whatever behavioral effect MSH or ACTH 4-10 has, Org 2766 has the same effect when given at doses a thousand times smaller.

The delay of extinction of conditioned taste aversion by ACTH and ACTH 4-10 was confirmed by Levine et al. (32). Thus it was very tempting to conclude that ACTH-like peptides will always delay extinction, independently of the type of test. However, in the same paper Levine showed that administration of ACTH during acquisition facilitates extinction. This is supported by findings of Gray and Garrud (27), using maze running behavior and by results of Sandman's group (2, 6) showing facilitation of reversal. So opposite effects on extinction can probably be obtained depending on the timing of the peptide treatment. This example shows us how dangerous it is to make hasty generalizations about peptide effects on behavior or to criticize other investigators when experimental findings do not seem to be consistent.

Conclusions

The examples discussed demonstrate that:

1. Because small peptides are metabolized so quickly, the results of structure-activity studies are more probably governed by the rules of their metabolism than by the rules of receptor interaction.
2. Simple relations between plasma concentrations and behavioral activity may not exist.
3. Giving a high dose of a peptide, assuming that one

will then pick up the effect of the substance, is a very dangerous procedure. A wide dose range should be studied.
4. Structure-activity studies should not be based on one test. Peptides with different profiles, perhaps acting on different receptors, may produce similar effects in a given test.
5. Generalizations should be made with great reservation.

PHYSIOLOGICAL ROLE OF PEPTIDES IN BEHAVIOR

Most of the peptides studied today are natural hormones, releasing factors, etc., their fragments, or, are close analogues made synthetically. Of course, questions arise about the physiological role of these peptides. Do the large quantities used to elicit effects mimic the natural behavioral response, or do they result from interaction with other receptors, so called pharmacological effects? Another question is whether these effects result from direct interaction with neuron receptors or are mediated via other hormones, effects on metabolism of natural transmittors, etc.

Direct or Indirect Effects

The latter question is usually "solved" by studying behavioral effects and endocrine or monoamine effects simultaneously in the same conditions. As an example, Endröczi (16) has correlated ACTH effects on behavior with increased catecholamine turnover in the brain. McGaugh's group has also postulated an intermediary role for the catecholamines in the effect of ACTH and ACTH 4-10 on consolidation (34). ACTH 4-10 indeed increases catecholamine turnover but Org 2766 which is behaviorally more potent, was inactive with respect to brain catecholamines (29, 31). Leonard (30) showed very convincing evidence of changes in hippocampal serotonin in relation to the anti-amnesic effects of ACTH 4-10. However, after long intervals the anti-amnesic effect was still present, while the effect on hippocampal serotonin could not be shown. We should never forget that correlations do not always mean direct, causal relationships.

Physiological or Pharmacological Effect

Assumptions that ACTH and vasopressin have effects on behavior in physiological conditions are largely based on studies of hormone deficient animals. A vast literature about the effects of hypophysectomy or partial hypophysectomy was recently completed by studies of animals with genetic deficiencies of pituitary hormones. Convincing evidence exists that deficiency of

ACTH or vasopressin causes behavioral defects. These
defects could not be cured by corticosteroid administration and only partially by a "cocktail" of adrenal,
thyroid, and gonadal hormones which "completely" cured
the peripheral endocrinological defects.

However, ACTH, MSH, growth hormone, and vasopressin
administration each restore the ability of such animals
to acquire shuttle-box avoidance conditioning (11, 60).
The fact that many hormones restore normal acquisition
of shuttle-box conditioning in hypophysectomized rats
should not be interpreted as evidence that they completely restore normal behavior. Probably these hormones affect the CNS in different ways. Though all
result in normal shuttle-box conditioning, other deficiencies may still exist, and be different with different treatments.

It is clear that the question of the physiological
action must be solved separately for each peptide hormone. The case for vasopressin is rather clear:

1. Vasopressin deficiency causes well described defects
   of behavior, and vasopressin administration restores
   these behaviors to normal (62).
2. Vasopressin is present in the CNS as are systems for
   its distribution, like peptidergic neurons, as shown
   by Renaud et al. (42) or cerebrospinal fluid as
   shown by Sterba (55), van Wimersma Greidanus et al.
   (62).

The method of using hormone deficient animals is not
so easily applied to the study of hypothalamic releasing factors. Even though the possibility exists of
lesioning the areas where these hormones are produced,
the damage to nerve networks will be so extensive that
it is hardly possible to assume that any resulting defects are purely due to the hormone deficiency which
has been produced. Recent work of Van Wimersma Greidanus suggests a more acceptable approach. In order to
obtain support for the assumptions that vasopressin is
necessary for normal acquisition of step-through passive avoidance and that vasopressin reaches its CNS
receptors by cerebrospinal fluid circulation, he injected specific vasopressin antibodies into the cerebral ventricles of rats. He showed that this treatment
produces the same behavioral deficiency as seen in genetically vasopressin deficient rats, although these
animals have a normal peripheral vasopressin level,
shown by the fact that they produce normally concentrated urine (60, 62).

Local injection of antibodies to peptide hormones
may be a way of producing specifically deficient animals for behavioral testing similar to the models produced by 6-OHDA injections which are used to produce
local and specific catecholamine depletion. Such a

technique may also be of use in experimental attempts to locate the site of action of these hormones.

Pharmacological Effects

Even in the case of vasopressin it is not at all definite that all the effects seen after its administration mimic the physiological functions of vasopressin.

Peripherally or centrally administered peptides may reach brain areas, which are never reached by such concentrations in normal conditions. Knowing that the CSF contains a few pg of vasopressin per ml (13) and that 10 pg vasopressin intracerebroventricularly consistently mimics the effect of vasopressin on extinction behavior (12), then it is unrealistic to assume that an effect which shows up only after 0.5 to 10 µg of vasopressin administered intracerebroventricularly, like the excitation seen by Dunn et al. (14) and Gispen et al. (21), are physiological effects of this peptide.

When pharmacological effects are contrasted against physiological effects, one usually means effects produced by doses which induce higher concentrations at the receptor than are assumed to occur under physiological conditions. With peptides the administered dose may seem excessively high, but because of their rapid metabolism the concentration at the receptor may still be in the physiological range. We have, however, other criteria. When, for instance, the s.c. dose of one µg of ACTH 4-10 produces an effect on extinction or amnesia, which lasts 4 to 6 hr, then the results of a study by Prange, where 10 mg ACTH 4-10 is needed to produce analeptic effects, suggests that the configuration of ACTH 4-10 is probably not the most optimal peptide structure to produce that analeptic effect, since ten thousand times more is needed than for the other effects (4, 40). I would call that effect a pharmacological effect and assume that that effect is probably not physiological.

Such pharmacological effects may be useful in conditions where the natural agonist is not available to produce the desired effect. However, one should expect many side effects of such "therapy."

Conclusions

It is not easy to determine whether a particular peptide-induced effect is a physiological function. Criteria to consider are that its effects are produced at physiological concentrations, that the substance can reach that receptor from its site of production, and that deficiency causes defective behavior which can be normalized by substitution of the hormone.

Evidence is still lacking or incomplete for most of the peptide hormones, except for vasopressin, where the evidence is rather clear.

SITE OF ACTION STUDIES

Behavioral pharmacologists have not given up the hope of being able to localize the site of action of a drug and thus understand the mechanisms by which it produces its effects in a simple way. Recently they have turned their hopes to biochemical systems instead of anatomical sites. Neither approach has been very successful, however.

The ability to mimic, with much lower doses by intra-cerebral application, the effects produced by peripheral administration argues strongly for a direct CNS effect and against an indirect effect via a peripherally evoked reflex. The dosage must be in the order of what can be expected to reach the brain after systemic administration.

When the effect is seen only after application of the substance to a particular brain region and not to other areas, it is suggestive that the activity is localized to that area.

Several localizing studies have been done with ACTH 4-10 and MSH. Local injection of the substance in the posterior thalamic area around and in the nucleus para-fascicularis produce the same effects as peripheral injections. This effect could not be produced by injections in other brain regions. Destruction of this area made peripheral peptide injections inactive. Destruction of the hippocampus also prevents peptide effects on behavior as do rostral septal lesions (59, 61). Distribution studies with radio-labeled MSH showed it to be concentrated in the posterior thalamic area (38). The synthetic analogue Org 2766, however, is concentrated in the septal area (64).

Additional support for localization studies may come from studies of effects on local blood flow, like the one by Goldman et al. (25, 26), of effects on local cerebral oxygen consumption, the study by Panksepp et al. (37), or from electrophysiological studies like those of Urban and de Wied (56, 57), and Lichtensteiger (33). In the case of the ACTH/MSH-like peptides these studies made things more complicated, as MSH-effects on blood flow indicated the visual cortex and those on oxygen consumption the locus ceruleus as possible sites of action. The studies of Urban and de Wied point to the reticulolimbic arousal system, those of Lichtensteiger to the l. ceruleus. It is probable, however, that the peptide receptors are located on cells that activate or inhibit other brain areas. Such secondary effects may cause the local blood flow or oxygen

consumption changes, that were reported to occur after
MSH.

SPECIFICITY OF PEPTIDE EFFECTS

Hormones are usually quite specific in their endocrine effects. Therefore one would expect that the effects of peptide hormones on behavior should be very
specific too.

How can this be reconciled with the demonstration of
many different behavioral effects? Two points should
be made here. The first is that when reviewing peptide
effects, it is usual to forget about the doses needed
to obtain such effects. It is well-known, however, that
at (very) high doses substances begin to interact with
other than their specific receptors. We know that
there are α-and β-adrenergic receptors and muscarinic
as well as nicotinic acetylcholine receptors in the
brain. There may also be different types of MSH receptors or vasopressin receptors, each differentially
sensitive to slightly different natural peptides and
both sensitive to our crude attack with injected synthetic materials. Many different behavioral effects
like improved acquisition, improved reversal, delayed
extinction, etc. may in fact be caused by one and the
same underlying mechanism, e.g., improved attention or
improved information processing.

Dose Related Lack of Specificity

Plotnikoff et al. (39) used mg dosages in the classical neuropharmacological test battery to evaluate the
peptides TRH, MSH, and MIF. They found them to have a
large number of effects. The profiles, however, did
not seem to be very specific.

Van Ree and Gispen found that μg doses of MIF facilitate the development of tolerance to the analgesic effect of morphine and accelerate the induction of physical dependence. MIF is more active than oxytocin or
vasopressin, which have the same effect (22, 58). MIF,
like vasopressin, facilitates consolidation of memory,
while TRH and MSH are inactive (47). MIF has no effect on extinction of conditioned taste aversion,
while vasopressin facilitates and ACTH-like peptides
delay extinction of conditioned taste aversion (47).

Org 2766, when given at doses 100 times those which
facilitate retrieval, can be shown to have an effect
on consolidation similar to that of vasopressin (46).

One may conclude from these examples that like other substances peptides have reasonable specificity
when given in low doses. At higher doses they may exert effects on other receptors as well and lose specificity. Hypotheses about their physiological functions
should be based only on effects seen at the lowest
doses.

Interaction with more than one Receptor Type

Peptide reaction with different types of receptors should be seriously considered. Peptide analogues do not necessarily have to have the same profile of receptor interaction. ACTH, MSH, ACTH 4-10 and Org 2766 all have a very similar effect on the process of extinction of conditioned behavior. Whichever behavioral test system is chosen, the potency ratio between ACTH, MSH, ACTH 4-10 and Org 2766 remains the same. All four peptides facilitate retrieval after amnesic treatments. However, the 7-D-Phe analogue of ACTH 4-10 (Org OI 64) which in most behavioral tests has opposite effects to ACTH 4-10 itself, facilitates retrieval like the "all-L" peptide (44). This strongly suggests that the receptors involved in retrieval facilitation have different structural requirements than those determining the delay of extinction.

Sex as a Cause of Differences

Sandman has repeatedly shown that the effects of ACTH 4-10 may differ in male and female rats. The differences were mainly quantitative (50, 53). Recent work in humans with ACTH by Cowley et al. (7) demonstrated that ACTH lowers testosterone production in normal and castrated males, but that in the presence of estrogens ACTH increases the production of testosterone in the adrenal glands, thus providing a firm basis for further studies of differences of effects of ACTH-like peptides in the sexes.

Conclusion

From the examples given, one might conclude that peptides probably bind to specific receptors. These receptors may be of different types, however. This may be a disaster for the investigator who takes a single test as a parameter of biological activity during purification of natural peptides or in a peptide synthesizing program, in order to find a peptide with a specific behavioral effect. It may turn out to be the wrong system to monitor the success of his efforts. However, it is also our hope for the future, as it may be possible to find substances with high affinity to only one receptor type, thus eliminating side effects.

HUMAN PHARMACOLOGY

We are all aware of the difficulties one runs into, when testing a substance in humans. Again, basically, two approaches are possible. One is to evaluate the effects of peptides in patient groups. The work with MIF, TRH, and LHRH demonstrates convincingly that this

approach does not lead to simple straightforward conclusions (15, 65).

It is for this reason that we chose a completely different approach to evaluate the effects of ACTH 4-10 in
humans. It is the task of the animal pharmacologist to
produce testable hypotheses about the action and indication of the substance in humans. On the basis of
animal pharmacology, our hypotheses were that either
the substance had an effect to improve concentration
(selective attention) and/or it would enhance memory
retrieval functions (better access to stored information). In collaboration with Miller and co-workers,
we designed experiments which would evaluate the first
hypothesis and together with Wagenaar and Gaillard the
second (20, 35, 36, 48, 51, 52, 54, 64).

Miller (35) found that the EEG habituation of arousal, when subjects perform a "go - no go" discrimination
task, is delayed and that selectively the arousal response to the "go" condition is maintained.

Gaillard et al. (20) showed that during prolonged
performance of a complicated serial reaction time task,
the average reaction time of the placebo treated volunteers did not improve very much due to the appearance
of lapses in performance due to inattention. The ACTH
4-10 treated group showed less and shorter periods of
inattention and made fewer mistakes. These and other
findings supported the first hypothesis made on the
basis of animal experiments.

There were inconsistencies, however. Wagenaar et al.
(64) performed a functional learning experiment and
tried to evaluate the knowledge obtained by looking at
the interference of functional learning by a previously
learned function. He found in one experiment that placebo treated volunteers showed great interference, but
that the ACTH 4-10 group, which performed better on the
first task, also performed better on the second task.
They shifted easier. This is consistent with the attention hypothesis. However, in the replication of the
experiment he found that the placebo group did not seem
to have any difficulty at all with the shift and the
ACTH 4-10 group, if anything, performed worse. This is
also consistent with the attention hypothesis. When
dimensional attention is optimal, the only possibility
for a drug is to impair performance. However, why
were the placebo groups so different? Knowing that
personality traits may influence performance, they analyzed the scores obtained during the selection procedure and found that in the first experiment most of the
volunteers were introverts and that this group was responsible for the ACTH 4-10 effect. The second experiment by chance contained almost only extraverted persons. Eysenck (17) has shown that introverts and ex-

traverts react differently, and sometimes in opposite directions, to increased levels of vigilance. Recently it was demonstrated clearly that caffeine too has opposite effects on introverted and extraverted persons (43). So, the results were explainable. However, how many investigators take personality traits into account when doing drug studies in volunteers or in patients? How often are sex differences studied?

GOOD PHARMACOLOGICAL PRACTICE

Guidelines

1. Evaluate in different species of animals, using wide dose ranges and time intervals, the effect of the peptide and its solvent on behavior. Use male as well as female animals and use tests of spontaneous and conditioned behavior. Use approach as well as avoidance, inhibition as well as activation (go – no go) conditions. Effects should be consistent, and dose-dependent. Only the effects found at low dosages should be considered for follow-up.
2. Evaluate, using the same dosages and intervals, the endocrine effects, the autonomic effects, and the effects on perceptual and motor functions.
3. Formulate the smallest number of hypotheses, which can explain the results and try to predict what other effects the substance would produce if the hypotheses were true. Test the hypotheses.
4. Design experiments to determine the site of action in the CNS. Determine whether the drug acts directly or whether the effects are dependent on known transmitters or hormones.
5. Extrapolate from the animal data as to the possible utility of the peptide for man.

None of these rules are new; neither are they complete. However, they are so frequently violated that it is necessary to draw continuous attention to them.

REFERENCES

1. Ader, R. and de Wied, D. (1972): Effects of lysine vasopressin on passive avoidance learning. *Psychon. Sci.*, 29:46–48.
2. Beckwith, B. E., Sandman, C. A., and Kastin, A. J. (1976): The influence of three short-chain peptides (MSH, MSH/ACTH 4-10, M.I.F. I) on dimensional attention. *Pharmacol. Biochem. Behav.* *(Suppl.)*, 5:11–16.
3. Berger, F. M. (1975): Depression and antidepressant drugs. *Clin. Pharm. Ther.*, 18:241–248.

4. Bissette, G., Nemeroff, C. B., Loosen, P. T., Prange Jr., A. J., and Lipton, M. A. (1976): Comparison of the Analeptic Potency of TRH, ACTH 4-10, LHRH and Related Peptides. *Pharmacol. Biochem. Behav. (Suppl.)*, 5:135-138.
5. Bradburry, A. F., Smith, D. G., and Snell, C. R. (1976): The C-fragment of lipotropin: an endogenous peptide with high affinity for brain opiate receptors. *Pharmacol. Biochem. Behav. (Suppl.)*, 5.
6. Champney, T. F., Sahley, T. L., and Sandman, C. A. (1976): Effects of neonatal cerebral ventricular injection of ACTH 4-9 analog and subsequent adult injections on learning in male and female albino rats. *Pharmacol. Biochem. Behav. (Suppl.)*, 5:3-10.
7. Cowley, T. H., Brownsey, B. G., Harper, M. E., Peeling, W. B., and Griffiths, K. (1976): The effect of ACTH on plasma testosterone and androstenedion concentrations in patients with prostatic carcinoma. *Acta Endocrinol.* 81:310-320.
8. De Nijs, H. (1976): *Personal communication.*
9. de Wied, D. (1969): Effects of peptide hormones in behavior. In: *Frontiers in Neuroendocrinology*, edited by W. F. Ganong and L. Martini, pp. 97-140. Oxford University Press, New York.
10. de Wied, D., Van Delft, A. M. L., Gispen, W. H., Weijnen, J. A. W. M., and Van Wimersma Greidanus, Tj. B. (1972): The role of pituitary-adrenal system hormones in active avoidance conditioning. In: *Hormones and Behavior*, edited by S. Levine, pp. 135-171. Academic Press, New York.
11. de Wied, D. (1976): Hormonal influences in motivation, learning and memory processes. *Hosp. Prac.*, 2:123-131.
12. de Wied, D. (1976): *Personal communication.*
13. Dogterom, J., Buys, R. M., and Van Wimersma Greidanus, Tj. B. (1975): Plasma vasopressin levels of rats as measured by radioimmunoassay. In: *Abstracts Symposia and Communications 16th Dutch Federative Meeting*, 1972. Stichting Federatie Med. Biol. Ver. in Nederland, Nÿmegen.
14. Dunn, A. J., Rees, H. D., and Iuvone, P. M. (1976): Behavioral and biochemical responses of mice to the intraventricular administration of ACTH peptides or lysin vasopressin. *Pharmacol. Biochem. Behav. (Suppl.)*, 5:139-146.
15. Ehrensing, R. H., and Kastin, A. J. (1976): Clinical investigations for emotional effects of neuropeptide hormones. *Pharmacol. Biochem. Behav. (Suppl.)*, 5:89-94.
16. Endröczi, E. (1976): Brain mechanisms involved in ACTH-induced changes of exploratory activity and conditioned avoidance behavior. *(This volume.)*
17. Eysenck, H. J. (1975): The measurement of emotion: psychological parameters and methods. In: *Emotions, Their Parameters and Measurement*, edited by Lennart Levi, pp. 439-468. Raven Press, New York.
18. Feldberg, W. (1976): The C-fragment of lipotropin: an endogenous peptide with high affinity for brain opiate receptors. *(Personal communication).*

19. Flood, J. F., Jarvik, M. E., Bennett, E. L., and Orme, A. E.
    (1976): Effects of ACTH-peptide fragments on memory function.
    Pharmacol. Biochem. Behav. (Suppl.), 5:41-52.
20. Gaillard, A. W. K., and Sanders, A. F. (1975): Some effects
    of ACTH 4-10 on performance during a serial reaction task.
    Psychopharmacologia, 42:201-208.
21. Gispen, W. H., Wiegant, V. M., Greven, H. M., and de Wied, D.
    (1975): The induction of excessive grooming in the rat by
    intraventricular application of peptides derived from ACTH:
    structure-activity studies. *Life Sci.,* 17: 645-652.
22. Gispen, W. H., Reith, M. E. A., Schotman, P., Wiegant, V. M.,
    Zwiers, H., and de Wied, D. (1977): The CNS and ACTH-like
    peptides: Neurochemical response and interaction with opiates.
    (This volume.)
23. Gold, P. E., and McGaugh, J. M. (1977): Hormones and memory.
    (This volume.)
24. Gold, P. E. (1976): *Personal communication.*
25. Goldman, H., Sandman, C. A., Kastin, A. J., and Murphy, S.
    (1975): MSH affects regional perfusion of the brain. *Phar-
    macol. Biochem. Behav.,* 3:661-664.
26. Goldman, H., Skelley, E. B., Sandman, C. A., Kastin, A. J.,
    and Murphy, S. (1976): Hormones and regional brain blood
    flow. *Pharmacol. Biochem. Behav. (Suppl.),* 5:165-170.
27. Gray, J. A., and Garrud, P. (1977): Adreno-pituitary hor-
    mones and frustrative nonreward. *(This volume.)*
28. Greven, H. M., and de Wied D. (1973): The influence of pep-
    tides derived from corticotropin (ACTH) on performance. Struc-
    ture activity studies in drug effects on neuroendocrine regu-
    lation. *Progress in Brain Research Vol. 39, Drug Effects on
    Neuroendocrine Regulation,* edited by E. Zimmerman, W. H.
    Gispen, B. E. Marks, and D. de Wied, pp. 429-442. Amsterdam,
    Elsevier.
29. Leonard, B. E. (1974): The effect of two synthetic ACTH ana-
    logues on the metabolism of biogenic amines in the rat brain.
    Arch. Int. Pharmacodyn., 207:242-253.
30. Leonard, B. E., Ramaekers, F., and Rigter, H. (1975): Ef-
    fects of ACTH 4-10 heptapeptide on changes in brain monamine
    metabolism associated with retrograde amnesia in the rat.
    Biochem. Soc. Trans., 3:113-115.
31. Leonard, B. E. (1976): *Personal communication.*
32. Levine, S., Smotherman, W. P., and Hennessy, J. W. (1977):
    Pituitary adrenal hormones and learned taste aversion. *(This
    volume.)*
33. Lichtensteiger, W. and Lienhart, R. (1976): Central action
    of α-MSH and prolactin: simultaneous responses of hypothalamic
    and mesencephalic dopamine (DA) systems. *Cellular and molec-
    ular bases of neuroendocrine processes,* edited by E. Endröczi,
    pp. 211-221. Academio Kiado, Budapest.
34. McGaugh, J. L., Gold, P. E., van Buskirk, R., and Haycock, J.
    (1975): Modulating influences of hormones and catecholamines
    in memory storage processes. *Progress in Brain Research Vol.
    42, Hormone, Homeostasis and the Brain,* edited by W. H.
    Gispen and L. Martini, pp. 151-162. Amsterdam, Elsevier.

35. Miller, L. H., Kastin, A. J., Sandman, C. A., Fink, M., and van Veen, W. J. (1974): Polypeptide influences on attention memory and anxiety in man. *Pharm. Biochem. Behav.*, 2, 663-668.
36. Miller, L. H., Harris, L., Kastin, A., and van Riezen, H. (1975): A neuroheptapeptide influence on brain-behavior mechanisms. In: *Abstracts of short communications IVth Int. Congr. Int. Soc. Psychoneuroendocrinol.*, p. 39. Aspen, Colorado.
37. Panksepp, J., Reilly, P., Bishop, P., Meeker, R. B., and Vilberg, T. R. (1976): Effects of α-MSH on motivation, vigilance and brain respiration. *Pharmacol. Biochem. Behav. (Suppl.)*, 5:59-64.
38. Pelletier, G., Labrie, F., Kastin, A. J. and Schally, A. V. (1975): Radioautographic localization of radioactivity in rat brain after intracarotid injection of ^{125}I-α-melanocyte-stimulating hormone. *Pharmacol. Biochem. Behav.*, 3:671-674.
39. Plotnikoff, N. P. and Kastin, A. J. (1977): Neuropharmacological review of hypothalamic releasing factors. *(This volume.)*
40. Prange, A. J., Lipton, M. A., Bissette, G., Nemeroff, C. B., Breese, G. R., Loosen, P. T., Cooper, B., and Wilson, I. C. (1975): Behavioral effects of peptides in animals: further experience with pentobarbital antagonism. Presented at American College of Neuropsychopharmacology, San Juan, Puerto Rico.
41. Redding, T. W., Kastin, A. J., and Nikolics, K. (1977): The disappearance, excretion and metabolism of labelled α-MSH in man. *Proc. Endocrine Soc., (In press.)*
42. Renaud, L. P., Martin, J. B., and Brazeau, P. (1976): Hypothalamic releasing factors: physiological evidence for a regulatory action on central neurons and pathways for their distribution in the brain. *Pharmacol. Biochem. Behav. (Suppl.)*, 5:171-178.
43. Revelle, W., Amaral, P., and Turriff, S. (1976): Introversion/extraversion, time stress and caffeine: effect on verbal performance. *Science*, 192:149-150.
44. Rigter, H. (1973): Amnesia in the rat. Thesis, University of Utrecht, Department of Pharmacology, Utrecht, The Netherlands.
45. Rigter, H. and Popping, A. (1976): Hormonal influences on the extinction of conditioned taste aversion. *Psychopharmacologia*, 46:255-261.
46. Rigter, H., Janssens-Elbertse, R., and van Riezen, H. (1976): Reversal of amnesia by an orally active ACTH 4-9 analog (Org 2766). *Pharmacol. Biochem. Behav. (Suppl.)*, 5:53-58.
47. Rigter, H. (1976): *Personal communication.*
48. Sanders, A. F., Truyens, C. L. and Bunt, A. A. (1975): ACTH 4-10 and learning. Institute for Perception TNO-Soesterberg, Report No. 1975-4.
49. Sandman, C. A., Kastin, A. J., and Schally, A. V. (1969): Melanocyte-stimulating hormone and learned appetitive behavior. *Experientia*, 23:100-102.

50. Sandman, C. A., Kastin, A. J. and Schally, A. V. (1971): Behavioral inhibition as modified by melanocyte-stimulation hormone (MSH) and light-dark conditions. *Physiol. Behav.*, 6:45-48.
51. Sandman, C. A., George, J. M., Nolan, J. D., van Riezen, H., and Kastin, A. J. (1975): Enhancement of attention in man with ACTH/MSH 4-10. *Physiol. Behav.*, 15:427-431.
52. Sandman, C. A., and Kastin, A. J. (1976): Neuropeptide influences on behavior: a possible treatment for disorders of attention. *Pharmacol. Biochem. Behav. (Suppl.)*, 5:1-2.
53. Sandman, C. A., Kastin, A. J., and Miller, L. H. (1977): Central nervous system action of MSH and related short-chain peptides. In: *Clinical Neuroendocrinology*, edited by G. M. Besser and L. Martini. Academic Press, New York *(In press.)*
54. Sandman, C. A., George, J., Walker, B., Nolan, J. D., and Kastin, A. J. (1976): The heptapeptide MSH/ACTH 4-10 enhances attention in the mentally retarded. *Pharmacol. Biochem. Behav. (Suppl.)*, 5:23-28.
55. Sterba, G. (1974): Das oxytocinerge neurosekretorische System der Wirbeltiere. Beitrag zu einem erweiterten Konzept. *Z. J. Physiol.*, 78:409-423.
56. Urban, I. and de Wied, D. (1975): Differences in RSA during paradoxical sleep in heterozygous and homozygous brattleboro rats: effect of DG-AVP. In: *Abstracts Symposia and Communications 16th Dutch Federative Meeting*, p. 369. Stichting Federatie Med. Biol. Ver. in Nederland, Nÿmegen.
57. Urban, I. and de Wied, D. (1976): Changes in excitability of the theta activity generating substrate by ACTH 4-10 in the rat. *Exp. Brain Res.*, 24:325-334.
58. Van Ree, J. M., and de Wied, D. (1976): Neuropeptides and morphine: physical dependence (in Dutch). *Abstracts symposia and communications 17th Dutch Federative Meeting*, p. 332. Stichting Federatie Med. Biol. Ver. in Nederland, Nÿmegen.
59. Van Wimersma Greidanus, Tj. B., Bohus, B. and de Wied, D. (1974): Effects of peptide hormones on behavior. Differential localization of the influence of lysine-vasopressin and of ACTH 4-10 on avoidance behavior. A study with rats bearing lesions in the parafascicular nuclei. *Neuroendocrinology*, 14:280-288.
60. Van Wimersma Greidanus, Tj. B., Bohus, B., and de Wied, D. (1975): The role of vasopressin in memory processes. In: *Prog. Brain Res.*, 42, 135-141.
61. Van Wimersma Greidanus, Tj. B., and de Wied, D. (1976): Dorsal hippocampus: a site of action of neuropeptides on avoidance behavior. *Pharmacol. Biochem. Behav. (Suppl.)*, 5:29-34.
62. Van Wimersma Greidanus, Tj. B., and de Wied, D. (1977): The physiology of the neurohypophyseal system and its relation to memory processes. In: *Biochemical Correlates of Brain Function*, edited by A. N. Dawson, Academic Press, London.
63. Verhoef, J. and Witter, A. (1976): Distribution of a behaviorally highly potent ACTH 4-9 analogue in rat brain after intraventricular administration. *Proceedings 17th Dutch*

Federative meeting of medical and biological societies, Amsterdam, Abstracts and communications, p. 397.   Stichting Federatie Med. Biol. Ver. in Nederland, Nÿmegen.

64. Wagenaar, W. A.   (1976):   *Personal communication.*
65. Wilson, I., Prange, A. J., Lara, P. P., Loosen, P. T.   (1976): Pituitary responses to thyrotropin releasing hormone in depressed patients: a review.   *Pharmacol. Biochem. Behav. (Suppl.),* 5:95–102.
66. Witter, A., Greven, H. M., and de Wied, D.   (1975):   Correlation between structure, behavioral activity and rate of biotransformation of some ACTH 4–9 analogs.   *J. Pharmacol. Exp. Therap.,* 193:853–860.

Neuropeptide Influences on the Brain and Behavior, edited by L.H. Miller, C.A. Sandman, and A.J. Kastin. Raven Press, New York © 1977.

EEG and Evoked Potential Approaches to the Study of Neuropeptides

Charles Shagass

Temple University Medical Center, and Eastern Pennsylvania Psychiatric Institute, Philadelphia, Pennsylvania 19129

This chapter has two principle goals: one, to discuss the available electrophysiological evidence concerning central effects of neuropeptides in man, and two, to consider ways in which electrophysiological methods can be applied to future investigations.

Two main kinds of electrical brain activity can be recorded from the surface of the human head: the electroencephalogram (EEG), and a variety of event related potentials (ERP). The EEG can be displayed directly after amplification, but ERPs must usually be extracted from the EEGs by a process of averaging. The major kinds of ERP include: (a), sensory evoked potentials (EPs); (b), long-latency potentials which are related more to the psychological than the physical attributes of stimuli, e.g., the P300 wave described by Sutton et al. (87); (c), potentials associated with movement, or motor potentials (29); and (d), slow potentials, such as the contingent negative variation (CNV) (95).

Role of Electrophysiological
Methods in Behavioral Research

In our present state of knowledge, scalp recordings of brain electrical activity provide relatively limited information about detailed neuronal processes, but they can play an important role in relating statistical attributes of such processes to behavioral events. The main limitations of electrophysiological methods can be summarized as follows: (a), electrical signals recorded at the scalp reflect the essentially statistical resultant of a complicated mix of events taking place in large numbers of neurons; (b), these are recorded at a distance and distorted to an unknown degree by conduction through intervening tissues; (c), the recordings

contain an extremely large amount of information, adequately quantifiable only with computer assistance; and
(d), mathematical techniques for reducing the measurements to a small number of meaningful terms are still
under development. Although computer technology can
now handle many problems of quantification and data reduction, serious practical and conceptual problems remain in applying a variety of analytic methods.

The compensating advantages of electrophysiological
methods are: (a) they reflect brain activity; (b) they
can provide more or less continuous recordings in subjects capable of reporting and responding; (c) they are
totally noninvasive; and (d) it is possible to record
in animals electrical brain signals analagous to those
obtained in man, so that electrophysiological correlates of behavior determined in man can be used to
devise animal models. These attributes of electrophysiological methods render them particularly important
tools for investigating mechanisms underlying the actions of agents which influence human behavior, among
which the neuropeptides may be included. In investigations of psychoactive drugs, EEG and EP methods have
been used to provide classifications of psychoactive
agents, and to predict the effects of new agents (25,
34, 36, 61).

Electrophysiological methods can be used in neuropeptide studies for one or more of several possible
purposes. Stated in a general way, these purposes
are: (a) simply to demonstrate that an agent alters
brain electrical activity, i.e., no specific effects
are predicted; (b) to test specific hypotheses about
brain effects, e.g., that EP will occur sooner (shorter
latency) because synaptic delay is reduced: (c) to
test behavioral hypotheses by means of known electrophysiological correlates, e.g., that attention to a
sensory stimulus is augmented, with concomitant increase in the amplitude of EP components occurring
after 100 msec (63). Studies to date have involved the
first and third kinds of goals. The second kind of
goal depends upon the availability of detailed knowledge concerning neurophysiological significance of
brain potential events, such as the location of the
source of potentials; although there is now a fair
amount of information of this kind, much remains to be
learned. Realization of the third kind of goal is obviously contingent upon knowledge of electrophysiological correlates of behavior; the required psychophysiological information is far from complete and is currently the focus of much investigative effort. An additional goal, which could be encompassed under the
third, would be involved in therapeutic application of
neuropeptides to clinical syndromes, such as schizo-

phrenia; electrophysiological measures previously found deviant in schizophrenia (70) could be obtained concomitantly with clinical observations.

SOME METHODOLOGICAL ISSUES

Individual Differences; State and Trait

EEG and ERP characteristics vary greatly between individuals in the "resting" state, and also in the extent to which they are changed by environmental manipulations or drugs. As in drug studies, investigations of the neuropeptides will have to take into account pretreatment level, not only as a base line for measurement of change, but also as a possible indicator of individuality in reaction to the agent. In other words, the possibility needs to be considered that the electrophysiological response to neuropeptides may depend upon individual EEG and ERP characteristics, which are of a relatively enduring nature and can be considered as traits. There is ample evidence that, under standard conditions, EEG and EP measurements are relatively stable over time (37, 41, 65). This stability appears to depend to a large extent upon genetic factors (5, 23, 47, 60). Although reactivity to a drug may be entirely a correlate of change in state, it could also reflect trait, including genetic factors (2). The practical relevance of this point for neuropeptide studies is that, unless the subject population is quite homogeneous with respect to base line measurements, a large sample may be required to distinguish the interactions between state and trait phenomena.

Age and Sex

Age and sex are major factors influencing EEG and ERP characteristics. Because of EEG variations with the menstrual cycle, Itil (34) found it useful to restrict his EEG investigations of drugs to males. However, once effects are demonstrated in males, it is still necessary to determine whether they occur in females. In normal subjects, interactions between age, personality (introversion-extraversion), and EP amplitude have been demonstrated (77). In psychiatric populations, we have found age and sex differences in EP characteristics, which were not present in normals (72, 73); such interactions can be demonstrated only by appropriate statistical designs.

Pharmacological Status

Most drugs with psychoactive effects influence EEG and ERP measurements (34, 67, 68). Although such drug

effects are generally recognized, it is less well
known that commonly used substances, such as caffeine
and tobacco, influence EEG and ERP measurements (31,
54). As might be expected from its psychoactive effects, alcohol also modified EEG and ERP, and the effects of different alcoholic beverages vary, depending
upon the congeners contained in them (48, 54). Experimental designs should also consider the fact that electrophysiological effects of short-term withdrawal from
alcohol and tobacco have been demonstrated (54, 90).

Level of Awareness

Changes in gross level of consciousness are associated with dramatic EEG and ERP alterations. Although
correlations with more subtle variations in levels of
attention and alertness may be less obvious, there is
much evidence that they occur (65). Such correlations
may, in themselves, be the focus of study, but controls
for the attentive state of the subject are required,
and may be difficult to implement. Many electrophysiological investigators attempt to achieve control over
state of alertness by recording within a task context,
e.g., reaction time (34) in order to reduce subject
"options" (86). When EEG and ERP phenomena related to
state of attention are the dependent variables, concomitant behavioral measures reflecting attentive processes are especially important.

Extracerebral Contaminants

EEG and ERP recordings are subject to contamination
by potentials of extracerebral origin, and the investigator must constantly deal with the possibility of this
kind of artifact. Potentials arising in the muscles
(EMG) and the orbit (electrooculogram) (EOG) are major
sources. Such contaminating potentials are usually
readily recognized in the EEG tracing, although it may
be difficult to distinguish between fast frequency
activity of brain and muscle origin. Visual screening
of records before computer quantification to remove
contaminated segments is mandatory, although obviously
not infallible. In ERP recordings, biological contam-
inants may present even more difficult problems of control, particularly with such phenomena as the microre-
flexes to which Bickford et al. (3) drew attention.

Instrumentation

Although a detailed discussion of instrumentation
issues is not warranted here, one requirement seems
worthy of emphasis. This is that frequency response
characteristics of amplifiers and tape recorders, and

the sampling rates used in averaging computers must be
such as not to distort or attenuate signals of interest. For example, upper frequency cutoffs at 3 KHz
are recommended to record early somatosensory EP
events (21), while a cutoff at 50 Hz is adequate for
later potentials. Conversely, slow potentials, such as
the CNV, require a long time constant (5 sec or more),
while a very short time constant will suffice for early EP events.

EEG

Functional Correlates

   The blocking of the alpha rhythm with opening of
eyes was perhaps the earliest observed EEG correlate
of change in functional state. Alpha-blocking, or reduction of alpha amplitude, may also accompany a large
variety of mental tasks, such as arithmetic performance.
Alpha frequency also generally increases with mental
work. Although these changes in EEG amplitude and frequency are usually taken as indicators of heightened
attention or "arousal," it should be noted that similar
changes occur in early stages of drowsiness or sleep,
which then need to be recognized by other indicators.
Another important factor influencing the significance
of changes in alpha activity with mental performance
is the nature of the imagery used in the task and the
subject's habitual style of imagery, i.e., verbal or
visual. Slatter (82) showed clearly that visual imagery is associated with reduction in the alpha rhythms,
whereas verbal imagery is associated with their persis-
tance. Furthermore, subjects with habitual visual
imagery tend to have low amplitude and intermittent
alpha, whereas those with habitual verbal imagery tend
to have high amplitude and persistent alpha.
   The parallel between blocking of the alpha rhythm in
man, and the desynchronization of cortial activity by
stimulation of the mesencephalic reticular formation
in animals contributed in an important way to development of arousal theory. However, there has been little
success in attempts to correlate EEG measures of arousal with autonomic indicators, such as heart rate, pal-
mar conductance, and respiratory rate (66). This casts
doubt upon notions of generalized arousal, and prompts
caution in interpretation of EEG measures within this
conceptual framework. One source of evidence, which
does suggest that alpha frequency may depend heavily
upon the level of activity in the reticular formation,
is the sensory deprivation literature. Prolonged
sensory deprivation appears to result in slowing of the
alpha frequency persisting for several hours (97), sug-

gesting that constant sensory inputs are needed to
maintain reticular formation influences.

Several investigators have attempted to relate alpha
frequency to reaction time with varying results (4, 85).
The positive results indicate that faster reaction times
are associated with shorter alpha periods, i.e., faster
frequency (85). There is also some evidence that reaction time in a given individual will vary with the
phase of the alpha cycle upon which the stimulus im-
pinges (11, 12, 46).

There has been a great deal of interest in the functional specialization of the hemispheres, the left
hemisphere being thought to be predominantly involved
in verbal tasks, and the right hemisphere in nonverbal
tasks. Galin and Ornstein (26) used the relative
amount of alpha blocking in each hemisphere during performance of verbal and nonverbal tasks to provide EEG
evidence of hemispheric specialization, greater blocking occurring in the more active hemisphere. Recently,
Callaway et al. (15) utilized a measure of cortical
coupling, developed by Callaway and Harris (14), to
compare EEG effects of auditory and visual stimuli.
The coupling measure indicates the extent to which the
activities of different brain areas covary. Callaway
et al. (15) found that, normally, there is greater
coupling between EEGs from different parts of the
right hemisphere with visual stimuli than with auditory
stimuli, whereas auditory stimuli were associated with
greater coupling between left hemisphere recordings.
This difference in coupling related to sensory modality
was absent in a group of dyslexic subjects. Callaway's
method represents one approach to the important problem of interarea relationships between brain potentials. Although a number of workers have attempted to
relate measures of interarea relationships to mental
activity with interesting results, e.g., Darrow et al.
(20), Livanov et al. (49), Giannitripani (28), the
methods applied have been more laborious than the Callaway coupling measure and the work has seldom been
repeated by others.

Psychopathological correlates of EEG characteristics
have been investigated by a number of workers. Results
in schizophrenia and depression have recently been summarized (69). The findings of greatest interest are
that mean frequency is about 1 cycle lower in chronic
schizophrenics than in normals and that α-blocking to
light flash is of longer duration in severe depressions.

Neuropeptide Effects on the EEG

Itil (35) reported that the tripeptide (L-prolyl-L-
leucylglycinamide), commonly called MIF (melanocyte-

stimulating hormone inhibiting factor), produced EEG changes in normal volunteers. The MIF was compared with placebo and administered in dosages ranging from 50 to 1,500 mg in single oral administrations. The effects in subjects with slow EEGs differed from those with fast EEGs. The EEG effects of the 50 mg dose suggested that MIF may have sedative properties in this dosage, while the high doses produced a profile like that obtained with stimulants. Itil states that the computerized EEG profiles of MIF differed from those seen with minor tranquilizers, major tranquilizers, and thymoleptics. The main conclusion reached from this study was that it can be demonstrated that MIF goes to the brain after oral administration.

Kastin et al. (42) studied the effect of melanocyte-stimulating hormone (α-MSH) on the EEG, and noted some tendency toward slowing, although this was not significant. Miller et al. (53) found that ACTH 4-10 decreased EEG activity in the 3 to 7 Hz band, and increased it in the bands with frequencies of 7 Hz and up. ACTH 4-10 also appeared to diminish the habituation of the α-blocking response. Miller et al. (53) failed to find EEG effects with ACTH 1-24. More recently, Sannita et al. (62) and Small et al. (personal communication) failed to demonstrate EEG changes with ACTH 4-10.

The five subjects in the Kastin et al. (42) study included 2 patients hypophysectomized for acromegaly and 1 patient with Sheehan's syndrome, while the subjects in the Miller et al. (53) study were 20 healthy medical students, and those in the Small et al. study were psychiatric patients; the investigations obviously differed in important respects. On the other hand, the subjects in the Sannita et al. (62) study were 12 healthy students, and one would have expected this population to give results comparable to the Miller et al. findings. The results, however, are not as incompatible as they might seem, since in the Sannita et al. study there were significant increases in slow activity with saline placebo which did not occur with ACTH 4-10. This suggests that the neuropeptide prevented changes associated with drowsiness under the placebo condition. Both the Miller et al. (53) and Sannita et al. (62) studies attempted to maintain vigilance by engaging the subject in various tasks.

Clearly, much more data must be gathered before any conclusions can be reached about EEG effects of ACTH 4-10. The evidence suggests that some increase of alerting may be reflected in the EEG. Systematic dosage studies with ACTH 4-10 would be useful, since the results reported by Itil (35) with MIF might lead one to expect different EEG effects with different doses of

ACTH 4-10. Sannita et al. (62) refer to an unpublished study by Fink and Irwin, which employed 10, 15, and
20 mg doses, in which EEG changes of decreased amplitude of alpha activity and increased beta and theta
activity were observed. In other unpublished studies
mentioned by Sannita et al. 15 mg doses of ACTH 4-10
did not define a systematic EEG profile, and transient
EEG changes were seen at doses above 90 mg, approximately 15 min after ACTH 4-10 administration.

Future Investigations

   If neuropeptides become available in adequate quantity for investigative purposes, it would seem worth-
while to perform thorough investigations of their EEG
effects. Such investigations should include recordings from several electrodes on each side of the head
to give adequate anteroposterior sampling. In addition
to power spectrum or period analysis types of quantification, it may be most valuable to apply measures of
interarea relationships. These could include the cross-
spectral phase shift and coherence ratio measures described by Caille (10), as well as the Callaway and
Harris (14) coupling measure, and perhaps cross-corre-
lation. De Wied et al. (22) have reviewed evidence indicating that the thalamic area and the limbic forebrain are structures sensitive to the behavioral effects of neuropeptides. Bilateral lesions in the rostral septal area and in the dorsal hippocampus abolished the behavioral effects of vasopressin, and lesions
in the nuclei parafascicularis prevented the inhibitory
effect of α-MSH on extinction of a shuttle-box avoidance response. These and other findings in animals indicate that brain structures involved in integrative
activity are modulated by neuropeptide substances.
Consequently, it seems reasonable to expect that EEG
measures directed at revealing interrelationships among
brain areas, or the interplay among these areas, might
be more revealing of subcortical effects than the quantitative description of activity in any one area. What
is suggested is a dynamic EEG approach to investigation
of brain activity in studying effects of neuropeptides.

EVENT RELATED POTENTIALS

Description

   In describing ERPs, the convention will be followed
of designating individual peaks by polarity and usual
latency, e.g., N100 indicates a negative peak occurring about 100 msec after stimulus.

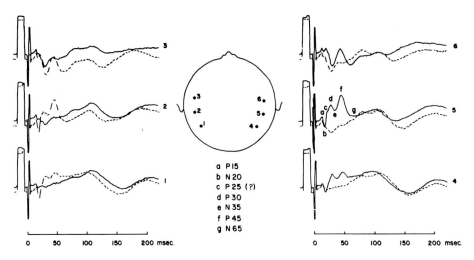

FIG. 1. Somatosensory potentials evoked by stimulating right (broken line) and left (solid line) median nerves with 0.1 msec square wave pulses 10 ma above sensory threshold. Tracings are group sums for 12 normal subjects. Scalp leads referred to linked ears. Positivity at scalp gives upward deflection. Square wave calibration preceding stimulus artifact, 5 uv. Note predominant contralateral location of early EP events (a to g). For further description, see text.

Somatosensory EP (SEP)

Figure 1 shows SEP to right and left median nerve shocks at an intensity 10 ma above sensory threshold; the traces are the group sum of 12 normal subjects. The early SEP events are seen in leads contralateral to the stimulated wrist. The letters a to g in the lead 5 tracings designate peaks P15, N20, P25, P30, N35, P45, and N65. P30 is not visible as a positivity in lead 6, which is anterior to the central sulcus, but is reversed in phase.

Allison et al. (1) have recently reviewed the neural origins of early SEP components. Integrating scalp EP data with results obtained from direct cortical recordings made in patients undergoing neurosurgery and in animal studies, they reached the following conclusions: (1), P15 is generated by the ascending afferent volley in cerebral lemniscal pathways. It corresponds to the large positive potential recorded in or near the venteroposterolateral (VPL) nucleus of the thalamus. P15 at the scalp thus represents some combination of lemniscal inflow to VPL, synaptic events in VPL itself, and the ensuing thalamocortial volley. P15 is recorded widely over the scalp because it is in essence a "far-field" potential. (2) N20, P25, and P30 reflect

initial cortical activity, or the primary SEP. There
are two separate generators in the postcentral gyrus.
One generator is located in the posterior bank of the
central sulcus and the dipole is oriented parallel to
the cortical surface; it gives rise to the N20-P30 SEP
in the posterior electrode (leads 2 and 5, Fig. 1) and
phase reversed N20-P30 in an anterior lead (leads 3 and
6, Fig. 1). The second generator produces the P25-N35
complex and is located in a restricted region of the
crown of the postcentral gyrus near the central sulcus.
Because the P25-N35 generator is oriented upward, no
phase reversal is observed. (3), The origins of P45
and N65 are not definitely established. They occur
only in contralateral cortex, and do not display a
phase reversal; they may reflect an upward oriented
generator like that of P25-N35. Although the P45, N65
generator may be the same as that of P25-N35, it appears to involve a more diffuse region of somatomotor
cortex.

The SEP events occurring later than N65 are better
visualized in Fig. 2, which shows the group sum SEP
tracings of 16 normal subjects recorded from 14 scalp
leads and one EOG lead. The later potentials are visible in recordings from leads over virtually the entire
head, although they are of greatest amplitude near the
vertex (Cz, F3X, F4X, C3X, C4X). The later peaks may
be designated as P90, N130, P180 and P280. Note that,
at Cz, P180 is of such high amplitude that the succeeding P280, although of relatively high amplitude, can
hardly be seen as a separate peak.

Goff et al. (30) have obtained evidence to indicate
the P90 wave reflects two sources, one of which is myo-
genic and probably in orbital structures; the other,
more posterior, source is in the brain. The anterior
P90 has not been seen in direct human brain recordings,
whereas the posterior P90 has been recorded by Goff et
al. (30); their evidence indicates that the posterior
generator of P90 is the same as that of N20-P30, i.e.,
in the posterior bank of the central sulcus.

The topographic studies conducted by Goff et al. (30)
indicate that the maximum amplitude of N130 and P180 is
at the vertex, as in Fig. 2; with depth electrodes,
N130 and P180 were found to reverse in phase at some
point below the cortical surface. The depth electrode
studies of Velasco et al. (92) indicate that these late
SEP components can be recorded from widespread subcortical regions, and that the nucleus ventralis anterior oralis is crucial in their production.

The SEP shown in Fig. 2 were obtained in a situation
in which several kinds of stimuli were presented in
pseudorandom order, and the subjects were required to
maintain eye fixation in anticipation of the visual

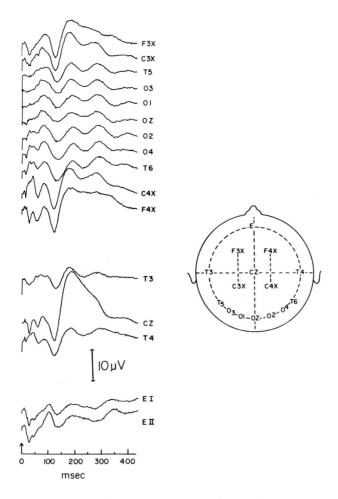

FIG. 2. Group sum EPs for 16 normal subjects (left median nerve stimuli). Linked ear reference, scalp positivity up. Note contralateral early response in lead C4X and maximal amplitude of later peaks (N130, P180, P280) in leads around vertex (Cz). EI and EII designate recordings from E lead taken in two separate runs.

stimulus, a checkerboard pattern. Such a situation may be considered capable of generating the P300 wave; P280 is probably an example of this event, which is associated with expectancy and some degree of uncertainty about the forthcoming stimulus (87).

Auditory EP (AEP)

By appropriate recording procedures, very early AEP events can be recorded from the scalp as "far-field"

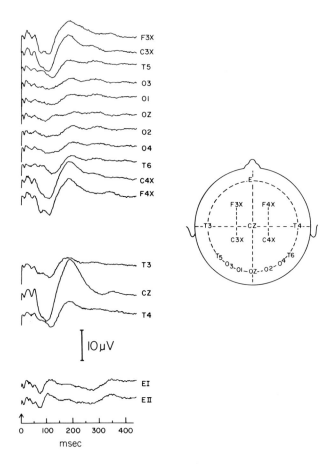

FIG. 3. Group sum potentials evoked by binaural clicks in 16
normal subjects. Recordings as in Fig. 2.

potentials (40). These can be designated as P1.5, N2,
P3, P4, P5, P6. Buchwald and Huang (9) have demonstrated that the generators of these early peaks are as
follows: P1.5, acoustic nerve; P3, cochlear nucleus;
P4, neurons of the superior olivary complex, activated
by projections crossing the midline; P5, neurons of the
ventral nucleus of the lateral lemniscus and preolivary
region, activated equally by crossed and uncrossed projections; P6, neurons of the inferior colliculus activated primarily by crossed projections.
  Figure 3 shows the later AEP events which can be
designated as P30, P50, N100, and P190. A small P360
is seen, most readily, in the Cz lead. Goff et al. (30)
have reviewed the evidence concerning which AEP peak
may reflect the primary response. They concluded that
none of the scalp-recorded AEP events meets the crite-

rion of a primary auditory response. Although this
renders interpretation of AEP findings difficult, the
conclusion seems reasonable in view of the fact that
Heschl's gyrus is located so far from the surface. It
is also of interest to note that, in depth electrode
studies, the AEP events appear to retain the same polarity in the depth as at the surface; this is quite
different from the observations made with SEP.

Visual Evoked Potentials (VEP)

Many VEP studies have been carried out using as stimuli relatively bright flashes, generated by strobo-
scopes. Cigánek's (17) description of the flash VEP
has been generally adopted; his peaks were as follows:
N40, P53, N73, P94, N114, P135, and N190. With eyes
closed, this sequence of components is often followed
by rhythmic waves of about 100 msec duration, which
have been referred to as the VEP after-rhythm or
"ringing." VEP are sensitive to many stimulus characteristics, such as intensity, color, pattern, contrast,
etc. (58). The primary visual response is probably the
very low amplitude P20 to 25 wave described by Cobb and
Dawson (18).

VEP latencies are generally longer with pattern
stimuli than with flash, and the potentials are greatly
influenced by the retinal location of the stimulus.
Jeffreys and Axford (38, 39) have described an initial
component with a latency of 65 to 80 msec, which appears to be of striate cortical origin, and a second
component at 90 to 100 msec latency which is extrastriate. Figure 4 shows the group sum VEP of 16 normal subjects, elicited by brief exposure of a checkerboard pattern subtending 8.5° to right and left of
central fixation. At the midline occipital (Oz) lead,
the components can be designated as N70, P90, N120,
and P225. In more anterior leads, there is a phase
reversal of the first 3 components, whereas the P225
lead maintains its polarity throughout; P225 appears to
be a "nonspecific" midline event. Evidence of a P300
wave can also be seen in most of the leads, the amplitude being greatest at Cz.

If the checkerboard flash stimulus is applied to one
or another visual half-field, the earlier VEP peaks
occur mainly in leads over the hemisphere contralateral
to the visual field stimulated. This is illustrated in
Fig. 5, which shows the group sum half-field VEPs to
checkerboard pattern onset in 13 normal subjects.
Peaks P125 and N175 are almost entirely contralateral,
whereas P225 is not lateralized. Spatial distribution
plots of the three peaks confirm the lateralization of
P125 and N175 (Fig. 6).

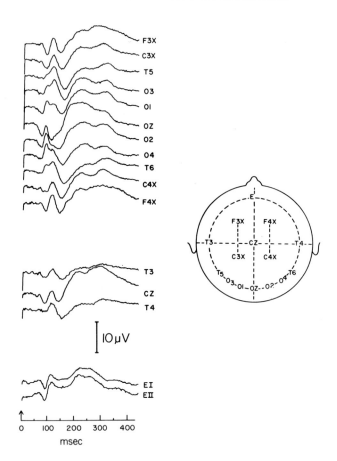

FIG. 4.   Group sum potentials evoked by full-field checkerboard flash (duration, 8 msec; intensity, 1.2 foot-lambert) in 16 normal subjects.   Recordings as in Fig. 2.

Motor Potentials

Kornhüber and Deecke (44) described a "readiness potential" which was enhanced by the "intentional engagement" of the subject to execute a motor act.   Gilden et al. (29) demonstrated additional aspects of cortical potentials associated with voluntary movement. The motor potential contains four main components: (a) starting about 1 sec before the onset of muscular contraction, a slow negative shift of the base line; (b) 50 to 150 msec prior to contraction a small positive deflection; (c) a large negative wave during the rising phase of the contraction; (d) about 150 msec after the start of the contraction a large positive wave. Vaughan et al. (91) consider the motor potential to originate over the Rolandic cortex, but Gerbrandt et al.

PATTERN-ONSET

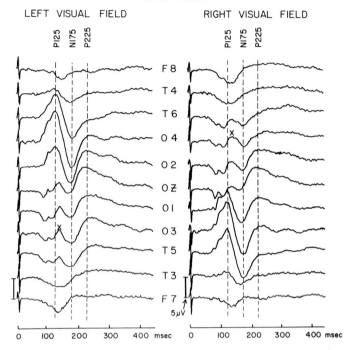

FIG. 5. Group sum potentials evoked by half-field checkerboard pattern onset stimuli in 13 normal subjects. F7 and F8 leads as in 10 to 20 system; remaining leads as in head diagram in preceding figure. Note that peaks P125 and N175 occur mainly in hemisphere contralateral to stimulated visual field. P140 peak marked by Xs in 03 and 04 tracings was an inconsistent event and represents an artifact of averaging across subjects.

(27) believe that the potential may, in part, be generated by sensory cortical events.

Long Latency Potentials

The long latency component designated as P300, or P3, has been referred to in descriptions of SEP, AEP, and VEP (Figs. 2 to 4). This component is recorded at maximum amplitude from the vertex, and is greatest when the nature of an expected forthcoming stimulus is least certain. Recently, it has been shown that there are at least two P3 waves, with different functional attributes and spatial distributions (19).

Contingent Negative Variation (CNV)

The CNV, the early slow negativity in the motor potential, and the readiness potential are slow potential

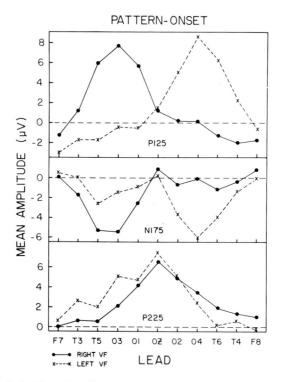

FIG. 6.   Spatial distributions of peaks P125, N175 and P225 in EPs
obtained with half-field checkerboard pattern onset (tracings in
Fig. 5).   Measurements substantiate lateralized distributions of
P125 and N175.

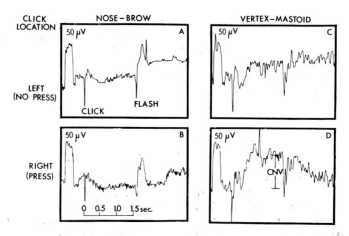

FIG. 7.   Contingent negative variation (CNV) tracings.   Experimental paradigm involved alerting clicks in left and right ears;
right ear click signaled that button press to succeeding flash
was required, whereas left ear click indicated no button press required.   Record D contains CNV, whereas record C does not.   Records A and B taken to monitor EOG artifact.

shifts. The CNV has been most investigated in a psychological context (88, 89). CNV is often measured in the framework of a reaction time paradigm; an alerting or warning signal precedes the delivery of an imperative stimulus to which the subject must make some kind of response, such as a button press. During the interval between stimuli, usually 1 to 2 sec, the CNV develops; a minimum interval of 0.5 sec is needed. The experiment may contain a control condition in which a similar signal without the same significance for a response is administered (Fig. 7). When a response is required, a slow negative potential deviation commences about 200 msec after the alerting stimulus, and continues to rise until there has been a response to the imperative stimulus; there is then a precipitous shift back toward the base line, or positivity. The CNV is generally symmetrically distributed and the maximum amplitude is near the vertex. CNV has been recorded from implanted electrodes in man (93) and in monkeys (50). Walter (94) states that implanted electrode studies indicate that only about 2% of frontal cortex is ordinarily involved in a CNV; this suggests that a great deal more cortex could be brought into play under appropriate conditions.

Functional Correlates

Early EP events are strongly determined by physical attributes of the stimulus. The EP is usually just detectable when stimulus intensity corresponds to sensory threshold; with increasing stimulus intensity, amplitude increases. Psychological manipulations, such as directions to focus attention, have little or no effect upon early EP components, whereas they can have a marked influence on components occurring after 100 msec. In Satterfield's (63) early experiment, the subject was stimulated alternately with click and nerve shock, and was asked to pay attention to one or the other. When attention was directed toward the click, the AEP contained a markedly augmented P180 component and the SEP did not; attention to shock produced reverse results. Näätänen (55) drew attention to the fact that experiments like Satterfield's did not really provide evidence of EP correlates of *selective* attention, in the sense that the response to one stimulus is augmented and that the other diminished; the increased P180 amplitude could be interpreted as evidence of preparatory activation preceding relevant stimuli. However, Eason et al. (24) were able to show that EP evidence of selective attention could be obtained providing stimuli were of low intensity and in the same sensory modality. The results of Eason et al. indicated that preparatory

activation was also a factor in increasing P180 amplitude.

The amplitude of the P300 wave is inversely related
to the probability of occurrence of a stimulus, so
that it was originally interpreted as an electrical
event signaling the resolution of stimulus uncertainty
(87). The P300 component may perhaps be most compre-
hensively understood in terms of orienting or dishabit-
uation. Ritter and Vaughan (59) found that the amplitude of P300 increased when the sensory discrimination
was very difficult, but that it was not correlated
with success in detecting the stimuli. After considering a number of possibilities, they concluded that P300
appears to be a correlate of central processes for cognitive evaluation of stimulus significance.

The CNV has been variously interpreted by different
workers as an electrical sign of expectancy, decision,
motivation, volition, preparatory set or conation, and
arousal. Tecce (88) pointed out that all of these conceptualized psychological states involve a heightening
of attention. CNV amplitude increases with concentration and decreases with distraction (51). There are
some data suggesting that CNV amplitude is greater with
faster reaction time, but this relationship has been
found only within some individuals (56).

A useful general interpretation of EPs is to regard
the early events as reflecting information transmission
and the later events as reflecting information processing activities. The early events are more neurophysiological, and the later events and slow potentials are
more psychophysiological in nature.

ERPs have been investigated in a variety of clinical
contexts (58, 65, 69). Practical application of AEP
recording has been made in audiometric examinations;
this is particularly valuable in subjects who are unable to respond verbally. VEPs can also be utilized
in the examination of vision; they can provide the
basis for accurate refraction. Recently, the VEP elicited by checkerboard reversal stimuli has been shown to
provide a useful diagnostic sign of multiple sclerosis
(32); prolonged P120 latency occurs in an eye with re-
trobulbar neuritis, even long after symptoms have abat-
ed. Correlations between EP measurements and various
kinds of psychological characteristics, such as intel-
ligence, have recently been thoroughly reviewed by Callaway (13).

Some special ways of measuring EP were developed
for the purpose of studying psychiatric populations,
although they have been applied in other contexts.
These measurements include: (a) curves relating response amplitude to stimulus intensity (8, 76); (b)
recovery cycles, determined by employing paired stim-

uli separated by varying intervals (74, 83); (c) recovery measurements employing trains of stimuli (64,
73); and (d) wave shape variability (16, 78). Studies employing these procedures have yielded a considerable amount of evidence indicating that EP characteristics of severely ill psychiatric patients differ
from normal (69, 70). Currently, in our laboratory,
we are employing a comprehensive EP approach to study
of psychiatric patients; we obtain, in a single experiment, EPs to right and left median nerve shocks,
checkerboard flash, and clicks. An initial evaluation
of results in schizophrenia confirmed previous findings that all later events of the N100, P200, and P300
type are much reduced from normal in schizophrenic
patients (80). In contrast, the amplitudes of early
SEP and AEP events were not attenuated, and there were
trends in agreement with previous findings (73) that
early SEPs were of greater amplitude and less variable
in chronic schizophrenics than in schizophrenics of
other types or in nonpatients. Discriminations between
subtypes of schizophrenia and depression have also been
yielded by the flash EP test of augmenting-reducing developed by Buchsbaum and Silverman (8), which measures
the intensity-response amplitude function (6, 45).

It should be apparent that ERP methods can be used
to demonstrate the effects of drugs or hormones in
either a neurophysiological or a behavioral context in
a large number of ways. Pharmacological studies of EP
have been reviewed fairly recently (61, 67). Within
the context of this conference, it is noteworthy that
EP amplitude characteristics have been shown to vary
with the state of thyroid, adrenal, and parathyroid
function. In hypothyroid patients, amplitudes are lower and average latencies prolonged; these differences
are eliminated by thyroid replacement therapy. Conversely, triiodothyronine (T3) increases EP amplitude
in normals (81, 84). T3 also increases the P200 wave
in an attention paradigm, but, interestingly, only when
the subject is asked to ignore the stimuli; the effect
was not noticed with stimuli to which the subject was
asked to attend (43). Carbohydrate-active steroids decreased the latency of VEP, particularly in the later
waves, but steroids which possess sodium-potassium activity did not (57). Recently, Buchsbaum and Henkin
(7) found that, in patients with adrenal cortical insufficiency, VEPs were of small amplitude and short
latency when the patient's steriod levels were low,
that amplitudes were even smaller when patients were
given ACTH, and that amplitudes were increased when
carbohydrate-active steroids were administered.

ERP Studies of Neuropeptides

Kastin et al. (42) observed a striking effect of α-MSH on SEP; the peptide increased the amplitude of P200 to a remarkable extent in 2 normal subjects and in 3 patients with absent or markedly reduced pituitary function. The changes were observed during both relaxation and attention, but were greater during attention. However, when the subject was distracted by psychological testing, MSH caused no increase in SEP amplitude. Also, the early components and the afferent nerve potential were not altered by α-MSH.

Miller et al. (53) recorded CNV and EEG during a disjunctive reaction time task in 20 normal subjects, half of whom were given ACTH 1-24 and the other half a placebo. An additional group of 20 subjects received ACTH 4-10 or placebo. No significant changes in CNV were observed with either drug, although ACTH 4-10 produced the EEG changes described earlier.

Recently, Miller et al. (52) recorded VEP to the relevant and irrelevant stimuli of a continuous performance task (CPT) and compared ACTH 4-10 with placebo. They observed diminished amplitude and delayed latency of a VEP N200 peak. This was seen with both task relevant and task irrelevant stimuli. The task relevant stimuli were associated with a large P300 wave (actual latency about 450 msec), but this wave was not affected by ACTH 4-10. An interesting correlate of the ACTH 4-10 was the appearance of an N350 peak in the task relevant EP; this peak, which was seen in most subjects with ACTH 4-10, was not present under placebo conditions. Miller et al. speculated that their data reflected the activation of a highly specific central alerting mechanism, and reflected a pattern of neural activation that has been shown to accompany attention or vigilance behavior in animals.

The remarkable augmentation of P200 in the SEP shown by Kastin et al. (42) seems not to have been replicated in VEP by Miller et al. (52); indeed, the findings of the latter investigators seem contrary. The noncomparability of the subject populations could be one reason for the discrepancy, but differences in the experimental situation may also be relevant. The Kastin et al. SEPs were recorded under three conditions: (a) relaxation, i.e., subject passive; (b) attention, i.e., subject instructed to press a lever immediately after receiving each stimulus to the median nerve; (c) distraction, i.e., subject undergoing psychological tests. The VEP in the Miller et al. (52) study were recorded within the context of the continuous performance task (CPT), and the stimuli were those to which the subject had to attend in order to decide whether or

not to press a button. Such a discrimination was not
required from the subjects in the Kastin study; the
Kastin attention condition can be considered similar
to the one employed by Satterfield (63), who simply
asked his subjects to pay attention to the stimulus.
If a α-MSH increased level of alertness in a general
way, one might expect to observe the Satterfield-type
effect in the attention, and perhaps the relaxation,
conditions of the Kastin study. In contrast, when SEP
were recorded with the subject distracted, any atten-
tion-augmenting effect of α-MSH might be directed away
from the stimulus; this would leave the SEP unchanged.
It seems possible that the reduced amplitude and prolonged latency of N200, found by Miller et al. in VEP
during CPT performance, may represent a distraction effect, in the sense that the CPT decision process could
direct attention toward the motor response and away
from the immediate sensory aspects of the stimulus.
Although this suggestion would reconcile the findings
of the two studies, it is not in agreement with the
overall results of EP studies of attention (88).

Another possible interpretation of the ACTH 4-10 effects, in the Miller et al. study, would be that the
N200 changes could be mainly pharmacological in nature.
The amplitude reduction was as Buchsbaum and Henkin (7)
found with ACTH, and is similar to the effect found by
Wolthuis and de Wied (96) in the rat with both 7-l-phe
ACTH 4-10 and 7-d-phe ACTH 4-10. The appearance of an
N350 peak with ACTH 4-10 in those trials that elicited
a P300 component, is difficult to explain. It is reminiscent of the enhanced N35, describable as "unmasking
of negativity" found by us with a wide range of psychoactive drug treatments (75).

Future Investigations

ERP Studies

There are many kinds of ERP phenomena, and each
type can be modified and made more complex by varying
the stimulus conditions and other aspects of the experimental situation. This constitutes an embarassment of
riches for the investigator who does not have a specific neurophysiological hypothesis upon which ERP observations are to be brought to bear. Since this appears
to be generally the case, it would probably be best to
approach ERP studies of neuropeptides by using methods
likely to yield the broadest range of data that can be
interpreted with relative ease. One can hope that the
results obtained with a broad-scan approach will lead
to more specific hypotheses for focused testing.

The comprehensive EP procedure, involving several

sensory modalities, which we are currently using, is
one approach that yields a broad range of EP data within a single experimental session (80). The entire procedure is computer-controlled and EP are averaged on-
line to give data of the kind shown in Figs. 2, 3, and
4. Although 192 EEG samples were averaged for each EP
of an individual subject's contribution to these tracings, four subaverages comprising 48 sweeps were also
obtained. The approach provides information about:
(a) topography, including between hemisphere and within hemisphere relationships; (b) variability of wave
shapes in time; (c) the extent to which results are
specific to one sensory modality. Obviously, the method could be used to determine whether neuropeptides
alter a broad range of EP characteristics. Furthermore, since several averages are obtained for each condition, this provides an error term, which permits statistical testing of the significance of within subject
changes.

Figure 8 illustrates one kind of descriptive statistical analysis that we have developed for use with the
comprehensive EP procedure; it involves computing t-
tests to assess the significance of the differences between means of individual data points in EPs reflecting
either group of experimental condition results. Group
sum SEPs to left median nerve stimuli of 16 normals, as
in Fig. 2, are compared with those of 32 schizophrenic
patients of the same age and sex. The t-tests (right
column) are displayed so that they rise above base
line only when they achieve the .05 level of significance. The number of significant differences between
the two populations was large, particularly in activities after 100 msec. The same program can be applied
to EPs equated for amplitude to assess relative contributions of amplitude and latency to the data point differences; differences due entirely to amplitude should
then disappear, while those due to variations in latency will persist.

It is perhaps noteworthy that we can perform these
operations with a minicomputer (PDP 12). With efficient utilization of memory capacity, we have been able
to examine both earlier and later events in detail.
We can also apply more complicated analytic techniques,
such as factor analysis, multiple discriminant functions, and various kinds of cluster and pattern analyses to aspects of the data which the descriptive analyses reveal to be important.

Although perhaps "shotgun" in nature, the comprehensive EP approach may provide the most efficient
means of detecting significant effects of neuropeptides
that merit further, more focused study. This is because

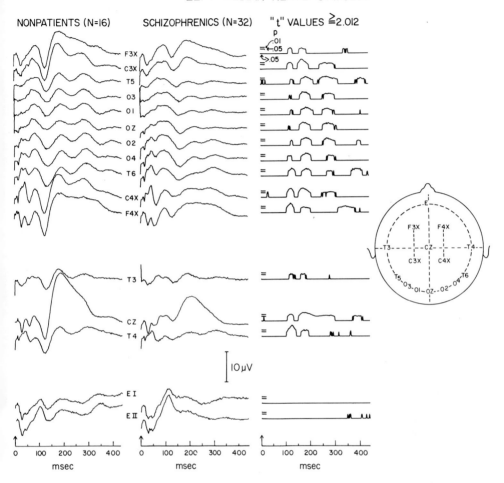

FIG. 8. Left and center columns: means EPs to left median nerve stimuli of 16 nonpatients and 32 schizophrenic patients matched for age and sex. Recordings as in Fig. 2. Right column indicates results of two-tailed *t*-tests performed on data points corresponding in time to those in EP tracings; when *t*-values were under 2.012 (*p*=.05), *t*-curve was kept at base line; values of 2.012 or greater plotted according to magnitude; .05 and .01 levels indicated by small parallel lines above left of *t*-curves.

so much information is obtained in every subject. The approach is, of course, not appropriate for testing specific hypotheses which require other experimental conditions. For example, a recovery function procedure would be needed to test a hypothesis about altered excitability, and several stimulus intensities would be

required to test augmenting-reducing, etc. However,
even when employing more complex stimulus procedures,
the investigator would do well to record from as many
leads as possible and to obtain more than one EP of
each kind.

EEG-Evoked Potential Relationships

Although one always records the EEG to obtain ERP,
the EEG taken during the stimulation period may not be
stored on analogue tape. It is desirable to do this
and also to record a few minutes of EEG in the "resting" state. This will permit the investigator to quantify the EEG data in various ways, to compare EEGs
taken during "resting" and stimulation conditions, and
to study the interrelationships between EEG and ERP
measurements. Investigation of EEG-ERP relationships
permits one to determine whether a measure of relationship predicts a criterion better than either EEG or ERP
alone; it can also provide leads concerning altered organization of brain activity. Relationships between
EEG and EP measurements have been found to be correlated with perceptual performance in normals (33, 71). We
have recently reported the results in the first study
of EEG-EP relationships in psychiatric patients (79).
We found that each of four major psychiatric diagnostic
groups tended to differ from normal in different ways
in terms of which kinds of EEG and EP variables yielded correlation differences. For example, SEP amplitude was positively correlated with EEG amplitude in
normals, while such correlations were negative in psy-
choneurotics (Fig. 9). Different combinations of EEG
and SEP variables yielded correlation differences for
three other groups: chronic schizophrenics, personality disorders, and depressed manic-depressives.

It will be apparent that considerable emphasis has
been placed here upon the need for investigating patterns of relationship between different kinds of brain
electrical events, and to take into account their topography and time course. The concept behind these
recommendations is that studies of electrophysiological
patterning will provide information about the functional organization of the brain. It seems reasonable
to believe that a pattern of physiological variables
has a greater probability of reflecting behavioral patterns than a single variable. If neuropeptides produce significant behavioral effects, they probably do
so by modifying organizational patterns of activity in
the brain, and methods used to study their brain effects should be oriented toward revealing these.

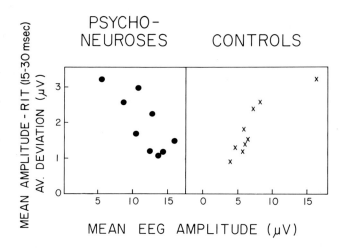

FIG. 9. Scatterplots for correlations between mean integrated EEG amplitude and amplitude of somatosensory EP during the epoch 15 to 30 msec after right median nerve stimulus. EP amplitude measured automatically as absolute mean deviation from epoch mean. Note positive correlation in controls and negative correlation in psychoneurotic patients.

SUMMARY

EEG and event related potential (ERP) phenomena were considered here from the standpoint of possible applications to investigations of the central effects of neuropeptides in man. These electrophysiological phenomena were viewed from the standpoint that they provide an accessible intermediate level of observation between behavior and detailed neuronal events. Several general methodological issues were discussed. An attempt was made to describe the EEG and ERP phenomena that may be pertinent to future neuropeptide studies and to consider their functional significance. Available data concerning electrophysiological effects of neuropeptides were also discussed. Suggestions for future research were made, which emphasized comprehensive recording of EEG and ERP phenomena to permit examination of the patterning of electrocerebral events.

ACKNOWLEDGMENTS

Research of the author supported, in part, by grant MH12507, from the U.S. Public Health Service.

REFERENCES

1. Allison, T., Goff, W. R., Williamson, P. D., and VanGilder, J. C. (1977): On the neural origin of early components of the human somatosensory evoked potential. In: *Proceedings of the*

International Symposium on Cerebral Evoked Potentials in Man.
Brussels, *(In press.)*

2. Ayd, F. J., Jr. (1975): Treatment—resistant patients: A
moral, legal and therapeutic challenge. In: *Rational Psycho-
pharmacotherapy and the Right to Treatment,* edited by F. J.
Ayd, Jr., pp. 37-61. Waverly Press, Baltimore, Maryland.

3. Bickford, R. G., Jacobson, J. L., and Cody, D. T. (1964):
Nature of average evoked potentials to sound and other stimuli
in man. *Ann. N.Y. Acad. Sci.,* 112:204-223.

4. Boddy, J. (1971): The relationship of reaction time to brain
wave period: A re-evaluation. *Electroencephalogr. Clin. Neurophysiol.,* 30:229-235.

5. Buchsbaum, M. S. (1974): Average evoked response and stimulus intensity in identical and fraternal twins. *Physiol. Psychol.,* 2:365-370.

6. Buchsbaum, M., Goodwin, F., Murphy, D., and Borge, G. (1971):
AER in affective disorders. *Am. J. Psychiatry,* 128:51-57.

7. Buchsbaum, M. S. and Henkin, R. I. (1975): Effects of carbohydrate-active steroids and ACTH on visually-evoked responses in patients with adrenal cortical insufficiency. *Neuroendocrinology,* 19:314-322.

8. Buchsbaum, M. and Silverman, J. (1968): Stimulus intensity
control and the cortical evoked response. *Psychosom. Med.,*
30:12-22.

9. Buchwald, J. S. and Huang, C. (1975): Far-field acoustic response. Origins in the cat. *Science,* 189:382-384.

10. Caille, E. J. (1974): Psychotropic drug-induced EEG changes
based on power spectrum analysis. In: *Psychotropic Drugs and
the Human EEG. Modern Problems in Pharmacopsychiatry, Vol. 8,*
edited by T. M. Itil, pp. 99-116. Karger, Basel.

11. Callaway, E. (1961): Day-to-day variability in relationship
between electroencephalographic alpha phase and reaction time
to visual stimuli. *Ann. N.Y. Acad. Sci.,* 92:1183-1186.

12. Callaway, E. (1962): Factors influencing the relationship
between alpha activity and visual reaction time. *Electroencephalogr. Clin. Neurophysiol.,* 14:674-682.

13. Callaway, E. (1975): *Brain Electrical Potentials and Individual Psychological Differences.* Grune & Stratton, New York.

14. Callaway, E. and Harris, P. R. (1974): Coupling between
cortical potentials from different areas. *Science,* 183:873-
875.

15. Callaway, E., Bali, L., and Gevins, A. (1975): Applications
of a new measure of cortical coupling. Presented at *Annual
Meeting of the American EEG Society,* Mexico City, Mexico.

16. Callaway, E., Jones, R. T., and Layne, R. S. (1965): Evoked
responses and segmental set of schizophrenia. *Arch. Gen. Psychiatry,* 12:83-89.

17. Cigánek, L. (1961): *Die Electroencephalographische Lichtrei-
zantwort Der Menschlichen Hirnrinde.* Slowakischen Akademie
Der Wissenschaften, Bratislavia.

18. Cobb, W. A. and Dawson, G. D. (1960): The latency and form
in man of the occipital potentials evoked by bright flashes.

J. Physiol., 152:108-121.

19. Courchesne, E., Hillyard, S. A., and Galambos, R. (1975): Stimulus novelty, task relevance and the visual evoked potentials in man. *Electroenchephalogr. Clin. Neurophysiol.*, 39: 131-143.

20. Darrow, C. W., Wilson, J. P., Vieth, R. N., and Maller, J. M. (1960): Acceleration and momentum in cerebral function reflected in EEG phase relations. In: *Recent Advances in Biological Psychiatry, Vol. II*, edited by J. Wortis, pp. 51-59. Grune and Stratton, New York.

21. Desmedt, J. E., Brunko, E., Debecker, J., and Carmeliet, J. (1974): The system bandpass required to avoid distortion of early components when averaging somatosensory evoked potentials. *Electroencephalogr. Clin. Neurophysiol.*, 37:407-410.

22. de Wied, D., Bohus, B., Gispen, W. H., Urban, I. and Greidanus, T. B. (1976): Hormonal influences on motivational, learning, and memory process. In: *Hormones, Behavior, and Psychopathology*, edited by E. J. Sachar, pp. 1-14. Raven Press, New York.

23. Dustman, R. E. and Beck, E. C. (1965): The visually evoked potentials in twins. *Electroencephalogr. Clin. Neurophysiol.*, 19:570-575.

24. Eason, R. G., Harter, M. R., and White, C. T. (1969): Effects of attention and arousal on visually evoked cortical potentials and reaction time in man. *Physiol. Behav.*, 4:283-289.

25. Fink, M. (1974): EEG profiles and bioavailability measures of psychoactive drugs. In: *Psychotropic Drugs and the Human EEG. Modern Problems in Pharmacopsychiatry, Vol. 8,* edited by T. M. Itil, pp. 76-98. Karger, Basel.

26. Galin, D. and Ornstein, R. (1972): Lateral specialization of cognitive mode: An EEG study. *Psychophysiology*, 9:412-418.

27. Gerbrandt, L. K., Goff, W. R., and Smith, D. B. (1973): Distribution of the human average movement potential. *Electroencephalogr. Clin. Neurophysiol.*, 34:461-474.

28. Giannitripani, D. (1971): Scanning mechanisms and the EEG. *Electroencephalogr. Clin. Neurophysiol.*, 30:139-146.

29. Gilden, L., Vaughan, H. G., Jr., and Costa, L. D. (1966): Summated human EEG potentials with voluntary movement. *Electroencephalogr. Clin. Neurophysiol.*, 20:433-438.

30. Goff, W. R., Williamson, J. C., VanGilder, J. D., Allison, T., and Fisher, T. C. (1977): Neural origins of long latency evoked potentials recorded from the depth and cortical surface of the brain in man. In: *Proceedings of the International Symposium on Cerebral Evoked Potentials in Man. Brussels, (In press).*

31. Hall, R. A., Rappaport, M., Hopkins, H. K., and Griffin, R. (1973): Tobacco and evoked potential. *Science*, 180:212-214.

32. Halliday, A. M. (1973): Evoked responses in organic and functional sensory loss. In: *Human Neurophysiology, Psychology, Psychiatry: Average Evoked Responses and Their Conditioning in Normal Subjects and Psychiatric Patients*, edited by A. Fessard and G. Lelord, pp. 189-211. Inserm, Paris.

33. Häseth, K., Shagass, C., and Straumanis, J. J. (1966): Per-

ceptual and personality correlates of EEG and evoked response measures. *Biol. Psychiatry,* 1:49-60.

34. Itil, T. M. (1974): Quantitative pharmaco-electroencephalography. In: *Psychotropic Drugs and the Human EEG. Modern Problems of Pharmacopsychiatry, Vol. 8,* edited by T. M. Itil, pp. 43-75. Karger, Basel.

35. Itil, T. M. (1975): New psychotropic drug trials in Turkey. *Psychopharm. Bull.,* 11:5-10.

36. Itil, T. M., Saletu, B., and Akpinar, S. (1974): Classification of psychotropic drugs based on digital computer sleep prints. In: *Psychotropic Drugs and the Human EEG. Modern Problems of Pharmacopsychiatry, Vol. 8,* edited by T. M. Itil, pp. 193-215. Karger, Basel.

37. Itil, T. M., Saletu, B., Davis, S., and Allen, M. (1974): Stability studies in schizophrenics and normals using computer-analyzed EEG. *Biol. Psychiatry,* 8:321-335.

38. Jeffreys, D. A. and Axford, J. G. (1972): Source locations of pattern-specific components of human visual evoked potentials, I. Component of striate cortical origin. *Exp. Brain Res.,* 16:1-21.

39. Jeffreys, D. A. and Axford, J. G. (1972): Source locations of pattern-specific components of human visual evoked potentials, II. Components of extrastriate cortical origin. *Exp. Brain Res.,* 16:22-40.

40. Jewett, D. L., Romano, M. N., and Williston, J. S. (1970): Human auditory evoked potentials: Possible brain stem components detected on the scalp. *Science,* 167:1517-1518.

41. Johnson, L. C. and Ulett, G. A. (1959): Stability of EEG activity and manifest anxiety, *J. Comp. Physiol. Psychol.,* 52:284-288.

42. Kastin, A. B., Miller, L. H., Gonzalez-Barcena, D., Hawley, W. D., Dyster-Aas, K., Schally, A. V., de Parra, M. L. V., and Velasco, M. (1971): Psycho-physiologic correlates of MSH activity in man. *Physiol. Behav.,* 7:893-896.

43. Kopell, B. S., Wittner, W. K., Lunde, D., Warrick, G., and Edwards, D. (1970): Influence of triiodothyronine on selective attention in man as measured by the visual averaged evoked potential. *Psychosom. Med.,* 32:495-502.

44. Kornhüber, H. H. and Deecke, L. (1965): Cerebral potential changes in voluntary and passive movements in man: Readiness potential and reafferent potential. *Pfluegers Arch.,* 284:1-17.

45. Landau, S. G., Buchsbaum, M. S., Carpenter, W., Strauss, J., and Sacks, M. (1975): Schizophrenia and stimulus intensity control. *Arch. Gen. Psychiatry,* 32:1239-1245.

46. Lansing, R. W. (1957): Relation of brain and tremor rhythms to visual reaction time. *Electroencephalogr. Clin. Neurophysiol.,* 9:497-504.

47. Lennox, W. G., Gibbs, F. A., and Gibbs, E. L. (1942): Twins, brain waves and epilepsy. *Arch. Neurol. Psychiatry,* 47:702-706.

48. Lewis, E. G., Dustman, R. E., and Beck E. C. (1970): The

effects of alcohol on visual and somatosensory evoked responses. *Electroencephalogr. Clin. Neurophysiol.,* 28:202-205.

49. Livanov, M. N., Gavrilova, N. A., and Aslanov, A. S. (1966): Reflection of some mental states in the spatial distribution of human cerebral cortex bipotentials. *Proceedings of 18th International Congress of Psychology,* Symposium No. 6, Moscow, pp. 31-38.

50. Low, M. D., Frost, J. D., Borda, R. P., and Kellaway, P. A. (1966): Surface-negative, slow potential shift associated with conditioning in man. *Neurology,* 16:771-782.

51. McCallum, W. C. and Walter, W. G. (1968): The effects of attention and distraction on the contingent negative variation in normal and neurotic subjects. *Electroencephalogr. Clin. Neurophysiol.,* 25:319-329.

52. Miller, L. H., Harris, L. C., Kastin, A. J., and van Riezen, H. (1976): Neuroheptapeptide influence on attention and memory in man. *Pharmacol. Biochem. Behav. (Suppl.),* 5:17-21.

53. Miller, L. H., Kastin, A. J., Sandman, C. A., Fink, M., and Van Veen, W. J. (1974): Polypeptide influences on attention, memory and anxiety in man. *Pharmacol. Biochem. Behav.,* 2:663-668.

54. Murphree, H. B. (1974): Electroencephalographic effects of caffeine, nicotine, tobacco smoking, and alcohol. In: *Psychotropic Drugs and the Human EEG. Modern Problems of Pharmacopsychiatry, Vol. 8,* edited by T. M. Itil, pp. 22-36. Karger, Basel.

55. Näätänen, R. (1967): Selective attention and evoked potentials. *Ann. Acad. Sci. Fenn.* (Biol), 151:1-226.

56. Näätänen, R. (1973): On what is the contingent negative variation (CNV) contingent in reaction-time experiments? In: *Human Neurophysiology, Psychology, Psychiatry: Average Evoked Responses and Their Conditioning in Normal Subjects and Psychiatric Patients,* edited by A. Fessard and G. Lelord, pp. 121-174. Inserm, Paris.

57. Ojemann, G. A. and Henkin, R. I. (1967): Steroid dependent changes in human visual evoked potentials. *Life Sci.,* 6:327-334.

58. Regan, D. (1972): *Evoked Potentials in Psychology, Sensory Physiology and Clinical Medicine,* Chapman and Hall, Ltd., London.

59. Ritter, W. and Vaughan, G., Jr. (1969): Averaged evoked responses in vigilance and discrimination: A reassessment. *Science,* 164:326-328.

60. Rust, J. (1975): Genetic effects in the cortical auditory evoked potential: A twin study. *Electroencephalogr. Clin. Neurophysiol.,* 39:321-327.

61. Saletu, B. (1974): Classification of psychotropic drugs based on human evoked potentials. In: *Psychotropic Drugs and the Human EEG. Modern Problems of Pharmacopsychiatry, Vol. 8,* edited by T. M. Itil, pp. 258-285. Karger, Basel.

62. Sannita, W. G., Irwin, P., and Fink, M. (1976): Personal communication.

63. Satterfield, J. H.   (1965):   Evoked cortical response enhance-
    ment and attention in man,   A study of responses to auditory
    and shock stimuli.   *Electroencephalogr. Clin. Neurophysiol.,*
    19:470-475.
64. Satterfield, J. H.   (1972):   Auditory evoked cortical response
    studies in depressed patients and normal control subjects.
    In: *Recent Advances in the Psychobiology of the Depressive
    Illnesses,* edited by T. A. Williams, M. M. Katz, and J. A.
    Shield, Jr., pp. 87-98.   U.S. Government Printing Office,
    DHEW Publication No. (HSM 70-9053), Washington, D. C.
65. Shagass, C.   (1972a):   *Evoked Brain Potentials in Psychiatry.*
    Plenum Press, New York.
66. Shagass, C.   (1972b):   Electrical activity of the brain.   In:
    Handbook of Psychophysiology, edited by N. S. Greenfield and
    R. Sternback, pp. 262-328.   Holt, Rinehart and Winston, Inc.,
    New York.
67. Shagass, C.   (1974):   Effects of psychotropic drugs on human
    evoked potentials.   In: *Psychotropic Drugs and the Human EEG.
    Modern Problems of Pharmacopsychiatry, Vol. 8,* edited by T. M.
    Itil, pp. 238-257.   Karger, Basel.
68. Shagass, C.   (1975):   Psychobiological measurement of change:
    Neurophysiological aspects.   In: *Neuropsychopharmacology*
    (Proceedings of IX Congress of the Collegium Internationale
    Neuropsychopharmacologicum), edited by J. R. Boissier and P.
    Pichot, pp. 176-185.   Excerpta Medica, Amsterdam.
69. Shagass, C.   (1975):   EEG and evoked potentials in the psy-
    choses.   In: *Biology of the Major Psychoses. A Comparative
    Analysis,* edited by D. X. Freedman, pp. 101-127.   Raven Press,
    New York.
70. Shagass, C.   (1976):   An electrophysiological view of schizo-
    phrenia.   *Biol. Psychiatry,* 11:3-30.
71. Shagass, C., Häseth, K., Callaway, E., and Jones, R. T. (1968):
    EEG-evoked response relationships and perceptual performance.
    Life Sci., 19:1083-1091.
72. Shagass, C., Overton, D. A., and Straumanis, J. J.   (1972):
    Sex differences in somatosensory evoked responses related to
    psychiatric illness.   *Biol. Psychiatry,* 5:295-309.
73. Shagass, C., Overton, D. A., and Straumanis, J. J.   (1974):
    Evoked potential studies in schizophrenia.   In: *Biological
    Mechanisms of Schizophrenia and Schizophrenia-like Psychoses,*
    edited by H. Mitsuda and T. Fukuda, pp. 214-234.   Igaku-Shoin
    Co., Ltd., Tokyo.
74. Shagass, C. and Schwartz, M.   (1961):   Reactivity cycle of
    somatosensory cortex in humans with and without psychiatric
    disorder.   *Science,* 134:1757-1759.
75. Shagass, C., Schwartz, M., and Amadeo, M.   (1962):   Some drug
    effects on evoked cerebral potentials in man.   *J. Neuropsy-
    chiatry,* 3:S49-S58.
76. Shagass, C. and Schwartz, M.   (1963):   Psychiatric disorder
    and deviant cerebral responsiveness to sensory stimulation.
    In: *Recent Advances in Biological Psychiatry, Vol. V.,* edi-
    ted by J. Wortis, pp. 321-330.   Plenum Press, New York.

77. Shagass, C. and Schwartz, M. (1965): Age, personality and somatosensory evoked responses. *Science,* 148:1359-1361.
78. Shagass, C., Soskis, D. A., Straumanis, J. J., and Overton, D. A. (1974): Symptom patterns related to somatosensory evoked response differences within a schizophrenic population. *Biol. Psychiatry,* 9:25-43.
79. Shagass, C., Straumanis, J. J., and Overton, D. A. (1975): Psychiatric diagnosis and EEG-evoked response relationships. *Neuropsychobiology,* 1:1-15.
80. Shagass, C., Straumanis, J. J., Jr., Roemer, R. A., and Amadeo, M. (1977): Evoked potentials of schizophrenics in several sensory modalities. *Biol. Psychiatry, (In press.)*
81. Short, M. J., Wilson, W. P., and Gills, J. P., Jr. (1968): Thyroid hormone and brain function. IV. Effect of triiodothyronine on visual evoked potentials and electroretinogram in man. *Electroencephalogr. Clin. Neurophysiol.,* 25:123-127.
82. Slatter, K. H. (1960): Alpha rhythms and mental imagery. *Electroencephalogr. Clin. Neurophysiol.,* 12:851-859.
83. Speck, L. B., Dim, B., and Mercer, M. (1966): Visual evoked responses of psychiatric patients. *Arch. Gen. Psychiatry,* 15:59-63.
84. Straumanis, J. J., Jr. and Shagass, C. (1976): Electrophysiological effects of triiodothyronine and propranolol. *Psychopharmacologia,* 46:283-288.
85. Surwillo, W. W. (1963): The relation of simple response time to brain-wave frequency and the effects of age. *Electroencephalogr. Clin. Neurophysiol.,* 15:105-114.
86. Sutton, S. (1969): The specification of psychological variables in an average evoked potential experiment. In: *Average Evoked Potentials - Methods, Results, and Evaluations,* edited by E. Donchin and D. Lindsley, pp. 237-297. National Aeronautics and Space Administration, Washington, D. C.
87. Sutton, S., Braren, M., and Zubin, J. (1965): Evoked-potential correlates of stimulus uncertainty. *Science,* 150:1187-1188.
88. Tecce, J. J. (1971): Attention and evoked potentials in man. In: *Attention: Contemporary Theory and Analysis,* edited by D. I. Mostofsky, pp. 331-365. Appleton-Century-Crofts, New York.
89. Tecce, J. J. (1971): Contingent negative variation and individual differences. *Arch. Gen. Psychiatry,* 24:1-16.
90. Ulett, J. A. and Itil, T. M. (1969): Quantitative electroencephalogram in smoking and smoking deprivation. *Science,* 164:969-970.
91. Vaughan, H. G., Jr., Costa, L. D., and Ritter, W. (1968): Topography of the human motor potential. *Electroencephalogr. Clin. Neurophysiol.,* 25:1-10.
92. Velasco, R., Velasco, M., Maldonado, H., and Munoz, H. (1976): Differential effect of thalamic and subthalamic lesions on early and late components of the somatic evoked responses in man. *Electroencephalogr. Clin. Neurophysiol.,* 40:329.
93. Walter, W. G. (1964): The convergence and interaction of visual, auditory, and tactile responses in human nonspecific

cortex. *Ann. N. Y. Acad. Sci.*, 112:320–361.

94. Walter, W. G. (1969): In: *Variations Contingentes Négatives*, edited by J. Dargent and M. Dongier, pp. 57–58, 76–77, 95–96. University of Liège, Belgium.

95. Walter, W. G., Cooper, R., Aldridge, V. J., McCallum, W. C., and Winter, A. L. (1964): Contingent negative variation: An electric sign of sensorimotor association and expectancy in the human brain. *Nature,* 203:380–384.

96. Wolthuis, O. L. and de Wied, D. (1976): The effect of ACTH-analogues on motor behavior and visual evoked responses in rats. *Pharmacol. Biochem. Behav.*, 4:273–278.

97. Zubek, J. P., Welch, G., and Saunders, M. G. (1963): Electroencephalographic changes during and after 14 days of perceptual deprivation. *Science,* 139:490–492.

*Neuropeptide Influences on the Brain
and Behavior,* edited by L.H. Miller,
C.A. Sandman, and A.J. Kastin.
Raven Press, New York © 1977.

CNS and ACTH-Like Peptides: Neurochemical Response and Interaction with Opiates

W.H.Gispen, M.E.A.Reith, P.Schotman, V.M.Wiegant, H.Zwiers,
and D.de Wied

*Division of Molecular Neurobiology, Rudolf Magnus Institute for Pharmacology,
and Laboratory of Physiological Chemistry, Medical Faculty, Institute of Molecular
Biology, Padualaan 8, Utrecht, The Netherlands*

INTRODUCTION

It is clear from many studies that peptide sharing sequences with the pituitary hormones ACTH and MSH have profound behavioral effects in animal and man.

Animal studies carried out either in the past or presently going on in our laboratories show that the behavioral effect of ACTH-like peptides becomes apparent in a variety of behavioral paradigms. At first the effects on acquisition and extinction of a conditioned avoidance response was found and extensively studied under both active avoidance (shuttle-box and pole jump box) and passive avoidance (elevated runway). These observations were then extended to experiments using an appetitive behavioral design, i.e., running for food and running of male rats in a straight runway for a receptive female. In addition, the peptides were found to facilitate reversal learning, increase resistance to a complex brightness discrimination task, reverse CO_2 retrograde amnesia and induce, after intraventricular administration, the display of excessive grooming, followed by stretching and yawning movements (10, 11, 12).

Despite the abundance of behavioral information indicating a direct interaction between ACTH-like peptides and the brain, the molecular aspects of such interaction are only sketchy and as yet not totally understood. This chapter aims to review neurochemical aspects of the interaction of ACTH-like peptides with nervous tissue, with some reference to their affinity to CNS opiate receptors.

THE PITUITARY AS SOURCE OF NEUROPEPTIDES

From a behavioral, neuroendocrine, and electrophysiological point of view, the CNS can be regarded as a

classical effector organ of peptides derived from pituitary hormones. In our opinion the designation of the
pituitary as the master gland for reasons of its trophic influences on a variety of endocrine and metabolic
processes in the organism also holds for the neurotrophic actions of these hormones. Despite recent evidence suggesting the existence of peptidergic neurons
(31,33) and putative transmitter induced synthesis of
brain oligopeptides (54) and the CNS effects of releasing hormones (51), the pituitary is an important potential source for neuropeptides. These peptides either
reach the brain effector cells through the circulation
or through a direct pituitary stalk-CSF channel (1).
With this in mind it is therefore reasonable to use hypophysectomized subjects in the search for neurochemical correlates of ACTH-like peptides. Such subjects
will be depleted from a large number of normally circulating pituitary peptides. Paralleling the work on
steroid receptor molecules in the brain which was facilitated by the use of adrenalectomized rats (9), it
was reasoned that in such a depleted animal substitution of a given peptide would lead to neurochemical
events which may be detected more readily than one
would expect to find under normal physiological conditions, i.e., in the intact organism. Removal of the
pituitary is known to lead to a dramatic disorder of
homeostasis that can be detected at almost all levels
of physiological analysis. The nature of the tissue
response of hypophysectomized animals to peptide treatment, however, may not be principally altered and only
be revealed in differences in sensitivity of the tissue
or the magnitude of the response studied. Therefore,
we shall treat neurochemical data obtained from studies
on hypophysectomized and intact subjects alike in order
to arrive at as complete a picture as possible with respect to the evidence available on neurochemical correlates of behaviorally active N-terminal fragments of
pituitary ACTH.

ACTH BRAINCELL SURFACE INTERACTION: CYCLIC NUCLEOTIDES

According to the prevailing point of view, ACTH (60),
and other polypeptide hormones (70) interact with a receptor on the surface of the plasma membrane of the effector cell resulting in increased production of intracellular cAMP; the cyclic nucleotide ("second messenger," see 70) mediates the information of peptide-cell
membrane binding and thus triggers the biochemical
train of events underlying the functional response of
the effector cell. Such mechanism of action is thought
to be involved in the CNS effects of ACTH-like peptides
(23, 65, 68) although definite experimental data are

not yet in hand. Because ACTH seems to act on rather
specific brain sites (47, 67, 76, 78) it might be difficult to identify the effects of ACTH on cyclic AMP
formation.

Bertolini et al. (3) reported that the behavioral
effect of intracranially administered ACTH (i.e., induction of SYS and sexual excitement, see below) could
be potentiated by theophylline blockade of brain phos-
phodiesterase (the enzyme which *in vivo* degrades cAMP to
the inert AMP). This observation would be in line with
the supposed cAMP mediation of ACTH-CNS effects. Contrary to such speculation are the negative results obtained on the action of ACTH on brain adenylcyclase (7)
and on cAMP accumulation in brain slices (18). Since
no detailed information was presented on the properties
of the adenylcyclase assay used (sensitivity, etc.) and
the effect of ACTH may be detected only in slices from
ACTH sensitive brain regions, it was decided to study
the effect of ACTH 1-10 on cAMP accumulation in slices
obtained from the rat posterior hypothalamus containing
the nucleus parafascicularis. These nuclei are essential to the expression of the behavioral activity of
the N-terminal ACTH analogs (5,78). Slices were preincubated for 30 min at 37°C in 2 ml Krebs-phosphate,
pH 7.4, under continuous gassing with pure oxygen. Incubation was started by adding 50 µl medium with or
without ACTH 1-10. After an incubation period of 15
min the slices were homogenized and the cAMP was purified basically according to Mao and Guidotti (46) and
determined by a protein binding assay according to Gilman (19). Basal levels of cAMP under these experimental conditions were in the order of 15 to 30 pmol/mg
slice protein. Incubation with 10^{-5} M resulted in a
circa 50% elevation of the basal level (82). These and
additional data were taken to indicate that ACTH-like
peptides affect brain metabolism through an increase in
the intracellular level of cAMP. Preliminary data on
the effect of intraventricular administration in conscious rats of ACTH 1-24 (1 µg/1 µl) on the levels of
cAMP in various brain regions 10 and 30 min after the
peptide injection suggest that there is a marked re-
gional effect of ACTH on brain cAMP content. The highest elevation was found in diencephalon and mesenceph-
alon and no effect in cerebral tissue (83). Thus,
using appropriate means of analysis the central effect
of ACTH on CNS tissue may be mediated through cAMP.

By assuming such a mechanism a peptide-brain plasma
membrane interaction must occur. Although for the neuropeptide TRH specific brain receptor binding has been
established (8) we have not yet been able to obtain
specific binding of radioactive-labeled ACTH fragments
with brain cell components. However, considerable af-

finity of these peptides for CNS opiate receptors has
been established (see below).

ACTH AND BRAIN RNA

By assuming that the first neurochemical events of
ACTH-like peptides are of the peptide-cyclic nucleotide
type, the following question then is what cellular process is affected by the second messenger. In a series
of experiments Jakoubek and co-workers have studied the
influence of stress on brain macromolecule metabolism
(39). In relation to stress they examined the effects
of exogenous ACTH on brain RNA metabolism in the mouse.
A single high dose of a purified ACTH preparation resulted in a transient inhibition of uridine incorporation into mouse brain RNA 60 min after the ACTH administration and 30 min after the uridine injection (38).
We subsequently studied the influence of two synthetic
ACTH analogs (ACTH 1-24 and ACTH 1-10) on RNA metabolism in rat brain after a single injection (65). ACTH
1-10 exerts the full behavioral activity without appreciable stimulation of the adrenal cortex *in vivo*. Both
intact and adrenalectomized rats were used to discriminate between extraadrenal and indirect, corticotrophic
effects of ACTH. ACTH 1-24 (5 IU/100 g body weight,
s.c.) was given 60 min before killing the rats. The
labeling of brain RNA was studied by injection of 100
μCi [5,^{3}H] uridine intraperitoneally 30 min before de-
capitation. In intact rats, injection of ACTH 1-24 led
to a small (-12%) but significant decrease in labeling
of brainstem RNA whereas the labeling of cerebral and
cerebellar RNA was not altered. The decrease in RNA
labeling was accompanied by a transient decrease in
brainstem RNA content 2.5 hr after the injection of
ACTH 1-24. These findings corroborate those of Jakoubek et al. (38). In adrenalectomized rats (36 hr after
surgery) similar treatment stimulated (+40%) instead of
inhibited uridine incorporation into brainstem RNA.
However, in adrenalectomized rats no alteration of
brainstem RNA content could be detected. The changes
in uridine incorporation could not be attributed to differences in brain precursor uptake or by gross changes
in precursor metabolism in brain tissue (22). ACTH 1-
10 was ineffective both in intact and in adrenalectomized rats. Chronic treatment of hypophysectomized
rats with ACTH 1-10 also fails to influence the labeling of messenger-like and ribosomal brainstem RNA (63)
and the content of brainstem polysomes (21). Reading
and Dewar (52) were also unable to detect an effect of
a related ACTH-like peptide ACTH 4-10 on the labeling
and content of mouse brain RNA. Although we do not fully understand the data, the corticotrophic effect of

ACTH 1-24 may be responsible for the differential action of this peptide in intact and adrenalectomized rats. Apparently, in intact rats the adrenal steroid production by ACTH 1-24 may have inhibited the stimulatory effect of ACTH on uridine incorporation. Depending on the experimental conditions, catabolic effects of glucocorticoids in this respect have been demonstrated (9). The ineffectiveness of ACTH 1-10 in stimulating uridine incorporation into brainstem RNA in the various experimental studies (intact, adrenex, hypox) may be explained by assuming that the transport of the peptide to the peptide-sensitive site in the CNS differs from that of ACTH 1-24 or that the sensitive site discriminates between the two sequences. Although in avoidance behavior the effects of ACTH 1-24 and ACTH 1-10 are of a similar nature, in other situations differences between these two peptides in interaction with the CNS were noted. ACTH 1-24 and ACTH 1-16 accelerate eye opening in neonatal rats, while ACTH 1-10 was ineffective (77) and intraventricular ACTH 1-24 induces grooming and stretching and yawning in the rat, while ACTH 1-10 and ACTH 4-10 even in massive doses are ineffective (27).

The data on brain RNA may suggest that the short N-terminal ACTH sequences (4-10 and 1-10) do not affect brain macromolecule metabolism at the level of transcription (uridine incorporation). Therefore, experiments were carried out to identify a peptide mediated influence on brainstem protein metabolism (see below).

ACTH AND BRAIN PROTEIN

Treatment of hypophysectomized rats during a 12-day period with ACTH 1-10 (20 µg s.c. zinc phosphate long-acting preparation, every other day) enhances the incorporation of [^{3}H] leucine into protein of the brainstem 5 min after injection of the precursor into the diencephalon, as measured on the day after the last peptide injection (63). Subcellular fractionation of the brainstem homogenate indicated that mainly cytoplasmic proteins were labeled in the 5 min incorporation period (62). An increase of 28% was found in the labeling of total brainstem protein. This experiment was replicated using another strain of rats and again a significant increase of overall labeling of brainstem protein was found (55).

The absolute increase in labeling of brain proteins is small. However, from the literature it can be derived that brain macromolecule metabolism responds only moderately to the effect of various causative stimuli (53). The hypophysectomized rat shows a decrement in brainstem protein labeling of 35%. Substitution of

ACTH 1-10 nearly completely restores the labeling to-
wards the level found in intact rats (63). In this
respect the effect is as large as one may possibly expect. It was subsequently decided to explore whether
labeling of specific proteins would be influenced by
peptide treatment or that the peptide effect would be
of a more general nature. In view of recent immuno-
neurochemical data on specific nervous tissue proteins
it was argued that a behaviorally active peptide may be
acting on brain protein metabolism by modulating the
presence of certain proteins which could be specific
for the brain or its function, i.e., behavior (23).
The incorporation of [^{3}H] leucine into rat brainstem
proteins was thus studied 5 min after the injection of
the precursor into the diencephalon of hypophysectomized rats chronically treated with ACTH 1-10 (similar
to procedure described above). The homogenate was se-
quentially extracted with a hypotonic buffer, a non-
ionic detergent (Triton X-100) and an anionic detergent
(SDS) resulting in a soluble and two particle bound
protein fractions. Analysis of these protein fractions
on polyacrylamide gels revealed that ACTH 1-10 enhanced
the incorporation into all proteins. Superimposed on
the general effect minor differences were found in two
low molecular weight protein bands (57). Thus, chronic
treatment with ACTH 1-10 interferes with overall protein metabolism rather than with certain protein species in particular. To substantiate this conclusion,
the effect of peptides on leucine incorporation into
brainstem protein *in vitro* was studied. Slices from the
posterior thalamus (see above) were preincubated for 30
min in Krebs phosphate buffer at 37°C in the presence
of various concentrations of ACTH 1-10. Subsequently,
the slices were incubated for another 30 min after adding [^{14}C] leucine. At the end of the incubation, the
slices were analyzed for incorporation of leucine into
slice proteins. ACTH 1-10 in concentrations of 10^{-5} M
and 5×10^{-7} M significantly enhanced leucine incorporation (39 and 34% respectively) while at 10^{-8} M a tendency to an enhanced incorporation was found [(13%,
Reith et al. (56)]. Lloyd (45) reported similar data
using ACTH 4-10 and rat brainstem slices. ACTH 4-10 in
doses of 0.5 and 10 μg/ml stimulated the incorporation
of [^{14}C] leucine into slice proteins which amounted to
about 90%. Several authors provided data on the effect
of ACTH-like peptides on brain protein metabolism consistent with the observations discussed above. Chronic
treatment of young rats with ACTH induced a complex
pattern of neurochemical changes including a biphasic
effect on brain protein content (49). Reading and
Dewar (52) reported that chronic ACTH 4-10 treatment of
intact mice stimulated the incorporation of labeled

amino acids into cerebral protein which was most pronounced when measured 48 hr after the injection of the
precursor. Rudman et al. (59) demonstrated that a single injection of either ACTH or β-MSH increases the
rate of accumulation of [^{14}C] valine into mouse brain
proteins by 20 to 100%, 6 to 24 hr after the intraperitoneal injection of the radioactive precursor. In addition Dunn and Rees (14) reported that incorporation
of [^{3}H] lysine into small mouse brain protein measured
10 min after subcutaneous injection of the precursor,
was enhanced by 10 to 20% by a single injection of
ACTH 1-24 or ACTH 4-10.

Various experiments were performed to determine
whether the peptides affected the incorporation process
per se or other variables which indirectly would account for the observed increased labeling. The possibility that an altered brain uptake of amino acids
after peptide treatment might contribute to the observed changes in incorporation into brain proteins was
investigated using [^{14}C] α-amino-isobutyric acid as a
metabolically inert amino acid analogue. No effects of
ACTH 1-10 on the uptake of this amino acid analogue
were found, neither *in vivo* after chronic treatment during 12 days, nor *in vitro* after the addition of the peptide (5 x 10^{-7} M) to the slice-incubation mixture.
These *in vitro* results were confirmed, using labeled
cycloleucine as amino acid analogue (64). In addition,
Rudman et al. (59) reported that ACTH and β-MSH do not
alter their precursor pool parameters. These authors
showed that treatment with ACTH did not affect the
brain uptake of valine, the concentrations of free
amino acids or the penetration of the metabolically inert amino acid analogue α-amino isobutyric acid.

STRUCTURE ACTIVITY: EFFECT ON BRAIN PROTEIN METABOLISM IN RELATION TO BEHAVIOR

Several behavioral studies indicate a difference in
response following application of either ACTH 1-10 or
[D-Phe^{7}] ACTH 1-10. Either the two analogues have opposite effects on the extinction of active avoidance
(10) or the D-isomer acts in a similar direction as the
L-isomer but is stronger or the influence lasts longer
(passive avoidance, grooming). It was therefore of interest to study the effect of the D-isomer on protein
metabolism. In our hands, chronic treatment with
[D-Phe^{7}] ACTH 1-10 led to a decreased incorporation of
leucine into total brainstem protein using hypophysectomized rats (55, 63). Thus, *in vivo* an effect of the D-
isomer was found opposite to that of the L-isomer.
Reading and Dewar (52) who reported a stimulation of
ACTH 4-10 on labeling of mouse cerebral proteins, how-

ever, failed to observe an effect of [D-Phe[7]] ACTH 4-10
under similar conditions. Under *in vitro* conditions using the slice preparation we were also unable to detect
an effect of [D-Phe[7]] ACTH 1-10 on leucine incorporation in doses ranging from 10^{-5} to 10^{-8} M (58). Lloyd
(45) had similar experiences with [D-Phe[7]] ACTH 4-10 on
the incorporation of [^{14}C] leucine into slice proteins
although the L-isomer was active in this respect.

At present we have no explanation for the ineffectiveness of the D-isomer under *in vitro* conditions, but
it may be that indeed the effect of the two isomers on
brainstem protein metabolism is not resulting from a
common mode of action. Interestingly, we found that
ACTH 1-24 exerts a stimulation of protein labeling *in
vitro* similar to ACTH 1-10 (58). Furthermore, the behaviorally inert sequence ACTH 1-24 was found to be
inactive with respect to leucine incorporation into
protein under both *in vivo* and *in vitro* conditions (58,
63). Thus, it would appear that the capacity of ACTH
analogues to influence active avoidance behavior parallels their effectiveness on brainstem protein synthesis *in vivo*.

ACTH AND NEUROTRANSMISSION

Do ACTH-like peptides modify CNS neurotransmission?
There is electrophysiological data which at best were
interpreted to assume a modulatory influence of peptides on transmission (40, 69, 75, 86). More than
twenty years ago it was reported that ACTH increases
acetylcholine synthesis in the neuromuscular junction
(74). Later it was found that ACTH in intact rats increases noradrenaline (NA) turnover in hypothalamus,
cortex and other parts of the brain (32). Since adrenalectomy also increased and hypophysectomy decreased
brain NA turnover (80), it was concluded that there is
a direct action of ACTH on brain noradrenergic mechanisms. Further studies revealed that ACTH 4-10 also increases NA turnover in the brain (43, 79). However,
[D-Phe[7]] ACTH 4-10 is not active in this respect. Although a correlation has been postulated between NA
turnover and the rate of extinction of a conditioned
avoidance response (32, 81), it is unlikely that the
behavioral effects of these peptides are mediated by
changes in brain NA turnover (80). Of course, the possibility remains that like TRH (31), posterior pituitary hormones (61), and substance P (34), the ACTH-like
peptides in fact may be produced in CNS neurons and may
themselves act as neurotransmitters in peptidergic synapses. At present there are no data to contradict nor
to support this speculation. Recently we found that
both ACTH 1-24 and ACTH 4-10 are capable of changing

the *in vitro* phosphorylation of rat brain membrane proteins as described elsewhere (88). Phosphorylation of membrane proteins is thought to alter membrane properties like ion permeability and may therefore underlie modulatory influences on neurotransmission as put forward by Greengard (29).

Finally, one may expect a modulatory influence of the peptides through the observed enhancement of protein synthesis. This may be responsible for changes in transmitter enzyme production, synaptic membrane protein renewal, or sprouting.

ACTH AND OPIATES

Neurophysiological Evidence

Krivoy and Zimmermann (41, 87) showed that ACTH-like peptides can antagonize morphine inhibition of spinal reflex activity. Using a Lloyd's preparation to measure spinal reflex activity in the anesthetized cat these authors found that morphine inhibits the amplitudes of evoked mono- and poly-synaptic reflex activity in a dose-dependent manner. β-MSH or ACTH 1-24 injected prior to morphine, prevented the depressant action of morphine on this reflex activity. Interestingly β-MSH enhanced reflex activity per se, while ACTH 1-24 only counteracted spinal reflex inhibition of morphine. These experiments were extended to elegant *in vitro* studies on reflex activity of the isolated spinal cord of the frog (87). Exposure of the *in vitro* preparation to 30 min of morphine (10^{-4} M) reduced the potential amplitude to about 70% of the control value. Incubation with ACTH 1-24 or with ACTH 1-24 in the presence of morphine failed to alter reflex activity. These *in vitro* data circumvent the problem of *in vivo* treatment with ACTH and are taken as strong support for an ACTH-morphine interaction at the CNS level.

Brain Opiate Receptors

Terenius and Wahlström (73) were the first to demonstrate the existence of an endogenous ligand of morphine receptors which was isolated from CSF. The factor appeared to be a peptide. Similar observations were made by others (35) and recently Hughes et al. (36) published the structure of two brain peptides with potent opiate activity which together were designated as enkephalin.

Terenius showed that ACTH 1-28 and ACTH 4-10 have appreciable affinity for the stereospecific opiate binding site in rat brain synaptosomal plasma membranes (71). These observations were confirmed and extended. Structure-activity studies pointed to an active site

around ACTH 4-10 with some indication that a second
affinity site might be present in a sequence adjacent
to 4-10 (72). The initial observation that ACTH 11-24
possessed affinity could not be replicated probably due
to the quality of the batch which was used (20). Both
the D-isomers of ACTH 4-10 and ACTH 1-10 were active.
Interestingly, α-MSH, vasopressin, DG-LVP, substance P,
MIF, and TRH were inactive (71, 72). The calculated
affinity constants were rather low (IC50 in the order
of 10^{-5} - 10^{-6} M) indicating that these ACTH analogs
cannot be regarded as powerful if at all endogenous
ligands for opiate receptors. Nonetheless the data
lend support to findings by Krivoy and Zimmermann (87)
that ACTH-like peptides interfere with morphine in the
CNS. This was further explored in experiments on morphine induced analgesia and grooming behavior.

Analgesia

Morphine is a potent profound activator of pituitary-
adrenal activity (13, 48, 66). Conversely interference
by hormones of this system with the analgesic action of
morphine on the CNS has been suggested (25, 50, 85).
It was found that purified ACTH and ACTH 1-24 can antagonize the analgesic effect of morphine in the presence of the adrenal gland (25, 50), Gispen et al. used
the response to unescapable footshock as a test system
for analgesic properties as suggested by Evans (16).
Not only sensoric properties are measured under these
circumstances but also CNS processes affecting the rat's
motor responses (24). Therefore, in a renewed approach,
the classical hot plate test according to Eddy and
Leimbach (15) was applied in order to further analyze
the role of ACTH-like peptides in counteracting morphine induced analgesia. A dose of 5 mg/kg morphine
i.p. 30 min prior to the hot plate trial was used. The
peptides were administered 60 min prior to the test
(100 µg/rat s.c.). Pretreatment with ACTH-like peptides (ACTH 1-24, ACTH 1-16, ACTH 4-10, and [D-Phe[7]]
ACTH 4-10) did not alter the rat's response latency on
the hot plate even if doses of 1 mg/kg were used. Morphine given alone, increased the response latency 13 to
16 sec. If, however, ACTH-like peptides were given
prior to the morphine treatment response latency was
reduced by approximately 50%, indicating that ACTH-like
peptides counteract the analgesic effect of morphine
(20). Since ACTH analogs devoid of corticotrophic activities, have similar effects, the postulated permis-
sive action of corticosteroids (25) might not be operating under these circumstances. Interestingly, it was
found that [D-Phe[7]] ACTH 4-10 was more potent than ACTH
4-10 and that ACTH 11-24 was inactive. These data then

seem to corroborate findings (71, 72) that ACTH-like peptides have an appreciable affinity for brain opiate receptors *in vitro*.

Induction of Excessive Grooming

As reported by several authors, ACTH-like peptides after intraventricular administration in the rat, produce excessive grooming (17, 27, 37). In a series of experiments a possible similarity between ACTH analogs and opiates in this respect was tested (26). First, it was shown that subcutaneous injection of 1 mg/kg naloxone, a specific opiate antagonist (4) completely suppressed the excessive grooming response elicited by intraventricular pretreatment of rats with 1 µg ACTH 1-24. Naloxone itself did not induce notable behavioral differences. This experiment was repeated by using another selective and powerful opiate antagonist, Naltrexone (4) in doses ranging from 0.1 to 1.0 mg/kg. Again a suppression of intraventricularly induced excessive grooming was found in all doses studied. In the last series of experiments morphine was injected intraventricularly in doses ranging from 0.05 to 0.5 µg per rat. These amounts of morphine induced a considerable grooming activity, both in intact and hypophysectomized rats, which upon detailed analysis appeared to be of a similar quality as that produced by ACTH 1-24 i.e., the dominant element observed being the head-body grooming movements. In doses higher than 0.5 µg/µl morphine depressed the overall behavior of the rat at least during the first hour after the injection. This is in agreement with findings by Ayhan and Randrup (2) who found that systemically given morphine in low doses to rats characteristically increased grooming activity. These data support at a behavioral level the notion that opiates and ACTH analogs may have a common denominator in their neurotrophic action.

Current research reveals the existence of endogenous peptides in brain and pituitary tissue which presumably are derived from β-LPH (6, 28, 30, 36, 42) with opiate-like effects and affinity for opiate receptors (enkephalin (LPH 61-65), α and β endorphin (LPH 61-76, LPH 61-91, C-fragment (LPH 61-91). Intraventricular injection of 0.3 µg LPH 61-91 elicited nearly maximal grooming activity (165 out of 200 possible positive scores). The effect appeared to be dose-dependent. A dose of 10 ng significantly induced grooming activity. LPH 61-91, therefore, has a higher potency than ACTH 1-24. It should be noted, however, that in contrast to ACTH-induced grooming, administration of LPH 61-91 in these low doses as used here, not only elicited grooming but also excitation in some rats as concluded from quick

movements of body and head, jumps, gnawing, and body
shakes. In a subsequent experiment the effect of subcutaneously administered naloxone on LPH 61-91-induced
excessive grooming was studied. Rats treated with 0.1
µg LPH 61-91 displayed excessive grooming prior to naloxone. However, after subcutaneous administration of 1
mg/kg naloxone excessive grooming was markedly sup-
ressed. Interestingly no overall behavioral differences were noted between saline/saline and saline/nal-
oxone treated rats, suggesting that naloxone itself did
not affect ongoing behavior. Apparently β-LPH itself
is practically devoid of activity in this respect. LPH
61-76 (γ-endorphin) was much less active than LPH 61-
91. The sequence LPH 61-69 seemed slightly less active
than LPH 61-76. LPH 61-65 and [Leu^{61}]LPH 61-65 hardly
exhibit grooming activity over the wide dose range tested. Similarly, LPH 65-69 was inactive. Previously it
was found that intraventricular injection of sheep β-
LPH in a dose of 25 µg/50 µl did not elicit grooming in
the rat unless an extremely high dose of 2.5 mg was
used (37). Since opiate antagonists suppress ACTH and
LPH induced behavior one is tempted to conclude that
the neural substrate for this behavior is sensitive to
ACTH fragments, LPH fragments, and opiates. Interestingly intraventricular administration of low doses of
morphine also induces excessive grooming to the same
extent of that found for LPH 61-76 (26).
    Structural differences exist between peptides which
induce excessive grooming, peptides which interact with
brain opiate receptors, peptides which act on ileum and
vas deferens preparations, and peptides with analgesic
properties. Yet, all these peptide-induced effects can
be blocked by naloxone or naltrexone. At best, the
data at present could be explained by assuming more
than one opiate receptor and more than one peptide receptor in the rat brain are involved in more than one
function of the CNS (12, 44, 84). Whether the "opiate
like" activity of these neuropeptides is the most important physiological effect remains to be elucidated.

CONCLUSION

    It is at present tempting to conclude that ACTH-like
peptides affect the brain in a manner similar to the
ACTH-peripheral effector cell interaction (Fig. 1).
Although definite evidence is not in hand, it is likely
that there are specific ACTH receptors in the CNS.
Binding to these receptors may stimulate adenylcyclase.
Subsequent changes in intracellular concentration of
cAMP induce changes in cAMP-dependent protein kinase
activity. The observed changes in membrane phosphorylation and in macromolecule metabolism by ACTH analogs,

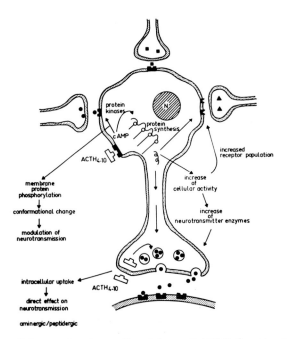

FIG. 1. Possible mechanism of action of ACTH fragments in the rat brain. The scheme represents a speculative synopsis assuming a similarity between ACTH-CNS and ACTH-peripheral effector cell interactions. In addition, the scheme includes a possibility assuming that small peptides may be taken up by neurons.

may result from these protein kinase activities and may be the basis of modulatory influences of neuropeptides on neurotransmission. So far, the behavioral effect of ACTH-like peptides is best correlated with their capacity to alter brainstem protein metabolism. Learning of new behavior in many instances is associated with the release of ACTH and other pituitary hormones. Increased availability of these hormones may provide a biochemical mediator by which protein metabolism is activated and plasticity in the nervous system facilitated necessary for the formation and maintenance of new behavior (See also Walter, *this volume.*).

From the differential effects found, using ACTH 1-24, ACTH 1-10, and [D-Phe[7]]ACTH 1-10 it is clear that we are only at the beginning of our understanding how peptides regulate brain function at the molecular level. The remarkable interaction between peptides and opiates at the receptor level which only recently became known, may assist us to improve our knowledge concerning the mode of action of ACTH analogs and other neuropeptides on the CNS.

ACKNOWLEDGMENTS

Part of the research discussed in this chapter was supported by grants from the Dutch Organization for the Advancement of Pure Research (ZWO), and from the Foundation for Fundamental Medical Research in The Netherlands (FUNGO).

REFERENCES

1. Allen, J. P., Kendall, J. W., McGilvra, R., and Vancura, C. (1974): Immunoreactive ACTH in cerebrospinal fluid. *J. Clin. Endocrinol.*, 38:586-593.
2. Ayhan, I. H. and Randrup, A. (1973): Behavioral and pharmacological studies on morphine-induced excitation of rats. Possible relation to brain catecholamines. *Psychopharmacology*, 29:317-328.
3. Bertolini, A., Vergoni, W., Gessa, G. L., and Ferrari, W. (1969): Induction of sexual excitement by the action of adrenocorticotrophic hormone in brain. *Nature (New Biol.)*, 221: 667-669.
4. Blumberg, H. and Dayton, H. E. (1973): Naloxone and related noroxymorphines. In: *Narcotic Antagonists,* edited by M. C. Brande, L. S. Harris, S. L. May, J. P. Smith and J. M. Villareal, pp. 33-43. *Advances in Biochemical Psychopharmacology, Vol. 8.* Raven Press, New York.
5. Bohus, B. and de Wied, D. (1967): Failure of γ-MSH to delay extinction of conditioned avoidance behavior in rats with lesions in the parafascicular nuclei of the thalamus. *Physiol. Behav.*, 2:221-223.
6. Bradbury, A. F., Smyth, D. G., Snell, C. R., Birdsall, N. M., and Haline, E. C. (1976): The C fragment of lipotropin: An endogenous peptide with high affinity for brain opiate receptors. *Nature,* 260:793-795.
7. Burkhard, W. P. and Gey, K. P. (1968): Adenylcyclase in rat brain. *Helv. Physiol. Pharmacol. Acta,* 26:197-198.
8. Burt, D. R. and Snyder, S. H. (1975): Thyrotropin releasing hormone (TRH): apparent receptor binding in rat brain membranes. *Brain Res.*, 93:309-328.
9. de Kloet, R. and McEwen, B. S. (1976): Glucocorticoid interactions with brain and pituitary. In: *Molecular and Functional Neurobiology,* edited by W. H. Gispen, pp. 257-307. Elsevier, Amsterdam.
10. de Wied, D. (1969): Effects of peptide hormones on behavior. In: *Frontiers in Neuroendocrinology,* edited by W. F. Ganong and L. Martini, pp. 97-140. Oxford University Press, New York.
11. de Wied, D. (1974): Pituitary-adrenal system hormones and behavior. In: *The Neurosciences,* 3rd Study Program, edited by P. C. Schmitt and F. C. Worden, pp. 653-666. MIT Press, Cambridge, Mass.
12. de Wied, D., Bohus, B., Gispen, W. H., Urban, I. and Wimersma

Greidanus, Tj. B. van (1975): Pituitary peptides on motivational, learning and memory processes. *Proc. of the VIth Int. Congress of Pharmacology, Helsinki, Finland,* edited by J. Tuomisto and M. K. Paasonen, 3:19-30.

13. de Wied, D., van Ree, J. M., and de Jong, W. (1974): Narcotic analgesics and the neuroendocrine control of anterior pituitary function. In: *Narcotics and the Hypothalamus,* edited by E. Zimmerman and R. Georde, pp. 251-268. Raven Press, New York.

14. Dunn, A. J. and Rees, H. D. (1975): Aminoacid incorporation into brain proteins: The role of hormones in behavior-related changes. *Fifth Int. Meeting I.S.N. Barcelona.* Abst. 383:477.

15. Eddy, N. B. and Leimbach, D. (1953): Synthetic analgesics II. Dithienylbutenyl and dithienylbutylamines. *J. Pharmacol. Exp. Ther.,* 107:385-393.

16. Evans, W. O. (1961): A new technique for the investigation of some analgesic drugs on reflexive behavior in the rat. *Psychopharmacologia,* 2:318-325.

17. Ferrari, W., Gessa, G. L., and Vargiu, L. (1963): Behavioral effects induced by intracisternally injected ACTH and MSH. *Ann. N. Y. Acad. Sci.,* 104:330-345.

18. Forn, J. and Krishna, G. (1971): Effect of norepinephrine histamine and other drugs on cyclic 3', 5'-AMP formation in brain slices of various animal species. *Pharmacology,* 5:193-204.

19. Gilman, A. G. (1970: A protein binding assay for adenosine 3'5'-cyclic monophosphate. *Proc. Nat. Acad. Sci.* (USA): 67:305-312.

20. Gispen, W. H., Buitelaar, J., Wiegant, V. M., Terenius, L., and de Wied, D. (1976): Interaction between ACTH fragments, brain opiate receptors and morphine-induced analgesia. *Eur. J. Pharmacol.,* 39:393-397.

21. Gispen, W. H., de Wied, D., Schotman, P., and Jansz, H. S. (1971): Brainstem polysomes and avoidance performance of hypophysectomized rats subjected to peptide treatment. *Brain Res.,* 31:341-351.

22. Gispen, W. H. and Schotman, P. (1976): ACTH and brain RNA: changes in content and labelling of RNA in rat brainstem. *Neuroendocrinol.,* 21:97-110.

23. Gispen, W. H. and Schotman, P. (1973): Pituitary-adrenal system, learning and performance: some neurochemical aspects. In: *Drug Effects on Neuroendocrine Regulation,* edited by E. Zimmerman, W. H. Gispen, B. H. Marks, and D. de Wied, *Prog. Brain Res.,* 39:426-442. Elsevier, Amsterdam.

24. Gispen, W. H., Van der Poel, A. M., and van Wimersma Greidanus, Tj. B. (1973): Pituitary-adrenal influences on behavior: responses to test situations with or without electric foot-shock. *Physiol. Behav.,* 10:345-350.

25. Gispen, W. H., van Wimersma Greidanus, Tj. B., Waters-Ezrin, C., Zimmerman, E., Krivoy, W. A. and de Wied, D. (1975b): Influence of peptides on reduced response of rats to electric

   footshock after acute administration of morphine. *Eur. J.*
   Pharmacol., 33:99-105.

26. Gispen, W. H. and Wiegant, V. M. (1976): Opiate antagonists
    suppress ACTH 1-24 induced excessive grooming in the rat.
    Neuroscience Lett., 2:159-164.

27. Gispen, W. H., Wiegant, V. M., Greven, H. H., and de Wied, D.
    (1975a): The induction of excessive grooming in the rat by
    intraventricular application of peptides derived from ACTH:
    structure-activity studies. *Life Sci.*, 17:645-652.

28. Gráf, L., Rónal, A. Z., Bajusz, S., Cseh, G., and Szekely, J.
    I. (1976): Opioid agonist activity of β-lipotropin frag-
    ments: a possible biological source of morphine-like sub-
    stances in the pituitary. *FEBS Lett.*, 64:181-184.

29. Greengard, P. (1975): Cyclic necliotides, protein phosphory-
    lation and neuronal function. *Advances in Cyclic Necleotide*
    Research, Vol. 5, edited by G. I. Drummond, P. Greengard, and
    G. A. Robison, pp. 584-601. Raven Press, New York.

30. Guillemin, R., Ling, N., and Burgus, R. (1976): Endorphines,
    peptides d'origine hypothalamique at neurohypophysaire a
    activite morphinomimetique. Isolement et structure molecul-
    aire d'α-endorphine. *C. R. Acad. Sci.* (Paris) [D.], 282:783-
    785.

31. Hökfelt, T., Elde, R., Johansson, O., Lupr, R., and Arimura,
    A. (1975): Immunohistochemical evidence for the presence of
    somatostatin, a powerful inhibitory peptide, in some primary
    sensory neurons. *Neurosci. Lett.*, 1:231-235.

32. Hökfelt, T. and Fuxe, K. (1972): On the morphology and
    neuroendocrine role of the hypothalamic catecholamine neurons.
    In: *Brain-Endocrine Interaction. Median Eminence: Structure*
    and Function, edited by K. M. Knigge, D. E. Scott, and A.
    Weindl, pp. 181-223. Karger, Basel.

33. Hökfelt, T., Fuxe, K., Johanssen, O., Jeffcoate, S. and White,
    N. (1975b): Thyrotropin releasing hormone (TRH)-containing
    nerve terminals in certain brainstem nuclei and in the spinal
    cord. *Neurosci. Lett.*, 1:133-139.

34. Hökfelt, T., Kellerth, J. O., Nilson, G. and Pernow, B.
    (1975c): Immuhohistochemical support for a transmitter role
    of substance P in primary sensory neurons and in central
    neuron systems. *Exp. Brain Res.*, 23 (suppl.): 90.

35. Hughes, J. (1975): Isolation of an endogenous compound from
    the brain with pharmacological properties similar to morphine.
    Brain Res., 88:295-308.

36. Hughes, J., Smith, T. W., Kosterlitz, H. W., Fothergill, L.
    A., Morgan, B. A., and Morris, H. R. (1975): Identification
    of two related pentapeptides from the brain with potent opiate
    agonist activity. *Nature*, 258:557-579.

37. Izumi, K., Donaldson, J., and Barbeau, A. (1973): Yawning
    and stretching in rats induced by intraventricularly admin-
    istered zinc. *Life Sci.*, 12:203-210.

38. Jakoubek, B., Buresova, M., Hajek, I., Etrychova, J., Parlik,
    A., and Dediciva, A. (1972): Effect of ACTH on the syn-
    thesis of rapidly labelled RNA in the nervous system of mice.

Brain Res., 43:417-428.

39. Jakoubek, B., Semiginovsky, B., Kraus, M., and Erdossova, R. (1970): The alteration of protein metabolism of the brain cortex induced by anticipation, stress and ACTH. *Life Sci.*, 91:1169-1179.

40. Krivoy, W. A. (1970): Effects of ACTH and related polypeptides on spinal cord. In: *Pituitary, Adrenal and the Brain*, edited by D. de Wied and J. A. W. M. Weyman. *Prog. Brain Res.*, 32:108-119. Elsevier, Amsterdam.

41. Krivoy, W. A., Kroeger, D., Taylor, A. N., and Zimmerman, E. (1974): Antagonism of morphine by β-melanocyte stimulating hormone and by tetracosactin. *Eur. J. Pharmacol.*, 27:339-345.

42. Lazarus, L. H., Ling, N., and Guillemin, R. (1976): β-lipotrophine as a prohormone for the morphinomimetic peptides, endorphins and enkephalins. *Proc. Natl. Acad. Sci.* (USA), 73:2156-2159.

43. Leonard, B. (1974): The effect of two synthetic ACTH analogues on the metabolism of biogenic amines in the rat brain. *Arch. Int. Pharmacodyn.*, 207:253.

44. Ling, N. and Guillemin, R. (1976): Morphinomimetic activity of synthetic fragments of β-lipotrophin and analogues. *Proc. Natl. Acad. Sci.* (USA), 73:3308-3310.

45. Lloyd, G. (1974): The action of neurotropic peptide analogues of the ACTH molecule. Thesis, University of Edinburgh, UK.

46. Mao, C. C. and Guidotti, A. (1974): Simultaneous isolation of adenosine 3', 5'-cyclic monophosphate (cAMP) and guanosine 3', 5'-cyclic monophosphate (cGMP) in small tissue samples. *Anal. Biochem.*, 59:63-68.

47. Motta, M., Mangoli, G., and Martini, L. (1965): A "short" feedback loop in the control of ACTH secretion. *Endocrinology*, 77:392-395.

48. Munson, P. L. (1973): Effects of morphine and related drugs on the ACTH-stress reaction. In: *Drug Effects of Neuroendocrine Regulation*, edited by E. Zimmerman, W. H. Gispen, B. H. Marks, and D. de Wied, *Prog. Brain Res.*, 39:361-372. Elsevier, Amsterdam.

49. Palo, J., and Savolainen, H. (1974): The effect of high doses of synthetic ACTH on the rat brain. *Brain Res.*, 70:313-320.

50. Paroli, E. (1967): Indagnini sull'effeto antimorfinicodell' ACTH. Relazioni corticosurrene ed i livelli ematici degli 11-OH steroidi. *Arch. Ital. Sci. Farmacol.*, 13:234-237.

51. Prange, A. J., Wilson, I. C., Breese, G. R., and Lipton, M. A. (1975): Behavioral effects of hypothalamic releasing hormone in animals and men. In: *Hormones, Homeostasis and the Brain*, edited by W. H. Gispen, Tj. B. van Wimersma Greidanus, B. Bohus, and D. de Wied, *Prog. Brain Res.*, 42:1-9. Elsevier, Amsterdam.

52. Reading, H. W. and Dewar, A. J. (1971): Effects of ACTH 4-10 on cerebral RNA and protein metabolism in the rat. *3rd Meeting I.S.N. Budapest*, edited by J. Domonkos, A. Fonyo, I. Huszák, and J. Szentágo, p. 199. Akadémiai Kaidó, Budapest.

53. Rees, H. D., Brogan, L. L., Entingh, D. J., Dunn, A. J., Shinkman, P. G. Damstra-Entingh, T., Wilson, J. E., and Glassman, E. (1974): Effect of sensory stimulation on the uptake and incorporation of radioactive lysine into protein of mouse brain and liver. *Brain Res.*, 68:143-156.

54. Reichelt, K. L. and Kvamme, E. (1973): Histamine-dependent formation of N-acetyl-Aspartyl peptides in mouse brain. *J. Neurochem.*, 21:849-859.

55. Reith, M. E. A. (1975): The effect of behaviorally active ACTH-like peptides on protein biosynthesis in the brainstem of hypophysectomized rats. Thesis, University of Utrecht, The Netherlands.

56. Reith, M. E. A., Schotman, P., and Gispen, W. H. (1974): Hypophysectomy, ACTH 1-10 and in vitro protein synthesis in rat brain slices. *Brain Res.*, 81:571-575.

57. Reith, M. E. A., Schotman, P. and Gispen, W. H. (1975): Incorporation of [H] leucine into brainstem protein fraction: The effect of a behaviorally active, N-terminal fragment of ACTH in hypophysectomized rats. *Neurobiology*, 5:355-368.

58. Reith, M. E. A., Schotman, P. and Gispen, W. H. (1975): The neurotropic action of ACTH: effects of ACTH-like peptides on the incorporating of leucine into protein of brainstem slices from hypophysectomized rats. *Neurosci. Lett.*, 1:55-59.

59. Rudman, D., Scott, J. W., Del Rio, A. E., Houser, D. H., and Sheen, S. (1974): Effect of melonatropic peptides on protein synthesis in mouse brain. *Am. J. Physiol.*, 226:687-692.

60. Sayers, G., Beall, R. J., and Seeliq, S. (1974): Modes of action of ACTH. In: *Biochemistry of Hormones*. edited by H. V. Rickenburg, M. T. P., H. L. Kornberg, and D. C. Philips. *Int. Rev. of Science, Biochemistry Series*, 8:25-60. Butterworths, London.

61. Scharrer, B. (1977): Neurosecretion - comparative and evolutionary aspects. *Prog. Brain Res.*, 45 *(In press.)*

62. Schotman, P. (1971): Macromolecular metabolism in the brainstem of the hypophysectomized rat in relation to the conditioned avoidance behavior. Thesis, University of Utrecht, The Netherlands.

63. Schotman, P., Gispen, W. H., Jansz, H. S., and de Wied, D. (1972): Effects of ACTH analogues on macromolecule metabolism in the brainstem of hypophysectomized rats. *Brain Res.*, 46:349-362.

64. Schotman, P., Reith, M. E. A., and Gispen, W. H. (1976): The influence of neuropeptides on protein metabolism in the central nervous system. *Abstract 17th Dutch Federation Meeting*, Amsterdam, p. 356.

65. Schotman, P., Reith, M. E. A., van Wimersma Greidanus, Tj. B., Gispen, W. H., and de Wied, D. (1976): Hypothalamic and pituitary peptide hormones and the central nervous system: with special reference to the neurochemical effects of ACTH. In: *Molecular and Functional Neurobiology*, edited by W. H. Gispen, 309:344. Elsevier, Amsterdam.

66. Selye, H. (1936): Thymus and adrenals in the response of the

organism to injuries and intoxications. *Br. J. Pathol.*, 17: 234-248.

67. Steiner, F. A. (1970): Effects of ACTH and cortiocosteroids on single neurons in the hypothalamus. In: *Pituitary, Adrenal and the Brain*, edited by D. de Wied and J. A. W. M. Weynen. *Prog. Brain Res.*, 39:102-107. Elsevier, Amsterdam.

68. Strand, F. L. and Cayer, A. (1975): A modulatory effect of pituitary polypeptides on peripheral nerve and muscle. In: *Hormones, Homeostasis and the Brain*, edited by W. H. Gispen, Tj. B. van Wimersma Greidanus, B. Bohus, and D. de Wied. *Prog. Brain Res.*, 42:102-107. Elsevier, Amsterdam.

69. Strand, F. L., Stobay, H., and Cayer, A. (1973/74): A possible direct action of ACTH on nerve and muscle. *Neuroendocrinology*, 13:1-20.

70. Sutherland, E. W. (1972): Studies on the mechanism of hormone action. *Science*, 177:401-408.

71. Terenius, L. (1975): Effect of peptides and aminoacids on dihydromorphine binding to the opiate receptor. *J. Pharm. Pharmacol.*, 27:450-452.

72. Terenius, L., Gispen, W. H., and de Wied, D. (1975): ACTH like peptides and opiate receptors in the rat brain: structure-activity studies. *Eur. J. Pharmacol.*, 33:395-399.

73. Terenius, L., and Wahlstrom, A. (1975): Morphine-like ligand for opiate receptors in human CSF. *Life Sci.*, 16:1759-1764.

74. Torda, C. and Wolf, H. G. (1952): Effect of pituitary hormones, cortisone and adrenalectomy on some aspects of neuromuscular systems and acetylcholine synthesis. *Am. J. Physiol.*, 169:140-149.

75. Urban, I., Lopes da Silva, F. H., Storm van Leeuwen, W. and de Wied, D. (1974): A frequency shift in the hippocampal theta activity: an electrical correlate of central action of ACTH analogues in the dog? *Brain Res.*, 69:361-365.

76. van Delft, A. M. L. and Kitay, J. I. (1972): Effect of ACTH on single unit activity in the diencephalon of intact and hypophysectomized rats. *Neuroendocrinology*, 9:188-196.

77. van der Helm-Hylkema, H. (1973): Effects of early neonatal injected ACTH and ACTH related peptides on the somatic and behavioral development of the rat. Thesis, University of Utrecht, The Netherlands.

78. van Wimersma Greidanus, Tj. B., and de Wied, D. (1974): Effects of peptide hormones on behavior. Differential localization of the influence of lysine vasopressin and of ACTH 4-10 on avoidance behavior. A study with rats bearing lesions in the parafascicular nuclei. *Neuroendocrinology*, 14:280-288.

79. Versteeg, D. H. G. (1973): Effect of two ACTH-analogs on noradrenaline metabolism in rat brain. *Brain Res.*, 49:483-485.

80. Versteeg, D. H. G., and Wurtman, R. J. (1976): Synthesis and release of monoamine neurotransmitters: Regulatory mechanisms. In: *Molecular and Functional Neurobiology,* edited by W. H. Gispen. pp. 201-234. Elsevier, Amsterdam.

81. Weiss, J. M., McEwen, B. S., Silva, M. T., and Kalkut, M.

(1970): Pituitary-adrenal alterations and fear responding. *Am. J. Physiol.*, 218:864–868.

82. Wiegant, V. M. and Gispen, W. H. (1975): Behaviorally active ACTH analogues and brain cyclic AMP. *Exp. Brain Res.*, 23 (suppl.):219.

83. Wiegant, V. M., Baer, L., and Gispen, W. H. *(unpublished)*.

84. Wiegant, V. M., Gispen, W. H., Terenius, L., and de Wied, D. (1977): ACTH-like peptides and morphine: interaction at the level of CNS. *Psychoneuroendocrinology*, 2, 63–69.

85. Winter, C. A., and Flataker, L. (1951): The effect of cortisone, desoxycortisone, and adrenocorticotrophic hormone upon the responses of animals to analgesic drugs. *J. Pharmacol. Exp. Therap.*, 101:93–105.

86. Zimmerman, E. and Krivoy, W. A. (1973): Antagonism between the morphine and the polypeptides ACTH, ACTH 1-24 and β-MSH in the nervous system. In: *Drug Effects on Neuroendocrine Regulation*, edited by E. Zimmerman, W. H. Gispen, B. H. Marks, and D. de Wied. *Prog. Brain Res.*, 39:383–394. Elsevier, Amsterdam.

87. Zimmerman, E. and Krivoy, W. A. (1974): Depression of frog isolated spinal cord by morphine and antogonism by tetracosactin. *Proc. Soc. Exp. Biol. Med.*, 146:575–579.

88. Ziers, H., Veldhuis, D., Schotman, P., and Gispen, W. H. (1976): ACTH, cyclic nucleoticles and brain protein phosphorylation *in vitro*. *Neurochemical. Res.*, 1:669–677.

Neuropeptide Influences on the Brain and Behavior, edited by L.H. Miller, C.A. Sandman, and A.J. Kastin. Raven Press, New York © 1977.

Neuropharmacological Review of Hypothalamic Releasing Factors

Nicholas P. Plotnikoff and Abba J. Kastin

Endocrinology Section of the Medical Service, Veterans Administration Hospital, and Department of Medicine, Tulane University School of Medicine, New Orleans, Louisiana 70146

INTRODUCTION

The effects of pituitary peptides on the central nervous system (CNS) have been studied for more than 20 years. Murphy and Miller (33), and Miller and Ogawa (31) have shown that administration of cortiocotropin (ACTH) resulted in resistance to extinction of a conditioned avoidance response. Krivoy et al. (28, 29) had looked at the actions of melanocyte-stimulating hormone (MSH) on spinal cord and electrical discharge, and Ferrari and co-workers (14, 17) had tested the effects of MSH and ACTH stretching activity and yawning. Later, de Wied (9) used a single aversive test in a series of studies which showed that MSH can have the same effect as ACTH and that the active sequence is ACTH/MSH 4-10 (10). Approaching the problem for the first time from a direct interest in MSH, several different behavioral tests in the rat and man as well as studies of electrical activity (EEGs) in the brain of these species were initiated in 1966 by Kastin and colleagues. The results from these investigations are consistent with the hypothesis that MSH results in improved visual memory and sustained levels of attention (24, 26, 27).

In an unrelated series of investigations, Prange and his co-workers (53) were studying the interactions of tricyclic antidepressants and thyroid hormones. Their early findings suggested that the time of onset of antidepressant activity was shortened by the use of thyroid hormone (53) (T3, triiodothyronine) as well as thyrotropin (TSH) (46), a pituitary hormone whose release is stimulated by thyrotropin-releasing hormone (TRH).

It therefore seemed logical to determine whether the relatively newly identified and isolated hypothalamic releasing and inhibiting factors (49), MIF-I (melanocyte-stimulating hormone release inhibiting factor, Pro-Leu-Gly-NH$_2$) and TRH had direct effects on the CNS. Later, other hypothalamic hormones like growth hormone release inhibiting hormone (GH-RIH; somatostatin) and luteinizing hormone (GH-RIH; somatostatin) and luteinizing hormone-releasing hormone (LH-RH) were also tested.

The first CNS activity to be reported for hypothalamic releasing factors was found with the Everett DOPA potentiation test (13) which is considered an indicator of central dopaminergic activity and possible psychotropic activity (34, 37, 40-45). These factors were MIF-I, LH-RH, and GH-RIF. In addition, MIF-I was found to actively antagonize the symptoms of oxotremorine in an animal model of parkinsonism (36, 38). Clinical studies suggested an effect of hypothalamic and pituitary peptides on the brain of man (25). In light of these early findings, it seemed advisable to learn more about the effects of the hypothalamic and pituitary peptides in a battery of neuropharmacological tests.

The rest of this report will describe our experiences using the following tests:

1. DOPA potentiation
2. Serotonin potentiation
3. Apomorphine potentiation
4. Deserpidine antagonism
5. Oxotremorine antagonism
6. Audiogenic seizures
7. Footshock-induced fighting
8. Maze performance
9. Methamphetamine antagonism
10. EEG effects in the rabbit

DOPA Potentiation Test

The Everett DOPA/pargyline potentiation test was used in the present study (12). The method consists of pretreating mice (17 to 22 g) with pargyline HCl orally (40 mg/kg), at least 2 hr before administering peptides. After pargyline and peptide treatment, d, L- DOPA (200 mg/kg) is given intraperitoneally and the animals (4 per cage) observed for one hr. Potentiation of the DOPA-induced response was scored as marked increase in irritability and reactivity, jumping, squeaking, and aggressive fighting. The Swiss albino mice used in these behavioral studies and ablated animals were obtained from the Charles River Laboratories and the Altech Laboratories, Madison, Wisconsin.

The original intent of the DOPA test was to charac-

terize the tricyclic antidepressant agents (12). The
activities of amitriptyline, imipramine and their de-
methylated products are marked in the dose range of 10
to 50 mg/kg by the oral route (Table 1). At the same
time, other psychotropic agents tested (such as methamphetamine, methylphenidate, pemoline, diazepam, and
clorazepate dipotassium) have also shown significant
activity.

Thus, it is apparent that the DOPA test is exceed-
ingly sensitive in detecting the CNS activities of a
large number of psychotropic agents. The large majority of these compounds have been reported to exhibit
various degrees of antidepressant and/or anti-anxiety
activities in man (48). However, it is interesting to
see that antiparkinsonian agents such as Artane and
Cogentin are also active in the DOPA test. Since these
agents presumably exhibit their activities through
dopaminergic systems, it is understandable that they
should be active in the Everett DOPA test (19).

It was of enormous importance to discover that the
hypothalamic releasing factors were markedly active in
the DOPA test (Table 2). A very potent peptide in this
test was found to be MIF-I. This tripeptide exhibited
significant activity in the dose range of 0.1 to 0.2
mg/kg. Another tripeptide, TRH, was also found to be
quite active in the DOPA test in a dose range of 0.2 to
0.4 mg/kg. By contrast, both GH-RIF as well as LH-RH
were considerably less active (1 to 2 mg/kg). There
appears to be approximately a 10-fold difference in
potency between MIF-I and TRH as compared to GH-RIF and
LH-RH. The differences in potency among these hypothalamic peptides in the Everett DOPA potentiation test
do not parallel their endocrine activity on the pituitary. Further evidence of CNS effects of the hypothalamic factors was demonstrated in hypophysectomized
animals. Thus, the activity of MIF-I, TRH, LH-RH, and
GH-RIF in hypophysectomized mice in the DOPA test demonstrated a direct effect on the brain independent of
any endocrine effects of the pituitary gland (Table 2).
These studies were the first demonstration of an extra-
pituitary, nonendocrine effect of the hypothalamic releasing factors - MIF-I, TRH, GH-RIF, and LH-RH. At
the same time, the pituitary hormones MSH as well as
TSH (and also T3 and T4) have been shown to exhibit
activity in the DOPA test. Therefore, the possibility
remains that in the intact animal receiving TRH, for
example, increased secretion of hormones like TSH (and
T3, T4) could further sustain the central effects of
the releasing factors.

In additional studies in mice, it was found that the
activity of TRH, MIF-I, and LH-RH is not lost in the
absence of a wide range of endocrine and even nonendo-

TABLE 1. *Activity of psychotropic agents
in the DOPA potentiation test*

	Dose (mg/kg) Oral route	Behavioral rating[a]	
Amitriptyline	5	2	(1 hr)
	10	3	
	20	3	
	30	2	
	5	2	(4 hr)
	10	3	
	20	3	
	30	3	
	50	3	
Nortriptyline	5	2	(1 hr)
	10	3	
	20	3	
	30	1	
	50	1	
	5	2	(4 hr)
	10	2	
	20	3	
	30	3	
	50	3	
Imipramine	5	2	(1 hr)
	10	3	
	20	2	
	30	3	
	50	3	
	5	1	(4 hr)
	10	2	
	20	3	
	30	3	
	50	3	
Desimipramine	5	2	(1 hr)

Table 1 continued

	Dose (mg/kg) Oral route	Behavioral rating[a]	
	10	3	
	20	2	
	30	3	
	50	3	
	5	3	
	10	3	
	20	3	
	30	3	
	50	3	
Clorazepate Dipotassium	0.3	1	(4 hr)
	0.6	2	
	1.25	2	
	2.5	2	
	5	3	
	10	3	
	20	2	
	40	2	
Diazepam	1.25	1	(4 hr)
	2.5	1	
	5	2	
	10	2	
	20	3	
	40	3	
Methamphetamine	1	3	(1 hr, i.p.)
	2	3	
Methylphenidate	25	1	(1 hr, p.o.)
	100	3	
Pemoline	5	1	(4 hr, p.o.)
	10	2	
	25	2	
	50	3	

Table 1 continued

	Dose (mg/kg) Oral route	Behavioral rating[a]	
Artane	25	2	(1 hr, i.p.)
	100	3	
Cogentin	2.5	1	(4 hr, p.o.)
	5	3	
	10	3	
	20	2	
	50	2	
	100	1	
Atropine	5	2	(1 hr, i.p.)
	10	3	
	20	3	
Scopolamine	5	1	(1 hr, i.p.)
	10	3	
	20	3	

[a]Behavioral rating in all tables: 1 = slight, 2 = moderate, 3 = marked.

TABLE 2. *DOPA potentiation test in hypophysectomized mice*

Dose (mg/kg, i.p.)	Response; 1 hr						
	MIF-I	TRH	LH-RH	GH-RIF	α-MSH	SP	Angiotensin I
0.1	3	2		1	2	1	2
0.2	3	3					
0.4	3	3	2				
1	3	3	2	2	2	1	1
2	3	3	3				
4	3		3				
8	3		3	2		2	

crine organs. The dopaminergic function of at least one hypothalamic peptide was further confirmed by use of α-methyl-p-tyrosine and Fla-63. With both compounds, TRH was still active in the DOPA test.

Other peptides tested in the DOPA test include MIF-II, substance P(SP), MSH, and tocinoic acid as well as TSH. All of these substances exhibited significant activity. Angiotensin I was inactive in a dose range of 0.1 to 1 mg/kg. The activities of MIF-I and TRH in the DOPA test were confirmed recently by Huidobro-Toro et al. (20).

Further comparative studies were carried out with a large number of analogs of MIF-I as well as TRH (Table 3). These particular analogs are less potent in their activity than the parent compounds, suggesting a strong degree of specificity in this test. This was recently confirmed by Burt and Snyder (4) in high-affinity binding studies in rat brain. It is interesting to note that Pro-Val-Gly-NH$_2$, and pGlu-Leu-Gly-NH$_2$ exhibited significant activity in the DOPA test but were less potent than Pro-Leu-Gly-NH$_2$ itself.

In Table 4 are shown analogs of TRH in the DOPA test. Again, it would appear that these analogs of TRH are less potent and of shorter duration of action than TRH itself. Several analogs, however, did exhibit significant activity, namely: boc-His-Pro-NH$_2$, pGly-His-Phe-histamide, pGly-His-Pro-NHEt, His-Pro-Tyr-NH$_2$, and pGlu-His(bis-DCM)-Pro-NH$_2$.

It can be seen that in the case of TRH as well as MIF-I there appears to be a high degree of specificity in terms of structure and activity.

Serotonin Potentiation Test

The hypothalamic releasing factors MIF-I and GH-RIF were found to be inactive in the mouse serotonin potentiation test in a dose range of 0.01 to 1.0 mg/kg. In contrast, TRH was active in a dose range of 0.2 to 0.8 mg/kg and LH-RH had slight activity at 8 mg/kg (Table 5).

Other peptides tested included SP, α-MSH and angiotensin I. All of these were found to be inactive. The intriguing CNS actions of MSH in the rat and man have been summarized elsewhere (23, 25, 26).

Apomorphine Potentiation

Hyperactivity in groups of rats was induced by medication with apomorphine at a dose of 5 mg/kg. The activity resulting was recorded on electromagnetic activity counters (Stoelting Co.) and also observed for behavioral changes. Pretreatment of the rats with MIF-I at doses of 1 to 2 mg/kg resulted in almost continuous mounting behavior and a reduction in random activity (Table 6).

TABLE 3. Analogs of *Pro-Leu-Gly-NH₂*

Structure	Dose (mg/kg)	DOPA potentiation test - 1 hr, i.p.	Oxotremorine antagonism	Serotonin potentiation
Pro-Leu-Gly-NH₂ (MIF-I)	1	3	+	0
Pro-Gly-tryptamine	10	1	0	-
Leu-Gly-NH₂	10	-	0	0
Pro-Gly-Gly-NH₂	10	-	0	-
Pro-Leu	10	-	-	-
Val-Gly-Gly-NH₂	10	2	-	-
Z-Pro-Leu-Gly-NH₂	10	-	0	0
Pro-Leu-Ala-NH₂	10	-	0	-
Pro-Ile-Gly-NH₂	10	2	0	+
Pro-Val-Gly-NH₂	10	2	-	-
Pro-Leu-β-Ala-NH₂	10	3	+	0
Pro-Leu-Gly-OEt	10	3	+	0
Pro-Leu-Gly-NH-Me	10	1	0	-
Pro-Leu-NH-Et	10	3	-	0
Pro-Leu-Val-NH₂	10	-	-	0
Pro-Leu-Phe-NH₂	10	-	0	0
Pro(3-OH)-Leu-Gly-NH₂	10	-	0	0
Leu-Val-Gly-NH₂	10	3	+	0

Compound				
Pro-Leu-NH-CH$_2$CN	10	3	+	o
Pro-Leu-Gly-OH	10	1	o	o
Val-Gly-NH$_2$	10	3	o	o
Pro-Leu-NHCH (CO-NH$_2$)$_2$	10	3	o	-
Boc-Leu-Gly-DAB(Z)-NH$_2$	10	1	-	-
Pro-Leu-Trp-NH$_2$	10	1	-	-
(Cyclo)-Leu-Pro	10	2	+	o
Pro-Leu-N-CH$_2$CH$_2$SCH-CO-NH$_2$ (DL)	10	3	o	o
Pro-Leu-N-CH$_2$CH$_2$SCH-CO-NH$_2$ (L)	10	1	o	o
Z-pGlu-Leu-Gly-NH$_2$	10	2	+	o
Z-Pro-Leu-D-Gly-NH$_2$	10	1	o	o
pGlu-Leu-Gly-NH$_2$	10	3	o	o
Pro-Leu-NH$_2$	10	3	o	o
Pro-Leu-D-Gly-NH$_2$	10	-	-	-
Z-Pro-Leu-NH$_2$	10	-	-	-
Cyclopentyl-CO-Leu-Gly-NH$_2$	10	2	o	+

Table 3 continued

Structure	Dose (mg/kg)	DOPA potentiation test - 1 hr, i.p.	Oxotremorine antagonism	Serotonin potentiation
Boc-Pro-D-Leu-Gly-NH$_2$	10	2	0	0
Pro-D-Leu-D-Gly-NH$_2$	10	3	0	+
Pro-D-Leu-Gly-NH$_2$	10	3	0	0
pGlu-His-Pro-Leu-Gly-NH$_2$	10	2	0	0
pGlu-Ser-Gly-NH$_2$	10	2	+	0

TABLE 4. *TRH analogs*

Structure	Dose (mg/kg)	DOPA potentiation test - 1 hr, i.p.	Oxotremorine antagonism	Serotonin potentiation
TRH	1	3	0	+
Boc-His-Pro-NH$_2$	10	3	0	0
Ser(C-O)-His-Pro-NH$_2$	10	2	0	0
pGlu-His-Phe-histamine	10	3	0	0
pGlu-(OMe)-His-Pro-NH$_2$	10	2	0	0
pGlu-His(3-Me)-Pro-NH$_2$	10	3	+	+
pGlu-His-Pro-NHEt	10	3	0	0
pGlu-His-Phe-His-NH$_2$	10	3	0	0

Compound				
CBZ-p-Glu-His	10	3	0	0
Ac-Ala-His-Pro-NH$_2$	10	3	0	0
D-L-D isomer of TRH	10	3	0	0
pGlu-His-Ala(N-Me)-NH$_2$	10	3	0	0
pGlu-His-Pro-Ala-NH$_2$	10	3	+	0
His-Pro-Tyr-NH$_2$	10	3	0	+
Pro-His-NH$_2$	10	3	+	0
Pyrrolidone-CO-His-Pro-NH$_2$	10	3	0	0
β-Ala-His-Pro-NH$_2$	10	3	0	0
pGlu-His(bis-DCM)-Pro-NH$_2$	10	3	0	0
pGlu-His-NEt$_2$	10	3	0	0
pGlu-His-N⟨S⟩—CONH$_2$	10	3	+	0
pGlu-Phe-Pro-NH$_2$	10	3	0	+

TABLE 5. *Serotonin potentiation test*

Dose (mg/kg, i.p.)	MIF-I	TRH	LH-RH	GH-RIF	SP	Angiotensin I
		Response; 1 hr				
0.1	0	1		0	0	0
0.4	0	2				
1	0	3	0	0	0	0
2	0		1			
4	0					
8			2			

TABLE 6. Apomorphine *potentiation*

	Dose (mg/kg)	Sensor counts
Apomorphine alone		17,239
plus		
MIF-I	1	12,633
MIF-I	2	14,664

Deserpidine Antagonism Test

Deserpidine-induced sedation in rodents has been described as an animal model of depression and parkinsonism by Everett and Toman (13). Antidepressants such as desimipramine and antiparkinsonian agents, like DOPA, reverse the behavioral and neurological effects of deserpidine in rodents.

The heavy sedative effect of deserpidine was reversed by both MIF-I and TRH in a dose range of 1 to 10 mg/kg (when pretreated with pargyline and DOPA). No significant reversal of the effects of deserpidine was seen with MIF-I and DOPA when the pargyline was omitted or with pargyline and DOPA alone (39) (Table 7).

Oxotremorine Antagonism Test

This animal model of parkinsonism was found to be quite sensitive to the protective actions of MIF-I. In a dose range of 1 to 16 mg/kg, MIF-I reduced the parkinsonian-like symptoms induced by oxotremorine. Furthermore, MIF-I was found to potentiate the effects of DOPA in reducing the symptoms of oxotremorine. Finally, MIF-I was active in reducing symptoms of oxotre-

TABLE 7. *Deserpidine antagonism in mice*

Dose of test agent (mg/kg)		Degree of antagonism of deserpidine
MIF-1	1	2
	5	3
	10	3
TRH	2.5	2
	5	2
	10	3
L-DOPA	25	0
	50	1
	100	2
	200	3
Desimipramine	25	3
	50	3
	100	3

morine in hypophysectomized mice in a further demonstration of the nonendocrine effects of MIF-I. In contrast to MIF-I, the other hypothalamic releasing factors, TRH, GH-RIF, and LH-RH were found to be inactive against oxotremorine.

Control animals receiving oxotremorine exhibited marked signs of parasympathetic stimulation consisting of tremors, head twitch, decreased activity, ataxia, lachrymation, salivation, and diarrhea. MIF-I, in a dose range of 2 to 16 mg/kg, reduced the tremor induced by oxotremorine in normal mice and blocked the peripheral effects as well (Table 8). MIF was also observed to potentiate the effects of L-DOPA in reducing the central and peripheral effects of oxotremorine. Thus, a minimally active dose of L-DOPA (100 mg/kg, i.p.) plus MIF-I (0.25 to 1 mg/kg) provided significant protection against the effects of oxotremorine (Table 9).

In hypophysectomized mice, oxotremorine was just as effective as in intact mice. In each group of animals, all the expected CNS and peripheral effects were seen. This finding extended the unpublished observations of one of us (AJK) made in 1969 that tremorine is effective in hypophysectomized albino rats. MIF-I was found to be as active in reducing the effects of oxotremorine in hypophysectomized mice as in intact mice (Table 10).

TABLE 8. *Oxotremorine antagonism by MIF-I in intact mice*

Dose (mg/kg, i.p.)	Tremors	Head twitch	Ataxia	Lachrymation	Salivation	Diarrhea
Oxotremorine						
0.5	3[a]	3	2	2	3	3
MIF-I + oxotremorine						
0.5	3	3	2	2	3	3
1	2	2	2	2	2	2
4	2	1	1	1	1	1
16	1	1	1	0	1	1

[a]Degree of oxotremorine effects after 1 hr: 3 = marked; 2 = moderate; 1 = slight; 0 = none

TABLE 9. *Oxotremorine antagonism by MIF-I and L-DOPA*

Dose (mg/kg, i.p.)	Tremors	Head twitch	Ataxia	Lachrymation	Salivation	Diarrhea
Oxotremorine						
0.5	3[a]	2	2	2	3	3
L-DOPA						
100	2	2	2	1	2	2
200	1	1	1	1	1	0

Dose (mg/kg, i.p.)	Tremors	Head twitch	Ataxia	Lachrymation	Salivation	Diarrhea
400	0	1	0	0	0	0
MIF-I + L-DOPA						
0.1 + 100	2	1	1	1	2	0
0.25 + 100	1	1	0	0	1	0
1.0 + 100	1	1	0	0	1	0

[a]Degree of oxotremorine effects: 3 = marked; 2 = moderate; 1 = slight; 0 = none.

TABLE 10. *Oxotremorine antagonism by MIF-I in hypophysectomized mice*

Dose (mg/kg, i.p.)	Tremors	Head twitch	Ataxia	Lachrymation	Salivation	Diarrhea
Oxotremorine						
0.5	3[a]	3	2	2	3	3
MIF-I + oxotremorine						
0.5	3	3	2	2	3	3
1	2	2	2	2	2	2
4	2	1	1	1	1	1
16	1	1	1	0	0	0

[a]Degree of oxotremorine effects after 1 hr: 3 = marked; 2 = moderate; 1 = slight; 0 = none.

TABLE 11. *Anticholinergic effects of MIF-I*
in the isolated guinea pig ileum

Dose MIF-I (μg/ml)	% Inhibition of ACh HCI (0.04-0.1 μg/ml)
5	11
10	8
50	4
100	36

No significant anticholinergic activity was observed with MIF-I when concentrations of 5, 10, and 50 μg/ml were added to the isolated guinea pig ileum. At the high concentration of 100 μg/ml, however, there appeared to be some inhibition of the spasm induced by acetylcholine (ACh) (Table 11).

Oral route. Substantial reduction of the effects of oxotremorine 1 hr after its administration was observed when MIF-I was administered by oral intubation (Table 12).

Intravenous route. MIF-I, given intravenously (i.v.) 1 hr earlier effectively antagonized the effects of oxotremorine at a dose of 10 mg/kg (score: 11), 20 mg/kg (score: 9), and 40 mg/kg (score: 7) as compared with controls (score: 22).

Subcutaneous route. MIF-I was also found to be effective in antagonizing the effects of oxotremorine 1 hr later when given by the subcutaneous route in a dose range of 10 to 40 mg/kg. This resulted in scores of 10-13.

Intraperitoneal route. MIF-I, as expected, was effective in reducing the responses induced by oxotremorine when administered by the i.p. route 8 and 24 hr earlier. Doses of 10 to 40 mg/kg reduced the scores from 22 to 9 to 12. This action was only slightly improved by administration of MIF-I for 5 consecutive days (score: 8-9).

Interactions with anticholinergic drugs. The effects of trihexyphenidyl hydrochloride (Artane) and MIF-I alone and in combination were tested. Scores resulting from the different mixtures of the two compounds are shown in Table 13. An analysis of variance followed by Duncan's multiple range test shows a significant effect of even the smallest dose (5 mg/kg) of trihexyphenidyl as well as one of MIF-I, but no significant interaction.

A similar analysis was also done on the effects of benztropine mesylate (Cogentin) with MIF-I. Table 13 shows the results. Benztropine, like trihexyphenidyl

TABLE 12. *Antagonism of oxotremorine by MIF-I
administered by the oral route*

Dose MIF-I (mg/kg)	1 hr
0	21
0.5	21
1	17
2	15
4	12
8	10
16	8
20	7
40	6

TABLE 13. *Antagonism of oxotremorine by MIF-I
and trihexyphenidyl or benztropine*

	Dose (mg/kg, i.p.)	Dose of MIF-I (mg/kg i.p.)			
		0	5	10	20
Benztropine	0	20	16	16	10
	1.25	6	6	6	6
	2.5	4	1	3	1
	5.0	0	1	2	0
Trihexyphenidyl	0	20	16	16	10
	5	11	7	8	10
	10	8	5	7	4
	20	6	1	0	1

(Artane), was found to have a significant dose-response
effect. MIF-I showed no significant combined effect
with benztropine.

Analysis of variance was also used to evaluate the
effects of scopolamine, MIF-I, and L-DOPA. The doses
and scores are given in Table 14. Scopolamine and MIF-
I each showed significant ($p < 0.01$) actions in antago-

TABLE 14. *Antagonism of oxotremorine by scopolamine, L-DOPA, and MIF-I*

Scopolamine	Dose (mg/kg, i.p.)		Score
	L-DOPA	MIF-I	
0	0	0	20
0.5	0	0	17
1.0	0	0	13
2.0	0	0	6
0.5	100	0	10
1.0	100	0	8
2.0	100	0	5
0	0	5	20
0	0	10	10
0	0	20	7
0.5	100	5	8
0.5	100	20	4

nizing the effects of oxotremorine. The interaction effect of administration of MIF-I together with L-DOPA tended ($p = 0.10$) to be greater than when either compound was injected by itself.

In studying numerous analogs of MIF-I in the oxotremorine test, it was found that all the ones tested were less potent than MIF-I in reducing the symptoms of oxotremorine. However, a number of analogs did exhibit activity. These included: Pro-Leu-B-Ala-NH$_2$, Pro-Leu-Gly-OEt, Leu-Val-Gly-NH$_2$, Pro-Leu-HN-CH$_2$CN, (Cyclo)-Leu-Pro, and Z-pGlu-Leu-Gly-NH$_2$. Castensson et al. (5) found pGlu-Leu-Gly-NH$_2$ to be more potent than the parent MIF-I.

Audiogenic Seizure Test

A sensitive method of detecting potential anticonvulsant activity involves the use of audiogenic seizures in mice (O'Grady strain) specially bred for susceptibility to audiogenic seizures. Groups of five mice were pretreated one hour before testing in an auditory stress chamber, and were observed for convulsions. Mice not having convulsions were considered protected.

Slight protection against audiogenic seizures was seen with the use of TRH, α-MSH and LH-RH but not with

TABLE 15. *Audiogenic seizure test*

	Dose (mg/kg)	Percent protection from seizures
MIF-I	25	10
	50	0
	100	10
TRH	25	0
	50	10
	100	30
GH-RIF	10	0
LH-RH	0.01	20
	0.1	40
	1.0	30
	10.0	30
α-MSH	0.01	20
	0.1	30
	0.0	30

MIF-I or GH-RIF (Table 15).

Footshock-Induced Fighting Behavior in Mice

The effects of the peptides on footshock-induced fighting behavior in mice were determined with a modified Tedeschi procedure which has been widely used to evaluate the effects of drugs on aggressive behavior. Paired mice were confined under a glass beaker (800 ml) placed on the grid floor of a Lehigh Valley fighting mouse apparatus. When electroshock was delivered to the grids, the mice responded with distinct and easily recognized aggressive and/or escape responses.

Mixed effects were observed with the use of the various peptides. Thus, MIF-I and TRH were observed both to increase and decrease slightly fighting behavior at various doses, while LH-RH and GH-RIF had no effect. α-MSH, on the other hand, was found to increase slightly fighting behavior (Table 16).

Maze Studies in Rats

A simple maze test was used to study the behavioral effects of MIF-I and TRH. Naive rats were trained to discriminate between light and dark compartments in a

TABLE 16.   *Mouse fighting test*

	Dose (mg/kg)	% change in fighting behavior
MIF-I	5	−23
	10	+ 9
	20	+30
TRH	5	+ 5
	10	+20
	20	−35
GH-RIF	10	0
LH-RH	0.1	+ 1
	1.0	− 6
	10.0	+12
α-MSH	0.01	+27
	0.1	+30
	1.0	+40

Y-maze. The correct response was for the test animal to escape to the lighted shock-insulated side of the maze after exposure to buzzer and footshock in the starting compartment. After ten acquisition trials on day one, ten extinction trials were conducted on the second day (with buzzer but no footshock). A significant difference between control animals and groups treated with MIF-I and TRH was observed during extinction (Table 17).

Methamphetamine Antagonism Studies in Rhesus Monkeys

Since Wilson and associates (53) reported that TRH appeared to reduce some of the symptoms of schizophrenia, it was of interest to try to find an animal model for this activity. We selected the one described by Snyder (50) which employs methamphetamine to produce increases in motor activity as well as stereotyped behavior in rhesus monkeys. This model is based on the finding that psychotic behavior can be induced in human beings with the amphetamines.

Rhesus monkeys were pretreated with TRH in a dose range of 2.5 to 80 mg/kg and then challenged 1 hr later with methamphetamine (5 mg/kg orally). A scale of 0 to 3 was used with 0 showing no effect, 1 slight, 2 moderate, and 3 marked protection against the symptoms of methamphetamine.

TABLE 17. *Rat maze study*

	Controls	MIF-I[a] (1 mg/kg)	TRH (1 mg/kg)
Day 1 Mean ten acquisition trials (sec ± SE)	8.4 ± 0.7	8.6 ± 0.6	8.0 ± 0.7
Day 2 Mean ten extinction trials	5.7 ± 0.8	2.9 ± 0.3[b]	3.1 ± 0.3[b]

[a]Eight rats per group

[b]$p < 0.05$ vs controls

TABLE 18. *Methamphetamine antagonism in monkeys*

TRH Dose (mg/kg)	2.5[a]	5	10	20	40	80
Hyperactivity	1[b]	1	1	1	2	3
Stereotyped behavior	1	1	1	1	3	3

[a]Two monkeys per dose

[b]Behavioral antagonism: 0 = no effect; 1 = slight; 2 = moderate; 3 = marked

EEG Effects in the Rabbit

Electroencephalographic activity of the rabbit was recorded from motor, somatosensory, and visual areas of the cerebral cortex as well as from the basal olfactory area and hippocampus. The background neocortical EEG activity was characterized by high voltage slow waves (2 to 4 Hz) and intermittent spindles (12 to 14 Hz) which resembled EEG patterns usually associated with behavioral sleep. Arousal or the EEG activation response resembled cerebral electrical activity in awake animals [activation or alerting was characterized by a low voltage, fast frequency pattern (12 Hz) in the neocortex and 5 to 7 Hz theta wave pattern in the hippocampus.]

At a dose of 1 mg/kg, i.v., MIF-I (35) and TRH elicited no significant changes in background EEGs of the rabbit. However, after 10 mg/kg of TRH and 30 mg/kg of

MIF-I, the neocortical background electrical activity changed from its sleep-like pattern to an EEG characteristic of continuous arousal.

DISCUSSION

These studies have shown that the hypothalamic-releasing factors (MIF-I, TRH, GH-RIF, and LH-RH) potentiate the behavioral effects of DOPA both in normal intact as well as hypophysectomized mice. Thus, it was demonstrated for the first time that the hypothalamic releasing factors have a direct action on the brain independent of peripheral endocrine effects. Furthermore, these studies suggest the possibility that hypothalamic and perhaps other peptides may have clinical effects on "mood" and some evidence exists to support this concept. Of the hypothalamic releasing factors, only TRH and LH-RH were active in the serotonin test. In reviewing a relatively large number of analogs of TRH as well as MIF-I, it was surprising that most of them were less active than the parent compounds. However, it is possible that potency alone may not be the only criterion for projection to clinical usage. Thus, it is extremely important to obtain additional clinical feedback on the effects of TRH and MIF-I in man in various psychiatric and neurological states. To date, several groups have reported on the potential use of TRH in depression and schizophrenia with mixed findings (7, 8, 11, 20, 21, 31, 32, 47, 52). However, a number of investigators are now beginning to report that TRH may be useful in characterizing subgroups of depression based on the diminished thyrotropin response to TRH (23, 51, 54). In addition, preliminary studies suggest that MIF-I may also have antidepressant activity (11). The animal models which supported these clinical studies include DOPA, apomorphine, and serotonin potentiation, stimulated EEG effects in the rabbit, as well as antagonism of the sedative effects of deserpidine. In this regard, Breese et al. (3) have also found that TRH can reverse the sedative effects of ethanol, chlorpromazine, and pentobarbital and this also has been confirmed by Kruse and Schacht (30), as well as Horita and Carino (18).

By far the most impressive clinical studies with MIF-I recently have been reported in the treatment of parkinsonism. Reduced symptomatology of tremor, akinesia, and rigidity was observed (1, 2, 6, 15, 16, 22).

Perhaps the various effects of the peptides reported in our animal models may eventually be found to have relevancy in other clinical conditions. For example, if a peptide could be demonstrated to have activity in reducing audiogenic seizures, it could possibly be found useful in the treatment of epilepsy. Reduction of behavioral responses to footshock-induced fighting by a peptide may be an index for reducing clinical anxiety and/or aggressive behavior. On the other hand, a peptide that increases fighting could possibly have antidepressant activity. Another exciting possibility is that peptides that improve maze performance may be found useful in the treatment of learning and memory disorders. Finally, a compound antagonizing the effects of methamphetamine might find application in the treatment of schizophrenia or other mental disease.

In conclusion, the most dramatic developments await the systematic development of new peptides. It is quite possible that new analogs will have more specific clinical effects with therapeutic utility. However, in the meantime, studies of the hypothalamic peptides should provide a sound basis for future investigations.

REFERENCES

1. Barbeau, A. (1975): Potentiation of levodopa effect by intravenous L-prolyl-L-leucyl-glycine amide in man. *Lancet*, 2:683-684.
2. Barbeau, A. and Kastin, A. J. (1975): Polypeptide therapy in Parkinson's disease - a new approach. 5th Int. Symp. on Parkinson's Disease, Vienna, edited by W. Birkmayer. Editions Roche, Paris.
3. Breese, G. R., Cooper, B. R., Prange, A. J., Cott, J. M., and Lipton, M. A. (1974): In: *The Thyroid Axis, Drugs, and Behavior*, edited by A. J. Prange, Jr., pp. 115-127. Raven Press, New York.
4. Burt, D. R. and Snyder, S. H. (1975): Thyrotropin-releasing hormone (TRH): apparent receptor binding in rat brain membranes. *Brain Res.*, 93:309-328.
5. Castensson, S., Sievertsson, H., Lindeke, B., and Sum, C. Y. (1974): Studies on the inhibition of oxotremorine induced tremor by a melanocyte-stimulating hormone release-inhibiting factor, thyrotropin releasing hormone and related peptides. *FEBS Lett.*, 44:101-105.
6. Chase, T. N., Woods, A. C., Lipton, M. A., and Morris, C. E. (1974): Hypothalamic releasing factors and Parkinson's disease. *Arch. Neurol.*, 31:55-56.
7. Coppen, A., Montgomery, S., Peet, M., and Bailey, J. (1974): Thyrotrophin-releasing hormone in the treatment of depression. *Lancet*, 2:433-435.
8. Deniker, P., Ginestet, D., Loo, H., Zarifian, E., and Cottereau, M. J. (1974): Etude preliminaire de l'action de la thyreostimuline hypothalamique (thyrotropine releasing hormone ou T.R.H.) dans les etats depressifs. *Ann. Med. Psychol.*, 1:249-255.
9. de Wied, D. (1965): The influence of the posterior and inter-

mediate lobe of the pituitary and pituitary peptides on the maintenance of a conditioned avoidance response in rats. *Int. J. Neuropharmacol.*, 4:157.

10. de Wied, D., Bohus, B., and Greven, H. M. (1968): Influence of pituitary adrenocortical hormones on conditioned avoidance behavior in rats. In: *Endocrinology and Human Behaviour*, edited by R. P. Michael, pp. 188-196. Oxford University Press, London, England.

11. Ehrensing, R. H., Kastin, A. J., Schalch, D. S., Friesen, H., Vargas, R., and Schally, A. V. (1974): Affective state and thyrotropin and prolactin responses after repeated injections of thyrotropin-releasing hormone in depressed patients. *Am. J. Psychiat.*, 161:714-718.

12. Everett, G. M. (1966): The DOPA response potentiation test and its use in screening for antidepressant drugs. Proc. 1st Int. Symp. Antidepressant Drugs. *Excerpta. Med. Int. Cong. Ser.* 122:164-167.

13. Everett, G. M. and Toman, J. E. P. (1959): Mode of action of rauwolfia alkaloids and motor activity. In: *Proceedings of the Society of Biological Psychiatry*. Grune & Stratton, New York, p. 76.

14. Ferrari, W., Gessa, G. L., and Vargiu, L. (1961): Stretching activity in dogs intracisternally injected with a synthetic melanocyte-stimulating hexapeptide. *Experientia*, 17: 90.

15. Fischer, P.-A., Schneider, E., Jacobi, P., and Maxion, H. (1975): Effect of melanocyte-stimulating hormone release (MIF) in Parkinson's syndrome. *Eur. Neurol.*, 12:360-368.

16. Gerstenbrand, V. F., Binder, H., Kozma, C., Pusch, S., and Reisner, T. (1975): Infusiontherapie mit MIF (melanocyte inhibiting factor) beim Parkinson-syndrom. *Wien. Klin. Wochenschr.*, 87:822-823.

17. Gessa, G. L., Pisano, M., Vargiu, L., Crabai, F., and Ferrari, W. (1967): Stretching and yawning movements after intracerebral injection of ACTH. *Rev. Can. Biol.*, 26:229-236.

18. Horita, A. and Carino, M. A. (1975): Studies on the analeptic action of thyrotropin-releasing hormone (TRH) in rabbits. *Pharmacologist*, 17:211.

19. Horn, A. S., Coyle, J. T., and Snyder, S. H. (1971): Catecholamine uptake by synaptosomes from rat brain: structure-activity relationships of drugs with differential effects on dopamine and norepinephrine neurons. *Mol. Pharmacol.*, 7:66-80.

20. Huidobro-Toro, J. P., Scotti de Carolis, A., and Longo, V. G. (1974): Action of two hypothalamic factors (TRH, MIF) and of angiotensin II on the behavioral effects of L-DOPA and 5-hydroxytryptophan in mice. *Pharmacol. Biochem. Behav.*, 2:105-110.

21. Itil, T. M., Patterson, C. D., Polvan, N., Bigelow, A., and Bergey, B. (1975): Clinical and CNS effects of oral and i.v. thyrotropin-releasing hormone in depressed patients. *Dis. Nerv. Syst.*, 36:529-536.

22. Kastin, A. J. and Barbeau, A. (1972): Preliminary clinical studies with L-prolyl-L-leucyl-glycine amide in Parkinson's disease. *Can. Med. Ass. J.,* 107:1079-1081.
23. Kastin, A. J., Ehrensing, R. H., Schalch, D. S., and Anderson, M. S. (1972): Improvement in mental depression with decreased thyrotropin response after administration of thyrotropin-releasing hormone. *Lancet,* 2:740-742.
24. Kastin, A. J., Miller, L. H., Nockton, R., Sandman, C. A., Schally, A. V., and Stratton, L. O. (1973): Behavioral aspects of melanocyte-stimulating hormone (MSH). In: *Progress in Brain Research,* Vol. 39, edited by E. Zimmermann, W. H. Gispen, B. H. Marks and D. de Wied, pp. 462-470. Elsevier, Amsterdam, The Netherlands.
25. Kastin, A. J., Plotnikoff, N. P., Hall, R., and Schally, A. V. (1975): Hypothalamic hormones and the central nervous system. In: *Hypothalamic Hormones: Chemistry, Physiology, Pharmacology and Clinical Uses,* edited by L. Martini, pp. 261-268. Academic Press, New York.
26. Kastin, A. J., Plotnikoff, N. P., Sandman, C. A., Spirtes, M. A., Kostrzewa, R. M., Paul, S. M., Stratton, L. O., Miller, L. H., Labrie, F., Schally, A. V., and Goldman, H. (1975): The effects of MSH and MIF on the brain. In: *Anatomical Neuroendocrinology,* edited by W. E. Stumpf and L. D. Grant, pp. 290-297. S. Karger, Basel, Switzerland.
27. Kastin, A. J., Sandman, C. A., Stratton, L. O., Schally, A. V., and Miller, L. H. (1975): Behavioral and electrographic changes in rat and man after MSH. In: *Progress in Brain Research, Vol. 42: Hormones, Homeostasis and the Brain,* edited by W. H. Gispen, Tj. B. van Wimersma Greidanus, B. Bohus and D. de Wied, pp. 143-150. Elsevier, Amsterdam, The Netherlands.
28. Krivoy, W. A. and Guillemin, R. (1961): On a possible role of β-melanocyte stimulating hormone (β-MSH) in the central nervous system of the mammalia: an effect of β-MSH in the spinal cord of the cat. *Endocrinology,* 69:170-175.
29. Krivoy, W. A., Lane, M., Childers, H. E., and Guillemin, R. (1962): On the action of β-melanocyte stimulating hormone (β-MSH) on spontaneous electric discharge of the transparent knife fish, G. eigenmannia. *Experientia,* 18:521-522.
30. Kruse, H. and Schacht, U. (1974): TRH-chlorpromazine-interaction. *J. Pharmacol.,* 5:53.
31. Miller, R. E. and Ogawa, N. (1962): The effect of adrenocorticotrophic hormone (ACTH) avoidance conditioning in the adrenalectomized rat. *J. Comp. Physiol. Psychol.,* 55:211-213.
32. Mountjoy, C. Q., Price, J. S., Weller, M., Hunter, P., Hall, R., and Dewar, J. H. (1974): A double-blind crossover sequential trial of oral thyrotrophin-releasing hormone in depression. *Lancet,* 1:958-960.
33. Murphy, A. V. and Miller, R. E. (1955): The effect of adrenocorticotrophic hormone (ACTH) on avoidance conditioning in rats. *J. Comp. Physiol. Psychol.,* 48:47-49.
34. Plotnikoff, N. P. (1975): Prolyl-leucyl-glycine amide (PLG)

and thyrotropin-releasing hormone (TRH): DOPA potentiation
and biogenic amine studies. *Prog. Brain Res.*, 42:11-23.

35. Plotnikoff, N. P. and Kastin, A. J. (1974): Pharmacological
studies with a tripeptide, prolyl-leucyl-glycine amide. *Arch.
Int. Pharmacodyn. Ther.*, 211:211-224.

36. Plotnikoff, N. P. and Kastin, A. J. (1974): Oxotremorine
antagonism by prolyl-leucyl-glycine-amide administered by different routes and with several anticholinergics. *Pharmacol.
Biochem. Behav.*, 2:417-419.

37. Plotnikoff, N. P., Kastin, A. J., Anderson, M. S. and Schally,
A. V. (1971): DOPA potentiation by a hypothalamic factor,
MSH release-inhibiting hormone (MIF). *Life Sci.*, 10:1279-
1283.

38. Plotnikoff, N. P., Kastin, A. J., Anderson, M. S., and
Schally, A. V. (1972): Oxotremorine antagonism by a hypothalamic hormone, melanocyte-stimulating hormone release-inhibiting factor (MIF). *Proc. Soc. Exp. Biol. Med.*, 140:811-
814.

39. Plotnikoff, N. P., Kastin, A. J., Anderson, M. S., and Schally,
A. V. (1973): Deserpidine antagonism by a tripeptide, L-
prolyl-L-leucylglycinamide. *Neuroendocrinology*, 11:67-71.

40. Plotnikoff, N. P., Kastin, A. J., and Schally, A. V. (1974):
Growth hormone release inhibiting hormone: neuropharmacological studies. *Pharmacol. Biochem. Behav.*, 2:693-696.

41. Plotnikoff, N. P., Minard, F. N., and Kastin, A. J. (1974):
DOPA potentiation levels in ablated animals and brain levels
of biogenic amines in intact animals after prolyl-leucylgly-
cinamide. *Neuroendocrinology*, 14:271-279.

42. Plotnikoff, N. P., Prange, A. J., Breese, G. R., Anderson, M.
S., and Wilson, I. C. (1972): Thyrotropin releasing hormone:
enhancement of DOPA activity by a hypothalamic hormone. *Science*, 178:417-418.

43. Plotnikoff, N. P., Prange, A. J., Breese, G. R., Anderson, M.
S., and Wilson, I. C. (1974): The effects of thyrotropin-
releasing hormone on DOPA response in normal, hypophysecto-
mized, and thyroidectomized animals. In: *The Thyroid Axis,
Drugs, and Behavior*, edited by A. J. Prange, Jr., pp. 103-113.
Raven Press, New York.

44. Plotnikoff, N. P., Prange, A. J., Breese, G. R., and Wilson,
I. C. (1974): Thyrotropin releasing hormone: enhancement of
DOPA activity in thyroidectomized rats. *Life Sci.*, 14:1271-
1278.

45. Plotnikoff, N. P., White, W. F., Kastin, A. J., and Schally,
A. V. (1975): Gonadotropin releasing hormone (GnRH): neuropharmacological studies. *Life Sci.*, 17:1685-1692.

46. Prange, A. J., Wilson, I. C., Knox, A., McClane, T. K., and
Lipton, M. A. (1970): Enhancement of imipramine by thyroid
stimulating hormone: clinical and theoretical implications.
Am. J. Psychiatry, 127:191-199.

47. Prange, A. J., Wilson, I. C., Lara, P. P., Alltop, L. B., and
Breese, G. R. (1972): Effects of thyrotropin-releasing hormone in depression. *Lancet*, 2:999-1002.

48. Sanghvi, I. and Gershon, S.   (1974):   Predicting clinical psy-
    chotropic drug activity from preclinical models (animal and
    human).   *Psychopharm. Bull.*, 10:20-22.
49. Schally, A. V., Arimura, A., and Kastin, A. J.   (1973):   Hypo-
    thalamic regulating hormones.   *Science,* 179:341-350.
50. Snyder, S. H.   (1973):   Amphetamine psychosis: a 'model'
    schizophrenia mediated by catecholamines.   *Am. J. Psychiatry,*
    130:61-67.
51. Takahashi, S., Kondo, H., Yoshimura, M., and Ochi, Y.   (1973):
    Antidepressant effect of thyrotropin-releasing hormone (TRH)
    and the plasma thyrotropin levels in depression.   *Folia Psy-
    chiatr. Neurol. Jpn.,* 27:305-314.
52. Takahashi, S., Kondo, H., Yoshimura, M., and Ochi, Y.   (1974):
    Thyrotropin responses to TRH in depressive illness: relation
    to clinical subtypes and prolonged duration of depressive
    episode.   *Folia Psychiatr. Neurol. Jpn.,* 28:355-364.
53. Wilson, I. C., Lara, P. P., and Prange, A. J.   (1973):   Thyro-
    trophin-releasing hormone in schizophrenia.   *Lancet,* 2:43-44.
54. Wilson, I. C., Prange, A. J., McClane, T. K., Rabon, A. M.,
    and Lipton, M. A.   (1970):   Thyroid hormone enhancement of
    imipramine in non-retarded depression.   *N. Engl. J. Med.,* 282:
    1063-1067.

*Neuropeptide Influences on the Brain
and Behavior,* edited by L.H. Miller,
C.A. Sandman, and A.J. Kastin.
Raven Press, New York © 1977.

Proposed Mechanisms of Action of Neurohypophyseal Peptides in Memory Processes and Possible Routes for the Biosynthesis of Peptides with a C-Terminal Carboxamide Group

Roderich Walter and P.L. Hoffman

*Department of Physiology and Biophysics, University of Illinois at the Medical
Center, Chicago, Illinois 60612*

INTRODUCTION

In this report we wish first to propose a biochemical model which attempts to explain the effects of neurohypophyseal hormones on memory processes, and second
to suggest a possible route for the biosynthesis of
peptide hormones which terminate in a carboxamide group.
By way of introduction earlier studies in the literature as well as more current papers are selectively reviewed. These reports formed the stimulus and helped
to produce the framework for the proposed hypotheses.
It should be noted at the outset that we have taken the
organizers of the conference literally in their invita-
tion to speculate freely.

PEPTIDES AS NEUROMODULATORS

The impact of some of the hypothalamic and pituitary
peptide hormones on various aspects of behavior and on
certain autonomic functions has been clearly demonstrated in recent literature (e.g., 35, 36, 76). The actions of the peptides in the central nervous system
suggest a role for these endogenous compounds either as
conventional neurotransmitters-i.e., factors which mediate short-term changes in neuronal excitability, or
as neuromodulators, which may participate in the long-
term regulation of neuronal excitability (2). Among
the peptides which appear to belong to the latter category are the neurohypophyseal hormones and substance
P(SP). The localization of SP in synaptosomal fractions, as well as its slow-in-onset and long-lasting
effects, support the suggestion that this peptide might

be a modulator of various mammalian neuron systems (2, 43). The neurohypophyseal peptides have not, in this connection, been studied in as great detail as SP, but several lines of evidence indicate their capacity to modify neuronal properties. Because iontophoretic application of vasopressin was found to depress the activity of neurons in the supraoptic nucleus (53), it was proposed that vasopressin might be released from recurrent collaterals of SON cells at synapses back on SON cells, to account for the recurrent inhibitory pathway found in this system (53). While recent evidence indicates that vasopressin is not directly responsible for the recurrent inhibition (2, 19), the inhibitory receptors on SON cells might provide for a feedback regulation of vasopressin release. On the other hand, other workers have found excitation of nerve cells in the paraventricular nucleus by iontophoretically applied oxytocin (52). Neurohypophyseal peptides have also been shown to have excitatory effects on certain invertebrate neurons (2). These neurons typically generate an endogenous bursting pacemaker potential (BPP) activity which is characterized by slow membrane potential oscillations on which is superimposed a burst of spikes (3). The primary actions of the peptides are initiation of BPP activity in cells from dormant (hibernating) snails, and enhancement of this activity in cells from active animals (2). The initiation of BPP activity is associated with a long-lasting change in the current-voltage relations of the neuronal membrane; as a result of this change, inhibitory and excitatory synaptic input that would normally produce small changes in potential and firing rate would now produce larger changes (2). Iontophoretic application of vasopressin to snail neurons produces changes in neuronal membrane properties which persist for some time after iontophoresis is terminated (2).

NEUROHYPOPHYSEAL PEPTIDES AND MEMORY

Neurohypophyseal hormones, especially vasopressin, have also been implicated in modification of various processes related to memory. These peptides delay extinction of an active avoidance response in intact rats (74, 78), and restore the ability of hypophysectomized rats to acquire such a response (5). Lysine vasopressin also inhibits extinction of passive avoidance behavior in intact animals (77). Rats with hereditary diabetes insipidus, that are unable to synthesize vasopressin, show enhanced extinction of a passive avoidance response, according to one study (77). According to another (6), the animals show difficulty in acquiring a conditioned avoidance response, but exhibit longer retention of the response than normal animals. In any case, the absence of vasopressin interferes with some aspect of learning or memory, as also evidenced by the fact that animals treated intraventricularly with anti-vasopressin antiserum fail to maintain a passive avoidance response (79). These actions of neurohypophyseal peptides can be dissociated from the peripheral, endocrinological effects of the hormones (78).

Furthermore, the compounds are much more potent when administered intraventricularly than systemically (76), indicating the central origin of the behavioral effects. An early study indicated that [des-9-glycinamide] lysine vasopressin (DGLVP) can also attenuate the amnesia caused by intracerebral injection of puromycin in mice trained in a Y-maze (42). More recently, we have examined the effect of vasopressin and several of its analogs and fragments on attenuation of this amnesia, and have concluded that the neurohypophyseal peptides modify consolidation of memory in such a way that expression or retrieval of memory becomes insensitive to puromycin (72). The work of de Wied and his colleagues also indicates that the neurohypophyseal peptides may affect consolidation of some aspect of memory, or enhance storage and/or retrieval of information (5, 74). An intriguing aspect of this work is the finding that the inhibition of extinction of an avoidance response caused by neurohypophyseal peptides is long-term, lasting for days or weeks (39, 75).

Thus, in several situations, the central effects of the neurohypophyseal hormones appear to involve some aspect of memory consolidation or information retrieval. Changes in neuronal excitability may be expected to have effects on various processes related to memory, so that the ability of these peptides to modify neuronal characteristics may well underlie their effects in the central nervous system. The neurochemical mechanism by which the compounds may regulate neuronal membrane properties, and the way in which this regulation is reflected in alterations of memory processes, is the subject of the hypothesis presented here.

NEUROCHEMICAL CORRELATES OF MEMORY PROCESS

The neurochemical events involved in the long-term memory processes we wish to consider, i.e., those which may be affected by neurohypophyseal peptides, have long been open to speculation and experimentation. Catecholamine theories of long-term memory have been suggested by several investigators (38, 57, 60). In particular, Kety has formulated a proposal in which catecholamines released in affective states may favor consolidation of learning by stimulating various chemical processes at recently activated synapses. This stimulation might then convert short-lived activity to a

more persistent increase in synaptic conductivity,
leading to a conditioned response (38). Much of the
experimental support for a theory of memory involving
catecholaminergic mechanisms comes from studies in
which lesions or pharmacological agents which deplete
brain catecholamines were shown to block memory measured in a given task. The dopamine β-hydroxylase in-
hibitor, diethyldithiocarbamate (DDC), decreases synthesis of norepinephrine (NE) in mouse brain (57).
When this drug was administered to animals before
training in a passive avoidance test, the retention of
the response was decreased (57). In another study, administration of DDC (or of dichloroisoproteronol, an α-
adrenergic blocking agent) to rats immediately after
training in a conditioned avoidance task also impaired
retention of the response (16). Drugs causing release
of norepinephrine have also been tested for their effects on memory. Treatment of rats with amphetamine
before training in a conditioned avoidance task resulted in better performance both during acquisition and
during recall of the response (61). Dismukes and Rake
(16) used reserpine to lower brain norepinephrine (NE)
levels after training of rats in a conditioned avoidance response, and found decreased recall of the response. The impairment of memory could be reversed by
post-training injections of L-DOPA but not 5-hydroxy-
tryptophan. All of these studies are compatible with a
role of NE in memory consolidation. Further evidence
for the role of catecholamines in memory processes is
available from studies using protein synthesis inhibitors. Barondes and Cohen (4) showed that mice treated
with a dose of cycloheximide which caused a 95% decrease in protein synthesis at the time of training
were able to remember an avoidance response for 3 hr,
but had impaired memory if tested 6 or more hr later.
This defect in "long-term" memory could be reversed by
footshock, amphetamine, or corticosteroids administered
3 hr after training, indicating to the authors that manipulations producing "arousal" can aid in the development of long-term memory. Roberts et al. (60) also demonstrated that a group of drugs which alters adrenergic
function was capable of restoring or improving memory
blocked by puromycin. Quartermain and Botwinick (56)
showed that the amnesia produced by pretraining injections of cycloheximide (in a food-motivated discrimination reversal task) could be blocked be pretesting
injections of monoamine oxidase inhibitors or amphetamine. Furthermore, α-methyltyrosine (α-MT) and DDC
were shown to produce amnesia very similar to that induced by cycloheximide. Since the amnesia produced by
cycloheximide may sometimes be spontaneously reversed
at 48 hr after training, the effects of the various

drugs which increase catecholamine levels or concentrations at the receptor were thought to be on memory retrieval or expression.

Biochemical evidence for mediation of the amnestic
action of protein synthesis inhibitors via adrenergic
mechanisms was presented by Flexner et al. (21) who
found an inhibition of rat brain tyrosine hydroxylase
activity caused by cycloheximide, although the conclusion that this enzyme inhibition has any effect on memory has been questioned (66). More recently, Flexner
and Goodman (20) have reported that cycloheximide, acetoxycycloheximide, puromycin, and anisomycin at dose
levels which cause amnesia in mice trained in a Y-maze,
all reduced the rate of accumulation of ^{14}C-dopamine
and ^{14}C-NE from ^{14}C-tyrosine (puromycin affected only
the synthesis of NE). While the time course of the decrease in accumulation did not correlate with time
course of the amnesia produced by these agents, a change
in catecholamine synthesis rate could conceivably affect memory at some time after the alteration was no-
ticeable.

A recent study by Stein et al. (67) demonstrated
that administration of NE (immediately after training)
into the lateral ventricle of rats which had been previously treated with DDC reversed the amnesia caused by
DDC in a passive avoidance test. In this study, short-
term memory (i.e., memory tested one min. after training) was not affected by DDC, while memory three days
after training was restored by NE. It has also been
shown that intraamygdaloid injections of 6-hydroxydopa-
mine, (6-HDA) which produce catecholamine depletion in
and around the amygdalae, inhibit acquisition as well
as retention of a conditioned avoidance response, in a
dose-related way (1). These results are compatible
with earlier studies in which intracisternal injections
of 6-HDA impaired acquisition and performance of a conditioned avoidance response (13). All of these studies
are consistent with the idea that adrenergic systems
are involved in the development or expression of long-
term memory, the processes that also appear to be affected by the neurohypophyseal peptides.

NEUROCHEMICAL HYPOTHESIS FOR NEUROHYPOPHYSEAL
PEPTIDE EFFECTS ON MEMORY

There have been some studies performed on the effects
of peptides on neurotransmitter synthesis, often with
conflicting results (e.g., 23, 41, 44, 68, 69). In the
case of neurohypophyseal peptides, Dunn (18) reported
no change in the rate of dopamine synthesis at one time
point after injection of ^{3}H-tyrosine in animals treated
with lysine vasopressin. The neurohypophyseal peptides

may affect noradrenergic systems by other means than
via direct effects on the synthesis of norepinephrine,
however, and while increased NE turnover might affect
memory consolidation, it would not easily explain the
long-term effects of neurohypophyseal hormones on memory, nor the long-term changes in neuronal excitability
which have been observed.

In order to propose a more comprehensive model of
peptide action at the neurochemical level, it is useful to review some of the available information regarding both the mechanism of action of the putative neurotransmitters and the molecular mechanism of action of
the neurohypophyseal hormones in their classical target tissues. Neurotransmitter molecules released from
the presynaptic terminals interact with postsynaptic
receptors to induce an electrical change, the postsynaptic potential. In the superior cervical ganglion,
it appears that the response to dopamine is mediated by
cyclic adenosine 3',5'-monophosphate (cAMP) (28). In
addition, the dopamine receptor in the caudate nucleus
has been suggested to be the dopamine-binding portion
of a dopamine-sensitive adenylate cyclas (37, 49). Adenylate cyclase systems sensitive to NE have also been
reported in the brain (40, 47). Stimulation of noradrenergic fibers reduces the firing rate of the cerebellar Purkinje cell, and this reduction can be mim-
icked by iontophoretic application of either NE or cAMP
(see 28). Thus, postsynaptic effects of NE may be mediated by cAMP, and these are likely to involve changes
in membrane permeability which will lead to generation
of postsynaptic potentials.

The antidiuretic effects of the neurohypophyseal
peptide, arginine vasopressin, and its analogs, have
been demonstrated to be mediated via cAMP in mammalian
kidney and in amphibian skin and bladder (e.g., 11, 17,
34, 54). Thus, these peptides induce changes in membrane permeability to Na^+ and water by activating hormone-sensitive adenylate cyclases in various tissues.
If the endocrine and extra-endocrine effects of neurohypophyseal hormones are mediated in similar manners,
it is not unreasonable to suppose that, in brain, these
peptides, released from centrally located peptidergic
neurons, may also act via stimulation of a specific
hormone-sensitive adenylate cyclase to induce changes
in neuronal membrane permeability. If this is the case,
there are several mechanisms by which the peptides
might affect noradrenergic transmission to modify neuronal excitability or synaptic efficacy (Fig. 1). If a
presynaptic hormone receptor exists, the increase in
cAMP could activate tyrosine hydroxylase, since this
enzyme has recently been shown to be sensitive to cAMP
(62), and thus lead to an increase in this rate-limiting

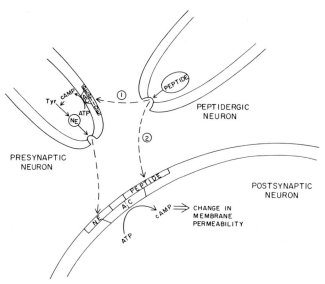

FIG. 1. Possible mechanisms of action of neurohypophyseal peptides for their central effects on memory. Peptides, released
from peptidergic neurons in the central nervous system, may interact with presynaptic receptors (1), to increase cyclic adenosine
3',5'-monophosphate (cAMP) levels and thereby stimulate tyrosine
hydroxylase and increase NE synthesis. Alternatively, or simultaneously, the peptides may interact postsynaptically (2), to alter membrane properties and/or cause a change in sensitivity of
NE-stimulated adenylate cyclase (AC).

step in norepinephrine synthesis. Alternatively—or simultaneously—by increasing cyclic AMP postsynaptically and inducing a change in membrane permeability the
hormone might mimic the effect of NE.
    Furthermore, the phenomena of super-sensitivity and
subsensitivity have been demonstrated in cyclase systems in brain responsive to NE stimulation (15, 22).
These phenomena may have some bearing on the effects of
the neurohypophyseal peptide on memory processes. For
example, stimulation of postsynaptic, cyclic-AMP generating receptors by the peptides could simulate increased NE at its postsynaptic receptor. The increased
stimulation would be expected to cause "subsensitivity"
of the norepinephrine receptor (15). Removal of the
peptide, by physiological processes, would then appear
as *decreased* stimulation and could result in "supersensitivity." In addition, it has been postulated that a
conformational change of the postsynaptic receptor can
alter the degree of receptor availability to the neurotransmitter. Interaction of the peptide hormone with a
receptor located at or near the norepinephrine receptor

site could induce such a change. Blockade of the NE
receptor by the peptide could also produce a situation
in which the postsynaptic receptor would be deprived of
norephinephrine, and supersensitivity could develop.
The change in sensitivity of the norepinephrine receptor would provide for the increased neuronal excitability which can be produced by neurohypophyseal peptides.
This change, occurring in the central noradrenergic system, could in turn contribute to enhanced consolidation
of memory as envisioned in catecholamine theories of
memory. More importantly, this mechanism suggests a
route by which the peptides may exert long-term effects
on memory, even after the compounds themselves have
been removed by physiological mechanisms.

It should be emphasized that this model is meant to
apply specifically to the neurohypophyseal peptides and
to their effects on memory processes. Each of the behaviorally active peptides appears to have a distinct
profile of activities (35) and each may prove to have a
unique biochemical mechanism of action, as well as specific neuronal receptors. Possibly one of the most important, and overlooked, parameters during testing of
peptide effects on memory and learning is the physiological state of the animal at the time the peptide is
released or administered. In female animals, it is
quite likely that the stage of estrus, and thus levels
of sex steroids, affect enzyme levels, enzyme activities, and perhaps receptor sensitivity. Experiments
testing peptide effects should therefore be carried out
either in male animals, or at known times during the
estrus cycle. Another perturbing influence lies in the
behavioral test chosen. Many such tests expose the
animal to stressful situations, which may be expected
to cause changes in responsiveness to peptides. Therefore the development of behavioral models which produce
minimal stress is critical. It is clear that in eval-
uating responses to behaviorally active peptides it is
necessary to characterize as fully as possible the milieu in which the peptide acts and ideally to maintain
this milieu constant.

A model similar to that presented here has been proposed for the central actions of ACTH and related peptides by Gispen et al. (25). This model must take into account the shorter-term actions of ACTH, and its
varied behavioral effects; however, it is also probable that the specificity of neuronal peptide receptors
may play an important role in determining their final
actions. It must also be pointed out that there is
most likely no one neurotransmitter which is solely involved in such complex processes as memory or learning.
For example, interactions between noradrenergic and
serotonergic (59), and noradrenergic and cholinergic

(46) neurons have been demonstrated both at the biochemical and behavioral levels.

Finally, it is apparent that postulating a role for
peptides as neuromodulators in memory processes is, in
a sense, begging the question. Although some peptides,
such as ACTH and vasopressin, are known to be released
into the systemic circulation in stressful situations,
it is not known, at present, whether stress also causes
increased brain levels of the peptides. In memory processes not connected to stressful situations, what is
the trigger for release of peptides from their neurons?
It is possible that the peptides are always present in
brain, and are responsible for subtle regulation of
neuronal properties involved in memory. In this case,
the effects of the peptides in intact animals or normal
humans may be difficult to detect.

Questions regarding the release, biosynthesis, mechanisms of action, termination of action, and physiological role of peptides as neuromodulators are all
critical to our further understanding of the role of
these compounds in the central nervous system. One of
these questions on which we would like to speculate is
the mode of biosynthesis of some of the centrally active peptides, i.e., those whose C-terminal amino acid
residue possess an amide moiety. One such peptide is
Pro-Leu-Gly-NH$_2$ (MSH-R-IF), the C-terminal tripeptide
of oxytocin, which inhibits *in vivo* and *in vitro* the release of MSH from rat pituitary (7, 9). This peptide
has also been recently shown to inhibit CRF-stimulated
release of ACTH from pituitaries *in vitro* (70) and, in
addition, the compound has a number of centrally-medi-
ated behavioral effects (for review, see 36). Thus,
MSH-R-IF potentiates the action of DOPA, reverses the
tremor caused by oxotremorine, and reduces the sedation
induced in monkeys and mice by deserpidine. The compound also induces stereotyped and compulsive behavior
in cats, and potentiates apomorphine-induced mounting
behavior in rats.

HYPOTHESIS ON BIOSYNTHESIS OF PEPTIDES
CONTAINING A C-TERMINAL CARBOXAMIDE GROUP

The finding that hypothalamic extracts partially de-
grade oxytocin and its C-terminal linear fragments to
give Pro-Leu-Gly-NH$_2$ (MSH-R-IF) (9 and for more detail
71), raised the intriguing and novel concept in endocrinology that a well-established hormone can serve as
a precursor for a factor(s) with a completely different
profile of biological activities. Thus, the biosynthesis of MSH-R-IF would involve the formation on ribosomes of a prohormone from which oxytocin is subsequently released by an enzymatic process (assuming the bio-

synthesis of oxytocin follows a similar route to that
of vasopressin [63]),which then in turn can serve as
substrate for the enzymatic formation of MSH-R-IF (71).

At about the same time Reichlin and his colleagues
proposed a totally different biosynthetic pathway for
the hypothalamic hormone TRH (50), which was a few
years later extended to include CRF, GRF, and PRF (for
summary see 58).   Since TRH synthesis was found to occur in the presence of protein synthesis inhibitors (29,
33, 51), it appeared that the biosynthesis of hypothalamic factors was nonribosomal and that the condensa-
tion of peptide bonds was mediated by ATP- and Mg^{++}
ion-dependent enzyme systems. Analogous biosynthetic
mechanisms had been established for the formation of
glutathione (< Glu-Cys-Gly) (48, 65) opthalamic acid,
norophthalamic acid (12) and bacterial antibiotics
(e.g., gramicidin; 24). However, using a cell-free
extract of newt brain it was recently found that while
the incorporation of [^{3}H]-proline into TRH was not
prevented by protein synthesis inhibitors, it was
blocked by pancreatic RNase (30). This suggests that
puromycin-induced truncated messenger-RNA molecules are
still capable of leading to the synthesis of low molecular weight peptides.

Neither of the above mechanisms, however, addresses
itself specifically to the issue of incorporation of
the primary carboxamide group into hypothalamic factors
and certain peptide hormones. One plausible mechanism
was recently suggested by Smyth (64). He postulated
that in such instances the conversion of the prohormone
to hormone may involve a transamidation reaction. Such
a reaction is in contrast to hydrolytic cleavage of the
peptide chain by trypsin-like enzymes.

We wish to suggest an additional route for the biosynthesis of peptides possessing a C-terminal amide
group, which might merit investigation. The scheme
involves the following steps (Fig. 2):

1. The hypothetical biologically active peptide-
   to-be would be synthesized on the ribosome;
2. The active peptide-to-be must be elongated
   at the C-terminus and the residue which is
   to bear the carboxamide function must be
   followed by a residue which can be enzymatically converted to a dehydroalanine residue. Cysteine or serine residues are excellent candidates. Dehydroalanine residues
   are not only native to such high-molecular-
   weight compounds as nisin (isolated from
   Streptococcus lactis) and subtilisin (from
   Bacillus subtilis [31]), but the metabolic conversion of specific cysteine residues to

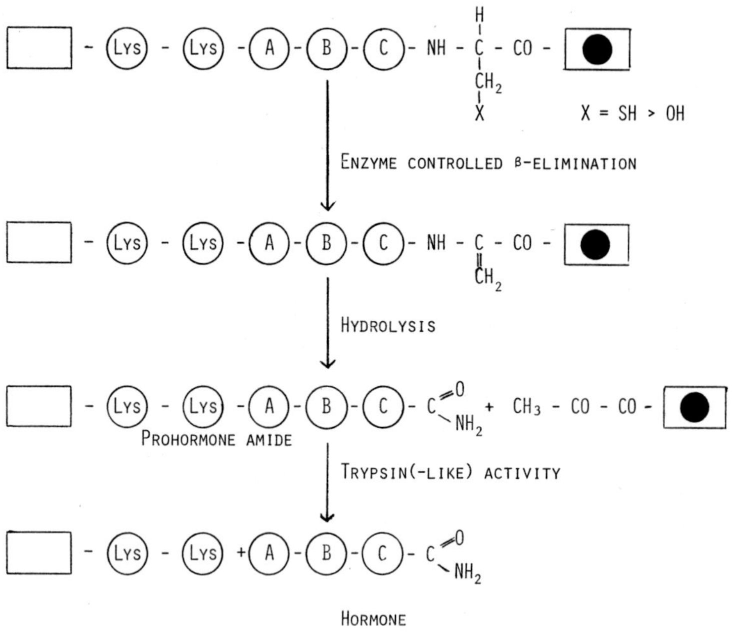

FIG. 2. Biosynthetic scheme for a hypothetical peptide possessing a C-terminal primary carboxamide group. The hypothetical hormone (A-B-C-CONH₂), formed on ribosomes as an inactive high-molecular weight compound, would be liberated enzymatically. A cysteine or serine residue located vicinal to residue C at the carboxyl side would be formally transformed via formation of a dehydroalanine residue to a primary carboxamide moiety, cleaving the peptide chain in the process. The peptide chain extending from the N-terminus of the hormone-to-be could either be liberated by the trypsin-like enzymes which recognize two neighboring basic residues as a site for cleavage (as illustrated in the Fig. by Lys-Lys, ref. 45) or by other enzyme systems, e.g., the one releasing MSH-R-IF from oxytocin (9, 71). The proposal leaves open the question of the sequence of liberation of N- or C-terminus. ☐ indicates peptide chain extension at the N-terminal side and ⬛ at the C-terminus.

dehydroalanine residues in certain enzymes (e.g., rat liver fructose diphosphatase, and rabbit muscle aldolase [14])produces dehydroalanyl enzymes (desulfo enzymes) which are as active or even more active than the native enzyme. In fact, evidence has been presented which was interpreted to suggest that a dehydroalanine residue actually is present in the "active site" of native histidine ammonia lyase isolated either from bacterial or mammalian sources (26, 27, 73);

3. Hydrolysis of the dehydroalanyl precursor
would result in the release of the peptide
amide, thus completing the formal conversion of the NH moiety of the cysteine residue to the C-terminal carboxamide. Gross
and his colleagues have already demonstrated the use of dehydroalanine-containing
polymer for the synthesis of biologically
active peptides terminating in the amide
function (32), and had reported earlier
that <Glu-His-Try-dehydroAla-Tyr-Gly-Leu-
Arg-Pro-Gly-NH$_2$, thought to be formed *in
situ* as an intermediate from an appropriately modified serine residue in position
3 of the luteinizing hormone, gives rise
to <Glu-His-Try-NH$_2$ (31).
4. The hormonally active part-to-be could be
elongated on its N-terminus and could be
liberated either by the trypsin-like, car-
boxypeptidase B-like enzyme system found
for the conversion of proinsulin and several other peptide hormone precursors to
the hormone (for a recent summary see 45),
or by the unknown enzyme system releasing
MSH-R-IF from oxytocin (9, 71).

Based on the above considerations, the C-terminal
amide of oxytocin could originate from a protein precursor of the following structure:

-Cys-Tyr-Ile-Gln-Asn-Cys-Pro-Leu-Gly-Cys-(or Ser)

in which the Cys (or Ser) at right is formally converted to an amide and the N-terminal of the Cys residue at
the left is liberated by peptide bond hydrolysis. The
oxytocin released could then be degraded stepwise to
form Pro-Leu-Gly-NH$_2$ as described (9, 71).
Previously we reported that Cys-Tyr-Ile-Gln-Asn-OH
was capable in ng amounts of stimulating the release of
pituitary MSH *in vivo* and *in vitro* (10). Subsequently,
it was found that in addition to Cys-Tyr-Ile-Gln-Asn-
OH, the two shorter fragments, Tyr-Ile-Gln-Asn-OH and
Ile-Gln-Asn-OH, exhibited MSH-releasing activity; in
fact all three peptides were equipotent on a molar basis, while Gln-Asn-OH was inactive (8). Application of
the above scheme suggested that breakdown of the hypothetical precursor

-Cys-Tyr-Ile-Gln-Asn- | Cys | -Pro-Leu-Gly-Cys(or Ser)

by liberation of the N-terminal of the Cys at the left
by hydrolytic cleavage of the peptide bond and conversion of the Cys residue following the Asn residue to an
amide, could give peptide amides which are more potent

in the release of MSH than the corresponding acids. Therefore we have recently prepared Ile-Gln-Asn-NH$_2$ (55) as well as the N-terminal penta- and tetra-peptide amides of the oxytocin sequence to be tested for their MSH-releasing activity.

ACKNOWLEDGMENT

This work was supported by U.S. Public Health Service Grant AM-18399.

REFERENCES

1. Ashford, J. and Jones, B. J. (1976): The effects of intra-amygdaloid injections of 6-hydroxydopamine on avoidance responding in rats. *Br. J. Pharmacol.*, 56:255-261.
2. Barker, J. L. (1976): Peptides: Roles in neuronal excitability. *Physiol. Rev.*, 56:435-452.
3. Barker, J. L., Ifshin, M., and Gainer, H. (1975): Studies on bursting pacemaker potential activity in molluscan neurons. III. Effects of hormones. *Brain Res.*, 84:501-513.
4. Barondes, S. H. and Cohen, H. D. (1968): Arousal and the conversion of "short-term" to "long-term" memory. *Proc. Natl. Acad. Sci. USA*, 61:923-929.
5. Bohus, B., Gispen, W. H., and de Wied, D. (1973): Effect of lysine vasopressin and ACTH 4-10 on conditioned avoidance behavior of hypophysectomized rats. *Neuroendocrinology*, 11:137-143.
6. Celestian, J. F., Carey, R. J., and Miller, M. (1976): Unimpaired maintenance of a conditioned avoidance response in the rat with diabetes insipidus. *Physiol. Behav.*, 15:707-711.
7. Celis, M. E., Hase, S., and Walter, R. (1972): Structure-activity studies of MSH-release-inhibiting hormone. *FEBS Lett.*, 27:326-327.
8. Celis, M. E., Nakagawa, S. H., and Walter, R. (1975): Release of pituitary melanocyte stimulating hormone by neurohypophyseal hormone fragments. In: *Peptides: Chemistry, Structure, Biology*, edited by R. Walter and J. Meienhofer, pp. 771-776. Ann Arbor Science Publishers, Ann Arbor, Michigan.
9. Celis, M. E., Taleisnik, S., and Walter, R. (1971): Regulation of formation and proposed structure of the factor inhibiting the release of melanocyte-stimulating hormone. *Proc. Nat. Acad. Sci. USA*, 68:1428-1433.
10. Celis, M. E. Taleisnik, S., and Walter, R. (1971): Release of pituitary melanocyte-stimulating hormone by the oxytocin fragment, H-Cys-Tyr-Ile-Gln-Asn-OH. *Biochem. Biophys. Res. Comm.*, 45:564-569.
11. Chase, L. R. and Auerbach, G. D. (1968): Renal adenyl cyclase: Anatomically separate sites for parathyroid hormone and vasopressin. *Science*, 59:545-547.
12. Cliffe, E. E. and Waley, S. G. (1958): Acidic peptides of the lens. IV. The biosynthesis of ophthalamic acid. *Biochem. J.*, 69:649-655.

13. Cooper, B. R., Breese, G. R., Grant, L. D., and Howard, J. L. (1973): Effects of 6-hydroxydopamine treatments on active avoidance responding: Evidence for involvement of brain dopamine. *J. Pharmacol. Exp. Ther.*, 185:359–370.

14. Cremona, T. T., Kowal, T. J., and Horecker, B. L. (1965): The mechanisms of action of aldolases. XI. *Proc. Natl. Acad. Sci. USA*, 53:1395–1402.

15. Dismukes, K. and Daley, J. W. (1974): Norepinephrine-sensitive systems generating adenosine 3',5'-monophosphate: Increased response in cerebral cortical slices from reserpine-treated rats. *Mol. Pharmacol.*, 10:933–940.

16. Dismukes, R. K. and Rake, A. V. (1972): Involvement of biogenic amines in memory formation. *Psychopharmacologia*, 23:17–25.

17. Dousa, T., Hechter, O., Schwartz, I. L., and Walter, R. (1971): Neurohypophyseal hormone-responsive adenylate cyclase from mammalian kidney. *Proc. Natl. Acad. Sci. USA*, 69:1693–1697.

18. Dunn, A. J., Iuvone, P. M., and Rees, H. D.: Neurochemical responses of mice to ACTH and lysine vasopressin. *Pharmacol. Biochem. Behav. (Suppl.)*, 5:139–146.

19. Dreifuss, J. J., Nordmann, J. J., and Vincent, J. D. (1974): Recurrent inhibition of supraoptic neurosecretory cells in homozygous Brattleboro rats. *J. Physiol.*, 237:25P.

20. Flexner, L. B. and Goodman, R. H. (1975): Studies on memory: Inhibitors of protein synthesis also inhibit catecholamine synthesis. *Proc. Natl. Acad. Sci. USA*, 72:4660–4663.

21. Flexner, L. B., Serota, R. G., and Goodman, R. H. (1973): Cycloheximide and acetoxycycloheximide: Inhibition of tyrosine hydroxylase activity and amnestic effects. *Proc. Natl. Acad. Sci. USA*, 70:354–356.

22. French, S. W., Palmer, D. S., Narod, M. E., Reid, P. E., and Rainey, C. W. (1975): Noradrenergic sensitivity of the cerebral cortex after chronic ethanol ingestion and withdrawal. *J. Pharmacol. Exp. Ther.*, 194:319–326.

23. Friedman, E., Friedman, J., and Gershon, S. (1973): Dopamine synthesis: Stimulation by a hypothalamic factor. *Science*, 182:831–832.

24. Gevers, W., Kleinkauf, H., and Lippmann, F. (1969): Peptidyl transfers in Gramicidin S. Biosynthesis from enzyme bound thioester intermediates. *Proc. Natl. Acad. Sci. USA*, 63:1335–1342.

25. Gispen, W. H., Reith, M. E. A., Schotman, P., Wiegant, V. M., Zwiers, H. (1977): The CNS and ACTH-like peptides: neurochemical response and interaction with opiates *(This volume)*.

26. Givot, I. L., and Abeles, R. H. (1970): Mammalian histidine ammonia lyase. *In vivo* inactivation and presence of an electrophilic center at the active site. *J. Biol. Chem.*, 245:3271–3273.

27. Givot, I. L., Smith, J. A., and Abeles, R. H. (1969): Studies on the mechanism of action and the structure of the electrophoretic center of histidine ammonia lyase. *J. Biol. Chem.*,

244:6341-6353.

28. Greengard, P. (1976): Possible role for cyclic nucleotides and phosphorylated membrane proteins in postsynaptic actions of neurotransmitters. *Nature,* 260:101-108 and references therein.

29. Grimm-Jorgensen, Y. and McKelvy, J. F. (1976): Control of the *in vivo* biosynthesis of thyrotropin releasing factor (TRF) in the red spotted newt (*triturus viridescens*). *Prog. Ann. Mtg. Endocrine Soc.,* 56th, Atlanta, p. A65.

30. Grimm-Jorgensen, Y. and McKelvy, J. F. (1976): TRF biosynthesis *in vitro:* Effect of inhibitors of protein synthesis. *Brain Res.,* 1:171-175.

31. Gross, E. (1972): Structural relationships in and between peptides with α,β-unsaturated amino acids. In: *Chemistry and Biology of Peptides,* edited by J. Meienhofer, pp. 671-678. Ann Arbor Scientific Publishers, Ann Arbor, Michigan.

32. Gross, E., Noda, K., and Nigula, B. (1973): Solid phase synthesis of peptides with carboxyl-terminal amides-thyrotropin releasing factor. *Angew Chemie Int. Ed.,* 12:664-665.

33. Guillemin, R. (1973): Biosynthesis of hypothalamic tripeptide-amide TRF. *Prog. 1st Annual Mtg. Soc. Neuroscience,* Washington, D.C., p. 70.

34. Jard, S. and Boeckart, J. (1975): Stimulus-response coupling in neurohypophyseal peptide target cells. *Physiol. Rev.,* 55: 489-536.

35. Kastin, A. J., Plotnikoff, N. P., Hall, R., and Schally, A. V. (1977): Hypothalamic Hormones and the Central Nervous System, (In press.)

36. Kastin, A. J., Plotnikoff, N. P., Sandman, C. A., Sprites, M. A., Kostrzewa, R. M., Paul, S. M., Stratton, L. O., Miller, L. H., Labrie, F., Schally, A. V., and Goldman, H. (1975): The effects of MSH and MIF on the brain. In: *Anatomical Neuroendocrinology,* edited by W. E. Stumpf and L. D. Grant, pp. 290-297. Karger, Basel.

37. Kebabian, J. W., Petzold, G. L., and Greengard, P. (1972): Dopamine-sensitive adenylate cyclase in caudate nucleus of rat brain, and its similarity to the "dopamine receptor." *Proc. Natl. Acad. Sci. USA,* 69:2145-2149.

38. Kety, S. S. (1970): The biogenic amines in the central nervous system: Their possible roles in arousal, emotion and learning. In: *The Neurosciences: Second Study Program,* edited by F. O. Schmitt, pp. 324-336. Rockefeller University Press, New York.

39. King, A. R. and de Wied, D. (1974): Localized behavioral effects of vasopressin on maintenance of an active avoidance response in rats. *J. Comp. Physiol. Psychol.,* 86:1008-1018.

40. Klainer, L. M., Chi, V. M., Friedberg, S. L., Rall, T. W., and Sutherland, E. W. (1962): Adenyl cyclase: Effects of neurohormones on the formation of adenosine 3',5'-phosphate by preparations from brain and other tissues. *J. Biol. Chem.,* 237: 1239-1243.

41. Kostrzewa, R. M., Kastin, A. J., and Spirtes, M. A. (1975):

α-MSH and MIF-I effects on catecholamine levels and synthesis in various rat brain areas. *Pharmacol. Biochem. Behav.*, 3: 1017-1023.

42. Lande, S., Flexner, J. B., and Flexner, L. B. (1972): Effect of corticotropin and desglycinamide 9-lysine vasopressin on suppression of memory by puromycin. *Proc. Natl. Acad. Sci. USA*, 69:558-560.

43. Leeman, S. E. and Mroz, E. A. (1976): Substance P. *Life Sci.* 15:2033-2044.

44. Leonard, B. E. (1974): The effect of two synthetic ACTH analogues on the metabolism of biogenic amines in rat brain. *Arch. Int. Pharmacodyn. Ther.*, 207:242-253.

45. Lernmark, A., Chan, S. J., Choy, R., Nathans, A., Carroll, R., Tager, H. S., Rubenstein, A. H., Swift, H. H., and Steiner, D. F. (1976): In: *Polypeptide Hormones, Molecular and Cellular Aspects*, CIBA Foundation Symposium #41, pp. 7-21. Elsevier, Amsterdam.

46. Levander, T., Jok, T. H., and Reis, D. J. (1975): Prolonged activation of tyrosine hydroxylase in noradrenergic neurons of rat brain by cholinergic stimulation. *Nature*, 258:440-445.

47. McCune, R. W., Gill, T. H., von Hungen, K., and Roberts, S. (1971): Catecholamine-sensitive adenyl cyclase in cell-free preparations from rat cerebral cortex. *Life Sci.*, 10 (Part 2): 43-450.

48. Mandeles, S. and Bloch, K. (1955): Enzymatic synthesis of γ-glutamyl cysteine. *J. Biol. Chem.*, 214:639-646.

49. Miller, R. J., Horn, A. S., and Iversen, L. L. (1974): The action of neuroleptic drugs on dopamine-stimulated adenosine cyclic 3', 5'-monophosphate production in rat neostriatum and limbic forebrain. *Mol. Pharmacol.*, 10:759-766.

50. Mitnick, M. and Reichlin, S. (1971): Biosynthesis of TRH by rat hypothalamic tissue *in vitro*. *Science*, 172:1241-1243.

51. Mitnick, M. and Reichlin, S. (1973): Enzymatic synthesis of thyrotrophin releasing factor (TRH) by hypothalamic "TRH synthetase." *Endocrinology*, 91:1145-1153.

52. Moss, R. L., Dyball, R. E. J., and Cross, B. A. (1972): Excitation of antidromically identified neurosecretory cells of the paraventricular nucleus by oxytocin applied iontophoretically. *Exp. Neurol.*, 34:95-102.

53. Nicoll, R. A. and Barker, J. L. (1971): The pharmacology of recurrent inhibition in the supraoptic neurosecretory system. *Brain Res.*, 35:501-511.

54. Orloff, J. and Handler, J. S. (1967): The role of adenosine 3',5'-phosphate in the action of antidiuretic hormone. *Am. J. Med.*, 42:757-768.

55. Orlowski, R. C., Walter, R., and Winkler, D. (1976): Study of benzhydrylamine-type polymers: Synthesis and use of *p*-methoxybenzhydrylamine resin in the solid phase preparation of peptides. *J. Org. Chem.*, 41:3701-3705.

56. Quartermain, D. and Botwinick, E. Y. (1975): Role of the biogenic amines in the reversal of cycloheximide-induced amnesia. *J. Comp. Physiol. Psychol.*, 88:386-410.

57. Randt, C. T., Quartermain, D., Goldstein, M., and Anagnoste, B. (1971): Norepinephrine biosynthesis inhibition: Effects on memory in mice. *Science,* 172:498-499.
58. Reichlin, S. and Mitnick, M. (1973): Biosynthesis of hypothalamic hypophysiotropic factors. In: *Frontiers in Neuroendocrinology,* edited by W. F. Ganong and L. Martini, pp. 61-88. Oxford University Press, New York.
59. Renaud, B., Buda, M., Lewis, and Pujol, J. F. (1975): Effects of 5',6'-dihydroxytryptamine on tyrosine hydroxylase activity in central catecholaminergic neurons of the rat. *Biochem. Pharmacol.,* 24:1739-1742.
60. Roberts, R. B., Flexner, J. B., and Flexner, L. B. (1970): Some evidence for the involvement of adrenergic sites in the memory trace. *Proc. Natl. Acad. Sci. USA,* 66:10-313.
61. Roffman, M. and Lal, H. (1971): Facilitatory effect of amphetamine on learning and recall of an avoidance response in rats. *Arch. Int. Pharmacodyn. Ther.,* 193:87-91.
62. Roth, R. H., Morgenroth III, V. H., and Salzman, P. M. (1975): Tyrosine hydroxylase: Allosteric activation induced by stimulation of central noradrenergic neurons. *Naunyn-Schmeidebergs Arch. Pharmacol.,* 289:327-343.
63. Sachs, H., Fawcett, P., Takatabake, Y., and Portanova, R. (1969): Biosynthesis and release of vasopressin and neurophysin. *Recent Prog. Horm. Res.,* 25:447-491.
64. Smyth, D. G. (1975): The peptide hormones: Molecular and cellular aspects. *Nature,* 257:89-90.
65. Snoke, J. E. and Bloch, K. (1952): Formation and utilization of γ-glutamyl cysteine in glutathione synthesis. *J. Biochem.,* 199:407-414.
66. Squire, L. R., Kuczenski, R., and Barondes, S. H. (1974): Tyrosine hydroxylase inhibition by cycloheximide and anisomycin is not responsible for their amnesic effect. *Brain Res.,* 82:241-248.
67. Stein, L., Belluzzi, J. D., and Wise, C. D. (1975): Memory enhancement by central administration of norepinephrine. *Brain Res.,* 84:329-335.
68. Versteeg, D. H. (1973): Effect of two ACTH-analogs on noradrenaline metabolism in rat brain. *Brain Res.,* 49:483-485.
69. Versteeg, D. H. and Wurtman, R. J. (1975): Effect of ACTH 4-10 on the rate of synthesis of [^{3}H] catecholamines in the brains of intact, hypophysectomized and adrenalectomized rats. *Brain Res.,* 93:552-557.
70. Voigt, K. H. Fehm, H. L., and Lang, R. E. (1977): The inhibition of ACTH release in isolated pituitary cells by somatostatin and by MSH-inhibiting factor (MIF). In: *Hypothalamic Hormones, Second European Colloquium,* edited by W. Voelter and D. Gupta. Verlagchemie, Weinheim. *(In press.) ibid: Horm. Metab. Res.,* Jan. 1977.
71. Walter, R. (1974): Oxytocin and other peptide hormones as prohormones. In: *Psychoneuroendocrinology,* edited by N. Hatotani, pp. 285-294. Basel, Karger.
72. Walter, R., Hoffman, P. L., Flexner, J. B., and Flexner, L. B.

(1975): Neurohypophyseal hormones, analogs and fragments: Their effect on puromycin-induced amnesia. *Proc. Natl. Acad. Sci. USA,* 72:4180-4184.

73. Wickner, R. B. (1969): Dehydroalanine in histidine ammonia lyase. *J. Biol. Chem.,* 244:6550-6552.

74. de Wied, D. (1971): Long-term effect of vasopressin on the maintenanance of a conditioned avoidance response in rats. *Nature,* 232:58-60.

75. de Wied, D. and Bohus, B. (1966): Long-term and short-term effects on retention of a conditioned avoidance response in rats by treatment with long acting pitressin and α-MSH. *Nature,* 212:1484-1486.

76. de Wied, D., Bohus, B., Urban, I., van Wimersma Greidanus, Tj. B., and Gispen, W. H. (1975): Peptides and memory. In: *Peptides: Chemistry Structure, Biology,* edited by R. Walter and J. Meienhofer, pp. 685-694. Ann Arbor Scientific Publishers, Ann Arbor, Michigan.

77. de Wied, D., Bohus, B., and van Wimersma Greidanus, Tj. B. (1975): Memory deficit in rats with hereditary diabetes insipidus. *Brain Res.,* 85:152-156.

78. de Wied, D., Greven, H. M., Lande, S., and Witter, A. (1972): Dissociation of the behavioral and endocrine effects of lysine vasopressin by tryptic digestion. *Br. J. Pharmacol.,* 45:118-122.

79. van Wimersma Greidanus, Tj. B., Dogterom, J., and de Wied, D. (1975): Intraventricular administration of anti-vasopressin serum inhibits memory consolidation in rats. *Life Sci.,* 16:637-644.

Neuropeptide Influences on the Brain and Behavior, edited by L.H. Miller, C.A. Sandman, and A.J. Kastin. Raven Press, New York © 1977.

Hormones and Memory

Paul E. Gold and James L. McGaugh

Department of Psychobiology, University of California, Irvine, California 92717

The results of an extensive series of studies indicate that memory processes are susceptible to modifying treatments for some time after a training experience (22, 32). The basic finding in this research is that, in general, the effect of a treatment on memory decreases as the time after training is increased. Traditionally, the time-dependent nature of posttrial effects on memory were interpreted as reflecting temporal characteristics of the underlying memory processes. It is a change in our thinking about this issue which led us to examine the effects of hormones on memory processes. In the present chapter, we will begin by discussing the significance of time-dependent effects on memory. Second, we will describe some recent data which focus on hormonal influences on memory. Third, we will describe a series of studies which suggest the possibility that a central biogenic amine response to hormonal treatments may mediate the hormonal influences on memory.

TIME-DEPENDENT EFFECTS ON MEMORY PROCESSES

All posttrial treatments which modify later retention of learned responses, except perhaps those treatments which permanently alter brain functions, have one characteristic in common. These treatments have their most profound influences on retention if administered shortly after training. At longer delays after training, the same treatment has no influence on retention. For the most part, those investigators who have examined retrograde amnesia and enhancement of memory processes have interpreted the time-dependent nature of these findings as reflecting temporal characteristics of underlying memory processes. In general, the time after training during which a treatment alters retention has been assumed to reveal the time required for

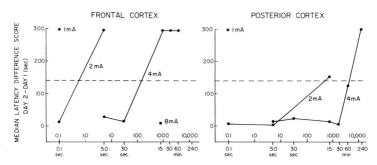

FIG. 1. Median latency difference score (day 2 minus day 1) for
crossing into shock compartment. All median latencies less than
140 sec (dotted line) are significantly lower than latencies for
animals receiving footshock only (median=300 sec) ($p<.05$, two-
tailed Mann-Whitney U-test).

the formation of a long-term memory process. This view
appears to be inaccurate on both logical and empirical
grounds. It has been recognized for some time that
retrograde amnesia gradients reveal only the time-
course of the disruptive influence of a treatment, rather than the time-course of memory trace formation (29,
38). Any specific statements based on the data of amnesia studies, regarding temporal properties of memory
fixation are highly inferential (13, 30).
    The findings of many studies now indicate that this
inference is incompatible with the data. For example,
in one study (11), we examined the effect of posttrial
electrical stimulation of the cortex on later retention
of an inhibitory (passive) avoidance task. In this experiment, the stimulation intensity, the stimulation
site (frontal or posterior cortex), and the training-
treatment interval were systematically varied. As
shown in Fig. 1, the findings indicate that the length
of a particular retrograde amnesia gradient varies with
the site of stimulation and, more important here, with
the intensity of the stimulation. For example, with 2
mA stimulation of frontal cortex, we observed an amnesia gradient of only 5 sec duration, while 4 mA stimulation produced a gradient of 15 min. A further increase in stimulation intensity (to 8 mA) produced amnesia even if delayed by 15 min. Thus, the threshold
intensity needed to produce amnesia increases with time
after training. The findings of many other studies are
also consistent with the view that the length of a retrograde amnesia gradient varies directly with the se-
verity of the amnestic treatment (1, 5, 11, 12, 20, 33).
The fact that many different amnesia gradients can be
obtained in animals trained in a single task indicates

that, although memory fixation may take some time, that
time is not directly reflected by a particular amnesia
gradient. A specific amnesia gradient, then, must reflect only the time-course of memory susceptibility to
impairment with a particular treatment.

HORMONAL MODULATION OF MEMORY PROCESSING

Although these findings indicate that a time-course
of memory fixation is not forthcoming from studies of
retrograde amnesia or enhancement of memory studies,
the findings do indicate that memory processes are de-
creasingly susceptible to modification with posttrial
treatments. The various theories of memory consolidation which have been proposed to account for the behavioral data assume that posttrial treatments act directly on the biological mechanisms underlying memory
formation (e.g., 2, 27, 28, 29). This general view remains a reasonable interpretation of the memory impair-
ing or enhancing effects of posttrial treatments. According to such a theoretical position, retrograde temporal gradients reflect a biological constraint on the
time required for memory formation. Thus, although the
specific time necessary for fixation may never be determined with retrograde amnesia studies, the possibility still exists that relatively long time periods are
required.

Recently, however, we suggested a different view of
the time-dependent nature of posttrial effects on memory (13, 15). If posttrial treatments are viewed as
modulators of memory storage processing, it becomes
possible to consider time-dependent effects on memory
to be a reflection of normal adaptive mechanisms which
promote or impair the storage of recent information.
The proposal that some treatments may modulate memory
storage predicts that there may be memory modulatory
systems which are activated by the treatments. Further,
an examination of the mechanisms underlying the effects
of various treatments on memory may reveal the nature
of biological factors which modulate retention in normal, untreated animals.

For these reasons, we began to think of possible responses to training which might function in this way.
Two classes of events readily emerged - arousal level
and hormonal responses. We focused on the hormonal responses primarily because we felt that it was difficult
to define or to manipulate "arousal level" in a manner
which would elicit general agreement.

Our initial studies were guided by the following ra-
tionale. If an animal is trained in a one-trial inhibitory (passive) avoidance task, retention performance
will vary directly with the footshock intensity. To

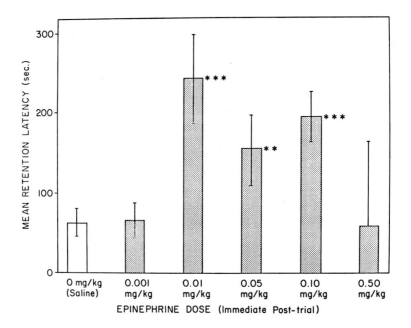

FIG. 2. Mean latencies to lick (and standard errors) for animals that received saline or epinephrine immediately after training. Within the dose range 0.01 to 0.1 mg/kg, retention performance was significantly facilitated. (***=$p<0.001$; **=$p<0.01$.)

what extent might the different retention performance be modulated by hormonal responses to training? The design we chose in these experiments was to train an animal with a weak footshock. Immediately after training, or at some delay up to several hr, we injected the animals with hormonal treatments which we felt might mimic the hormonal consequences of a stronger footshock. Remarkably enough, animals which receive an appropriate posttrial hormone injection have enhanced retention performance which is comparable to that observed after training with a stronger footshock.

In our first experiment of this nature, water-deprived rats were pretrained (one trial/day) to lick from a water spout at the end of a long alleyway. After latencies to lick reached a low baseline, each rat received a training trial. On this trial, a mild footshock (0.7 mA, 0.35 sec) was administered while the animal was drinking. Immediately after the footshock, animals were removed and were injected (subcutaneous) with saline or various doses of epinephrine. The latency to lick from the water spout on a test trial the next day was taken as the measure of retention.

The results are shown in Fig. 2. Note that those rats which received intermediate doses of epinephrine

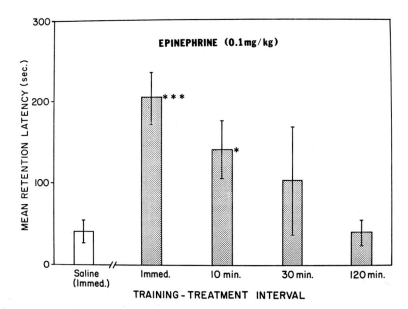

FIG. 3. Mean latencies to lick (and standard errors) for animals that received saline immediately after training or epinephrine (0.1 mg/Kg) at various delays after training. Note that the effectiveness of the drug in facilitating retention varied inversely with the training-treatment interval. (***=$p<0.001$; *=$p<0.05$.)

(0.01 to 0.1 mg/kg) had significantly enhanced retention performance. This effect on retention was time-dependent. In Fig. 3, note that injections delayed by 30 min or longer after training did not significantly affect later retention performance.

These findings are consistent with the view that hormonal responses to training may have a modulatory effect on memory processing, promoting storage of the information provided by an experience which would normally elicit the hormonal response. Of course, epinephrine is not the only hormone released following footshock. In fact, most, if not all, pituitary hormones are released by many stressors (26).

Therefore, under similar experimental conditions, we examined the effects of several posttrial hormone injections. Before detailing some of these findings, a summary is presented in Fig. 4. Note that posttrial injections of epinephrine and ACTH, and possibly also vasopressin, can either enhance or impair later retention (16). As will be described below, these differential effects are based on dose and footshock intensity interactions.

ENHANCEMENT	IMPAIRMENT	NO EFFECT
Epinephrine	Epinephrine	Growth Hormone
		Corticosterone
		Thyroid Hormone
		Thyroid Stimulating Hormone
Vasopressin (?)	Vasopressin	
ACTH	ACTH	
Norepinephrine		

FIG. 4.   Summary of effects of posttrial hormone injections on memory.

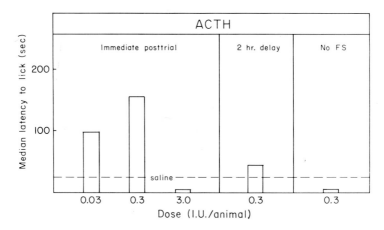

FIG. 5.   Retention performance of intact animals trained in a one-trial inhibitory (passive) avoidance task.   Rats were pretrained to lick from a water spout at the end of a shock compartment.   After 4 days of pretraining, the rats received a weak footshock while drinking.   Retention was measured as the latency to return to the water spout on the next day.   Note that the effects, on memory, of immediate posttrial injections of ACTH varied with the dose in an inverted-U manner.   Animals receiving the two lowest ACTH doses (0.03 or 0.3 IU/animal) had significantly enhanced retention performance; those animals which received 3.0 IU/animal had significantly impaired retention.   Delayed injections had no effect on later retention performance.

We will next detail some of the findings we have obtained with posttrial ACTH injections.   As shown in Fig. 5, injections of ACTH immediately after training in an inhibitory avoidance task can either enhance or impair later retention (17).   The effects of ACTH on later retention performance were dose-dependent.   An-

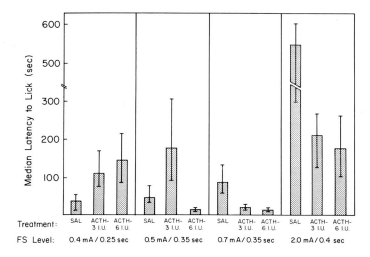

FIG. 6. Median retention latencies (and interquartile ranges) of
rats which were trained in an inhibitory (passive) avoidance task
and which received posttrial saline or ACTH (3 or 6 IU) injections.
Note that the 3 IU ACTH dose enhanced later retention of training
with the two lowest footshock levels, but disrupted retention of
training with the two highest footshock levels. The 6 IU ACTH injection significantly enhanced retention only of the lowest footshock level. This ACTH dose significantly impaired retention of
training with all other footshock levels.

imals which received injections of 0.03 or 0.3 ACTH
IU/animal had significantly enhanced retention performance. Those animals which received the highest ACTH
dose (3.0 IU/animal) displayed impaired retention,
i.e., these animals had retrograde amnesia. ACTH injections delayed by 2 hr after training had no effect
on later retention.

Therefore, posttrial ACTH effects on memory have an
inverted-U dose-response relationship with later retention. In another experiment, Gold and van Buskirk (17)
found that the inverted-U relationship between circulating ACTH levels and later retention could apparently
be generated by maintaining a constant dose of ACTH and
varying the footshock level. These findings are presented in Fig. 6. In this study, animals received posttrial injections of 3 or 6 ACTH IU/animal after inhibitory avoidance training with four different footshock
levels. Note that (a), both ACTH doses enhanced retention of training with the lowest footshock level; (b),
3 IU enhanced retention of training with a slightly
higher footshock level, but 6 IU impaired retention under this training condition; and (c), both doses impaired retention of training with either of the highest
footshock levels. Thus, the effect on retention of a

single dose of ACTH varies with the footshock level.
These findings support the view that there is an inverted-U relationship between posttrial circulatory
ACTH levels (endogenous ACTH + injected ACTH) and memory processing. It should be noted that the interaction between training-related stress and the effects on
memory of several posttrial treatments has been observed
in other studies as well. Epinephrine (18), pentylenetetrazol (25), and electrical stimulation of the midbrain reticular formation (4) or amygdala (8, 9) each
enhance retention of training under low stress conditions (e.g., appetitive training or low footshock) and
impair retention of training with strong footshock.
These findings thus suggest the intriguing possibility
that the biological dimension underlying the well-known
inverted-U relationship between stress and performance
(3, 21, 35) may be hormonally mediated, perhaps by ACTH
and epinephrine.
    If hormonal responses to training experiences are
important in promoting the storage of recent information, one might expect hypophysectomized rats to have
retention performance poorer than that of intact animals. Furthermore, retention deficits in these animals should be reduced in animals which receive posttrial hormonal injections. Recent evidence from our
laboratory is consistent with these predictions. For
example, in one study (10), intact and hypophysectomized rats were trained in an inhibitory avoidance task.
Each animal received one trial a day until it had a retention latency of 300 sec. Intact rats trained with a
very weak footshock required nearly three trials before
they avoided the shock compartment for 300 sec. As the
footshock intensity increased, most rats acquired the
learned response after a single footshock. However,
hypophysectomized rats had a different pattern of results. At all footshock intensities, hypophysectomized
rats required multiple trials (means = 2.6 to 2.8 trials) before successfully avoiding the shock compartment.
Thus, hypophysectomized rats did not show an improved
acquisition rate as the footshock level was increased.
Posttrial ACTH injections significantly enhanced retention in these animals. In Fig. 7, note that an ACTH
injection of 0.3 IU/animal resulted in one-trial acquisition of inhibitory avoidance training in hypophysectomized rats. Furthermore, the effects of ACTH were
time-dependent; delayed injections did not significantly enhance later retention performance.
    We have obtained comparable results with visual dis-
criminated-escape training (14). In this task, animals
receive six training trials (massed) in which they can
escape footshock by entering the illuminated area of a
Y-maze. On the test trials the next day, the number of

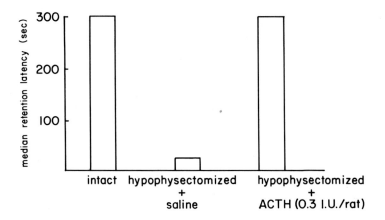

FIG. 7. Retention performance in a one-trial inhibitory avoidance
task. Rats received a footshock (0.4 ma, 0.4 sec) upon entering
the shock compartment. Retention was measured 24 hr later as the
latency to re-enter the shock compartment. Note that hypophysectomized rats showed a retention deficit compared to intact rats.
The hypophysectomized rats which received a single immediate posttrial injection of ACTH had retention latencies significantly higher than those of saline-injected hypophysectomized rats, and comparable to those of intact rats.

correct choices on the first six trials is taken as the
measure of retention. As shown in Fig. 8, intact animals perform quite well in this task, making nearly
five correct choices in the six test trials. Retention
performance of the hypophysectomized rats is significantly impaired (3.2 mean correct choices on six trials). If administered within 2 hr after training, a
single ACTH injection (0.03 to 3.0 IU/rat) significantly enhances later retention performance. ACTH injections administered 6 hr after training do not significantly enhance retention performance.
    Thus, our findings indicate that posttrial injec-
tions of any of several hormones, including ACTH, can
enhance or impair retention of intact animals. Furthermore, a single posttraining injection of ACTH can
apparently compensate for impaired retention observed
in hypophysectomized rats. These results are consistent with the view that hormonal responses to training,
which are normally posttraining events, may modulate
(i.e., promote or impair) the storage of information of
recent events. Of course, these hormonal influences
must be mediated by brain effects of the agents. In
the next section, we describe some evidence which suggests that the activity of central biogenic amine systems may be closely related to the behavioral findings
described thus far.

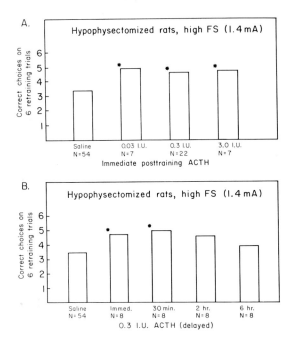

FIG. 8. Retention performance on a brightness discriminated avoidance Y-maze by saline-injected and ACTH-injected hypophysectomized rats. A. Hypophysectomized rats which received immediate posttraining injections of ACTH (at all doses tested) had retention performance significantly higher than that of the group which received saline injections. B. Hypophysectomized rats which received ACTH (0.3 IU/animal) had significantly enhanced retention performance if the injection was administered immediately or 30 min after training, but not if delayed by 2 hr or 6 hr after training. (*$p<0.05$ vs. saline injected controls.)

HORMONALLY-INITIATED CENTRAL BIOGENIC AMINE MODULATION OF MEMORY PROCESSES

We now have considerable evidence which indicates that hormonal responses to training have the potential, at least, of modulating memory storage processes. We next turned to the question of how peripheral hormone injections might act on the brain to enhance or impair retention of recent experiences. We chose central biogenic amine levels, and, in particular, norepinephrine levels as our neurobiological measure, for several reasons. First, we wanted to examine a neurobiological response which could be initiated by training conditions. For example, if we train an animal with a strong footshock, we should obtain evidence that the neural system shows a response. Our hope was that, if we enhance retention of training with weak footshock (using a hormonal injection), we should use a parallel change in the system. There is considerable evidence indicating that brain norepinephrine concentrations are sensitive to various stressors, including footshock (cf., 36). A second reason for choosing to examine brain norepinephrine responses was the evidence that several acute drug treatments which interfere with nor-adrenergic functioning at, or immediately after, the time of training may impair later retention (7, 20, 31, 34). Third, our choice of the central noradrenergic measure was influenced by the suggestions by Kety (23, 24) that this system may modulate memory processes, a possible function for brain norepinephrine which is conceptually quite similar to that which we attributed to hormonal responses to training.

In this series of experiments, then, we examined brain norepinephrine concentrations at various times after inhibitory avoidance training with no footshock, low footshock (0.7 mA, 0.4 sec), or high footshock (2.0 mA, 1.0 sec). The animals received immediate posttrial peripheral injections of any of several doses of epine-phrine or ACTH. Some animals were retained for behav-ioral testing the next day. Others were sacrificed 10 min, 30 min, 90 min, or 24 hr after the training-treat-ment manipulations. Because the major changes in nore-pinephrine concentrations were rapid and transient, on-ly the results obtained with a 10 min training-sacri-fice interval will be described in detail. First, in Fig. 9, note that high footshock training, without a posttrial treatment, resulted in a 20% decrease in brain norepinephrine concentrations, compared to either no footshock or low footshock conditions. Of course, the high footshock animals also had retention latencies significantly higher than those animals in either of the other footshock conditions. Of major interest here are the findings shown in Figs. 10 and 11. Note that, in each case, those doses of epinephrine or ACTH which enhance retention of weak footshock training also pro-duce a 20% decrease in brain norepinephrine levels. Lower doses of either drug do not significantly alter either the neurochemical or the behavioral measure. Higher doses produce a 40% decrease in norepinephrine concentrations and impair retention performance (i.e., produce amnesia).

The relationship between posttraining brain nore-pinephrine levels (with and without posttrial injec-tions) under several other conditions have been exam-ined. In each case, the general results fit the same pattern: the animals which have good retention perfor-mance are those which show approximately a 20% decrease in brain norepinephrine levels 10 min after training + treatment. The 20% decrease is observed in those ani-

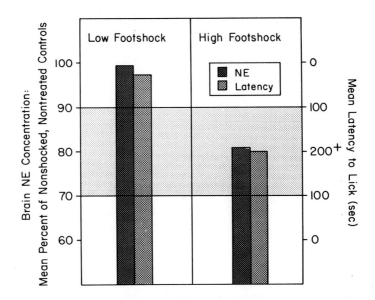

FIG. 9. Telencephalic norepinephrine concentrations as measured 10 min after training in a one-trial inhibitory avoidance task, and retention performance of animals trained in the same manner as measured 24 hr after training. The retention performance scale is bidirectional; this was required because, in later studies, low latencies (poor retention) could result from either poor training (with low footshock) or from amnesia (*cf.*, Figs. 10 and 11). Note that the high footshock resulted in good retention performance and resulted in a 20% decrease in norepinephrine concentration. The decrease in norepinephrine concentration was quite transient; if measured 90 min after training the levels did not differ from those of nonshocked control animals.

mals that receive either high footshock alone or that receive low footshock training followed by a memory enhancing treatment. Poor retention performance is seen in those animals which either do not have a change in norepinephrine concentration (e.g., low footshock + saline) or which have a 40% decrease in norepinephrine concentrations (e.g., high footshock + epinephrine or ACTH). Thus, it appears that posttraining brain norepinephrine levels are an excellent predictor of later retention performance for inhibitory avoidance training under many different conditions.

CONCLUSIONS

At the beginning of this chapter, we outlined several reasons for proposing that the time-dependent effects of posttrial treatments reflect modulatory influences on memory processes. This view suggested the

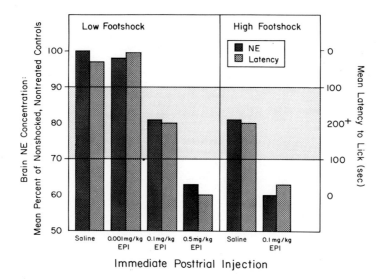

FIG. 10. Telencephalic norepinephrine concentration and retention performance of animals trained in an inhibitory avoidance task with low footshock followed by posttrial injections of saline or epinephrine (0.001, 0.1, or 0.5 mg/kg). The ordinates are the same as those in Fig. 9. Of particular significance, note that the dose-response curves for the neurochemical and behavioral effects of epinephrine are quite similar.

possibility that the relatively nonspecific consequences of training may modulate retention in normal, untreated animals as well. We believe our findings support the view that interacting classes of trophic responses to training may modulate later retention of the learned response. First, it is now clear that posttrial peripheral injections of some hormones, including epinephrine, norepinephrine, and ACTH can enhance retention of avoidance training with weak footshock in rats and mice. These findings are consistent with the view that the treatments act by mimicking a component of the normal hormonal responses to training with more intense footshock. It is important to note that hormonal responses to training are posttrial events in normal animals which follow the training experience with a relatively short latency. A second normal posttrial response to training is a transient decrease in brain norepinephrine. This decrease has been reported to follow many stressors (*cf*., 36). Our results suggest that the brain biogenic amine response to stress may be hormonally mediated; hormonal injections result in a decrease in brain norepinephrine concentrations comparable to that produced by footshock. Such findings are typically interpreted as reflecting the brain

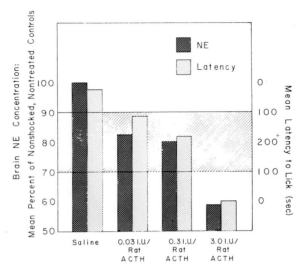

FIG. 11. Telencephalic norepinephrine concentrations and retention performance of animals trained in an inhibitory avoidance
task with low footshock followed by posttrial injections of saline
or ACTH (0.03, 0.3, or 3.0 IU/rat). The ordinates are the same as
those in Figs. 9 and 10. Note that the dose-response curves for
the neurochemical and behavioral effects of ACTH are very similar.

state following the release of norepinephrine prior to
its resynthesis via homeostatic mechanisms (cf., 6, 37).
Our recent findings suggest that the posttrial brain
norepinephrine concentration is a very good predictor
of later retention performance under a variety of conditions.

We interpret the hormonal and neurochemical findings
as suggesting that normal, relatively nonspecific physiological consequences of a training experience may be
important in modulating the storage and later retention
of the specific information provided by the experience.
The modulatory responses to training may help to explain the neurobiological bases underlying retrograde
amnesia and enhancement of memory storage with other
treatments as well. Furthermore, the time-dependent
nature of posttrial effects on memory may reflect the
natural synchrony between training experiences and the
modulatory events. It is important to note that hormonal and neurotransmitter responses to a training experience are normally posttrial events. It is possible
that as these systems developed a modulatory influence
on memory processes, the inherent time relationships
between the hormonal changes and the experience may

have been adapted to form a mechanism that functioned to select, from all experiences, those which should be committed to permanent memory storage.

ACKNOWLEDGMENTS

Supported by NIMH Research Grants MH 25384 and MH 12526, and by NSF Research Grant GB 52746

REFERENCES

1. Alpern, H. P. and McGaugh, J. L. (1968): Retrograde amnesia as a function of duration of electroshock stimulation. *J. Comp. Physiol. Psychol.*, 65:265-269.
2. Barondes, S. H. (1970): Multiple steps in the biology of memory. In: *The Neurosciences*, edited by F. O. Schmitt, pp. 272-278. Rockefeller University Press, New York.
3. Berlyne, D. I. (1966): Conflict and arousal. *Sci. Am.*, 215: 82-87.
4. Bloch, V. (1970): Facts and hypotheses concerning memory consolidation. *Brain Res.*, 24:561-575.
5. Cherkin, A. (1969): Kinetics of memory consolidation: Role of amnesic treatment parameters. *Proc. Natl. Acad. Sci. USA*, 63:1094-1101.
6. Costa, E. and Meek, J. L. (1974): Regulation of biosynthesis of catecholamines and serotonin in the CNS. *Annu. Rev. Pharmacol.*, 14:491-511.
7. Dismukes, R. K. and Rake, A. V. (1972): Involvement of biogenic amines in memory formation. *Psychopharmacologia*, 23:17-25.
8. Gold, P. E., Hankins, L. L., Edwards, R. M., Chester, J., and McGaugh, J. L. (1975): Memory interference and facilitation with posttrial amygdala stimulation: Effect on memory varies with footshock level. *Brain Res.*, 86:509-513.
9. Gold, P. E., Hankins, L. L., and Rose, R. P. (1976): Enhancement of memory processes with posttrial unilateral amygdala stimulation: Neuroanatomical localization. (In preparation.)
10. Gold, P. E., Hankins, L. L., and Rose, R. P. (1977): Impaired retention for inhibitory avoidance training in hypophysectomized rats. (In preparation.)
11. Gold, P. E., Macri, J., and McGaugh, J. L. (1973): Retrograde amnesia gradients: Effects of direct cortical stimulation. *Science*, 179:1343-1345.
12. Gold, P. E., McDonald, R., and McGaugh, J. L. (1974): Direct cortical stimulation: A further study of treatment intensity effects on retrograde amnesia gradients. *Behav. Biol.*, 10: 485-490.
13. Gold, P. E. and McGaugh, J. L. (1975): A single-trace, two-process view of memory storage processes. In: *Short-Term Memory*, edited by D. Deutsch and J. A. Deutch, pp. 355-378. Academic Press, New York.

14. Gold, P. E., Rose, R. P., Spanis, C. W., and Hankins, L. L. (1977): Retention deficit for avoidance training in hypophysectomized rats: Time-dependent enhancement with posttraining ACTH injections. *Horm. Behav., (In press.)*
15. Gold, P. E. and van Buskirk, R. B. (1975): Time-dependent memory processes with posttrial epinephrine injections. *Behav. Biol.,* 13:145-153.
16. Gold, P. E. and van Buskirk, R. B. (1976): Effects of posttrial hormone injections on memory processes. *Horm. Behav.,* 7:509-517.
17. Gold, P. E. and van Buskirk, R. B. (1976): Enhancement and impairment of memory processes with posttrial injections of adrenocorticotrophic hormone. *Behav. Biol.,* 16:387-400.
18. Gold, P. E. and van Buskirk, R. B. (1977): Posttraining brain norepinephrine concentrations: Correlation with retention performance of avoidance training and with peripheral epinephrine. (Submitted for publication.)
19. Haycock, J. W. and McGaugh, J. L. (1973): Retrograde amnesia gradients as a function of ECS-intensity. *Behav. Biol.,* 9, 123-127.
20. Haycock, J. W., van Buskirk, R., and McGaugh, J. L. (1977): Effects of catecholaminergic drugs upon memory storage processes in mice. *Behav. Biol. (In press.)*
21. Hebb, D. O. (1966): *A Textbook of Psychology.* W. B. Saunders, Philadelphia.
22. Jarvik, M. E. (1972): Effects of chemical and physical treatments on learning and memory. *Am. Rev. Psychol.,* 23:453-486.
23. Kety, S. S. (1970): The biogenic amines in the central nervous system: Their possible roles in arousal, emotion, and learning. In: *The Neurosciences,* edited by F. O. Schmitt, pp. 324-336. Rockefeller University Press, New York.
24. Kety, S. S. (1972): Brain catecholamines, affective states and memory. In: *The Chemistry of Mood, Motivation and Memory,* edited by J. L. McGaugh, pp. 65-80. Plenum Press, New York.
25. Krivanek, J. (1971): Facilitation of avoidance learning by pentylenetetrazol as a function of task difficulty, deprivation and shock level. *Psychopharmacologia,* 20:213-229.
26. Mangili, G., Motta, M., and Martini, L. (1966): Control of adrenocorticotrophic hormone. In: *Neuroendocrinology,* Vol. 1, edited by L. Martini and W. Ganong. Academic Press, New York.
27. McGaugh, J. L. (1966): Time-dependent processes in memory storage. *Science,* 153:1351-1358.
28. McGaugh, J. L. (1969): Effects of analeptics on learning and memory in infrahumans. In: *Drugs and the Brain,* edited by P. Black, pp. 241-250. The Johns Hopkins Press, Baltimore.
29. McGaugh, J. L. and Dawson, R. G. (1972): Modification of memory storage processes. In: *Animal Memory,* edited by W. K. Honing and P. H. R. James, pp. 215-242. Academic Press, New York.
30. McGaugh, J. L. and Gold, P. E. (1974): Conceptual and neurobiological issues in studies of treatment affective memory

storage.   In: *The Psychology of Learning and Motivation*, Vol. 8, edited by G. H. Bower, pp. 233-262.   Academic Press, New York.

31. McGaugh, J. L., Gold, P. E., van Buskirk, R. B., and Haycock, J. W.   (1975):   Modulating influences of hormones and catecholamines on memory storage processes.   In: *Hormones, Homeostasis and the Brain* (Progress in Brain Research, Vol. 42), edited by W. H. Gispen, Tj. B. van Wimersma Greidanus, B. Bohus and D. de Wied, pp. 151-162.   Elsevier, Amsterdam.

32. McGaugh, J. L. and Herz, M. J.   (1972):   *Memory Consolidation.* Albion Publishing Company, San Francisco.

33. Miller, A. J.   (1968):   Variations in retrograde amnesia parameters of electroconvulsive shock and time of testing.   *J. Comp. Physiol. Psychol.*, 66:40-47.

34. Randt, C. T., Quartermain, D., Goldstein, M., and Anagnoste, B.   (1971):   Norepinephrine biosynthesis inhibition: Effects on memory in mice.   *Science,* 172:498-499.

35. Selye, H.   (1950):   *The Physiology and Pathology of Exposure to Stress.*   Acta, Inc., Montreal, Canada.

36. Stone, E. A.   (1975):   Stress and catecholamines.   In: *Catecholamines and Behavior*, Vol. 2, edited by A. G. Friedhoff, pp. 31-72.   Plenum Press, New York.

37. Weiner, N.   (1970):   Regulation of norepinephrine biosynthesis. *Annu. Rev. Pharmacol.*, 10:273-312.

38. Weiskrantz, L.   (1966):   Experimental studies of amnesia.   In: *Amnesia,* edited by C. W. M. Whitty and O. L. Zangwill, pp. 1-35.   Butterworths, London.

Neuropeptide Influences on the Brain and Behavior, edited by L.H. Miller, C.A. Sandman, and A.J. Kastin. Raven Press, New York © 1977.

Some Properties of Substrates of Memory

Donald R. Meyer and Michael S. Beattie

Department of Psychology, The Ohio State University, Columbus, Ohio 43210

Memory was among the very first of the functions which are commonly regarded as mental to have been proposed to be interpretable in terms of operation of the nervous system. It was so regarded by Descartes (9), who found the supposition essential to his concept that mental processes are always conscious. Descartes believed that knowledge of things are momentary, but they leave their traces behind them as changes in the walls of the cavities within the brain's cerebral hemispheres. Today, we can comfortably conclude that his model of memory formation was wrong, but we also can forgive him for his errors in view of the fact that his work is over three centuries old.

We can also forgive him for his errors on the grounds that our own understandings of the substrates of memory are not especially clear. We do have our theories of the properties of traces, and we also have some very powerful procedures for studying learning and for altering or observing events within the central nervous system. However, we have found that it is easier to form a habit than it is to catch an engram, and thus far, engrams have managed to elude us for approximately 100 years.

The most important reason why we are still unable to identify the substrates of memory is that we have yet to discover a procedure that, beyond any doubt, will selectively destroy those substrates. This isn't because we haven't tried. Thus, at the beginning of the present century, Pavlov (33) was already studying the effects of enormous cerebral ablations, and was finding that the habits he established with his methods would thereafter be lost, but had a way of coming back once again. By 1950, that had been the observation of many experimental surgeons; and Lashley (25), after decades of studies of the problem, had ruefully concluded that he just couldn't see how learning was possible at all.

At that time, many young neuroscientists concluded
that there had to be some other, better way of accom-
plishing the feat. Experiments were then performed in
which large or small electrical currents were passed
through the brain; in which the animals were trained
and then subjected to radical reductions of their core
temperatures; in which the functions of the cortex were
suppressed through induction of spreading depression;
in which the animals were given a variety of just bare-
ly sublethal doses of poisons; and in which various
kinds of antibiotics were employed in the hope that
they would block the synthesis of putative memory molecules.

Possibly, by one procedure or another, the carriers
of memory will eventually be shown to be polypeptide or
protein molecules. If such a supposition should prove
to be correct, then at least we already know that the
molecules are tough customers. We know this because
the memories for which they would serve as the substrates are tough, and are simply not as pictured by
Salvador Dali in his painting, *The Persistence of Memory*.
They have thus far resisted the effects of an almost
incredible array of interventions, and although some
workers have from time to time concluded that they
haven't always done so, the proofs of those yieldings
are extremely tenuous at best.

Although our many efforts to rob the memory bank
have not been particularly successful, we have learned
many other things about the nervous system in the process. We believe that for students of the functions of
peptides in memory and related processes, the most important message to have come from these studies is that
memory is stable but that access to memory is not (28).
We now know of many ways of interfering with an animal's remembrances of habits, and the outcomes can be
so profound and so persistent as to lead us to believe
that the subject has lost its memory. That fact has
led many theorists of memory to come to erroneous conclusions, and the trap that it presents has caught some
great thinkers, including Karl Lashley himself.

As a first illustration of the nature of the trap,
we will next describe experiments concerning the determinants of one of Lashley's classical results. Lashley
(24) found that rats prepared with extirpations of the
posterior portion of the dorsal pallial cortex will
show no postoperative retention of a habit of choosing
the lighter of a pair of exits from an apparatus. However, they will nonetheless relearn the habit, and
their rate of relearning will be about the same as the
rate at which the habit is learned by rats that haven't
been given preoperative training. This is a result
that is easy to confirm, and it has been replicated in

our laboratory in studies of very large groups of animals (12, 15, 19).

The finding has for many years been thought to imply that the loss was a memorial impairment, that is, that the operations served to destroy the engrams which the rats that were given preoperative training had previously formed. However, such impairments are not memorial deficits but rather are impairments which at least in large part are due to failures of the operated rats to remember. The first proof of this was given by Braun et al. (4) who observed that if rats are first trained on the habit, then subjected to posterior neocortical ablations, and then tested for retention of the habit while being treated with *dl-*amphetamine, they will relearn the habit at a relatively rapid rate (Fig. 1). Moreover, a dosage that produces this effect (1 mg/kg) has no effect upon the rate at which the habit is learned by preoperatively-naive rats (Fig. 2). Hence the result was a facilitation of retrieval or remembering of the habit, and it showed that a component of the traces which were formed by the preoperatively-trained rats had evidently survived the operation.

Another proof that memories of this kind can seem to be completely gone when they have only been forgotten has been recently supplied by a study of LeVere and Morlock (26). In their investigation, one group of rats was trained on black-white discrimination problems and were then tested for retention of the habits following posterior decortications. Other groups were similarly trained and were given the same kinds of surgical treatments, but were subsequently tested for reversals of the habits that had been established prior

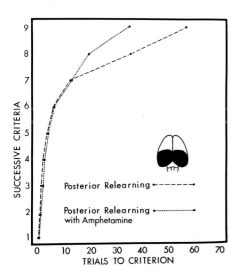

FIG. 1. Mean relearning trials to each of 9 successive criteria required by rats with posterior cortical ablations which received injections of either saline or of 1 mg/kg *dl*-amphetamine. Both groups had been trained to a 9/10 criterion on the black-white habit prior to surgery.

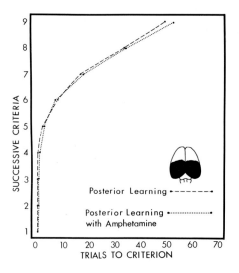

FIG. 2. Mean learning trials to each of 9 successive criteria required by rats with posterior cortical ablations which received injections of either saline or 1 mg/kg *dl*-amphetamine. Neither group received preoperative training on the black-white habit.

to surgery. As was expected, the subjects which were given the conventional relearning tests failed to show retention of the habits. However, the rats which were postoperatively trained on reversals of the habits were very slow to learn the reversals (Fig. 3). Therefore the study showed that rats which will not ordinarily exhibit any signs of retention of a habit that was learned prior to surgery nonetheless have engrams which will interfere with postoperative learning of a contradictory discrimination.

Another demonstration of the fact that a trace can be present when it doesn't seem to be is detailed in the recently completed study of Beattie et al. (3). The study was concerned with the performance of rats which had undergone extensive simultaneous bilateral destructions of the dorsal pallial cortex. We knew from a previous investigation of Meyer et al. (29) that such preparations are essentially incapable of learning the Miller-Mowrer two-way shuttle-avoidance task. However, Meyer et al. also observed that isodecorticated subjects will learn the problem quickly if, in addition, they are also prepared with electrolytic lesions of the forebrain septum. Since septal ablations had been shown to facilitate shuttle-box performances in otherwise-intact animals (22, 29), and inasmuch as treatments with amphetamines had had similar effects in normal subjects (2, 35) it seemed appropriate to ask if the drug would also facilitate shuttle-box learning by rats with dorsal pallial ablations.

The results from the initial phase of the study seemed to indicate that such effects are modest at best. Thus, both decorticated rats which were treated with

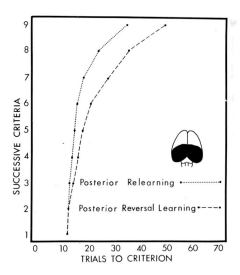

FIG. 3. Mean trials to each of 9 successive criteria required by rats with posterior cortical ablations which either relearned a preoperatively established black-white habit, or learned a reversal of the original habit.

amphetamine and others which were given injections of saline performed very poorly during ten days of shuttle-box training at 30 trials per day (Fig. 4). The treated rats exhibited significantly higher levels of performance than the control rats, but their levels of correct avoidances were not maintained. Thus the treated subjects, after having attained moderate performance levels during the first three to four days, thereafter began to stop avoiding and would rarely do so by the tenth day of training. Also, when these animals were subsequently trained to avoid while they were being given saline, less than half the rats showed more than one avoidance response during ten further days of testing. And finally, when once again treated with amphetamine, these subjects performed somewhat better but, once again, their levels of performance were not what one could term spectacular.

However, a very different picture emerged when the rats which were first trained while being given saline were trained for an additional 300 trials after daily pretraining injections of *d*-amphetamine. These animals, which showed very few signs of learning during their initial 300 trials of training, began to perform very quickly when treated with the drug. They reached very high final levels of performance, but those levels were amphetamine-dependent; thus, when they were once again injected with saline, they once again became very poor performers during 10 final sessions of training on the task.

The effects of the treatments were thus the most pronounced when given to decorticated subjects that had previously shown very few signs of learning during

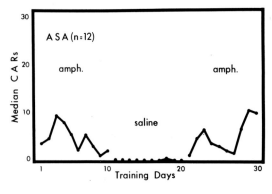

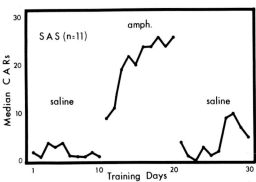

FIG 4. Median number of conditioned avoidance responses (CARs) achieved by decorticated rats in groups ASA and SAS over the 30 days of shuttle-box training. Injections of either saline or *d*-amphetamine sulfate (1 mg/kg) were given i.p. 30 min prior to each daily session.

their initial 300 training trials with saline. Hence the observations implied that the training taught them something, for they then learned the habit at a rate that was astounding when compared with the desultory progresses of rats which had sustained exactly the same operations, but whose treatments with amphetamine began when they were first exposed to the training situation. We interpret this outcome as another striking instance of facilitation of retrieval, and as further support for a suspicion that amphetamines have much more powerful effects upon remembering than they have upon processes of learning (5, 13, 35).

We think it is of interest that the subjects which were trained under saline conditions first and then were given treatments, responded to the treatments by exhibiting avoidances at somewhat faster rates than the rates which are observed when normal rats are first given shuttle-box training (Fig. 5). While this is an imperfect comparison because the normal rats did not receive the drug, we think that it is nonetheless a fair comparison because the normal subjects had the benefits of cerebral cortices. At any rate, the study showed that very small doses of amphetamine, if given

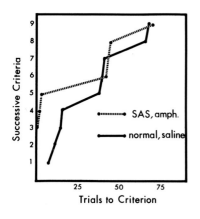

FIG. 5. Median trials to each
of 9 successive criteria required by normal rats during
initial training, and by decorticated rats in group SAS
when trained under amphetamine
conditions after 10 days of
initial training with saline.

to bilateral dorsal pallial preparations, will elicit
performances that otherwise are not seen in isodecorticated rats.

What we don't understand about the findings as yet
is why it is that training under saline conditions following training during treatments with amphetamine does
not permit retrievals of shuttle-box learning when amphetamine is given thereafter. However, the decline of
performance that is seen when dorsal pallial subjects
are transferred from second-stage amphetamine conditions to saline conditions are state-dependency phenomena. In Figs. 6 and 7, we present the results that we
obtained from two rats with isocortical ablations which
were first given training under saline conditions, were
thereafter given training while being treated with amphetamine, and then, after having reached very high
levels of shuttle-box performance, were given saline
and then amphetamine or saline on alternating days.

Alternations of the treatments resulted, at first,
in dramatic alternations of the animal's levels of performance. Thereafter, when the subjects were given
further training while the doses of amphetamine were
gradually reduced, they eventually were able to sustain,
when given saline, reasonable levels of avoidance.
These levels were not the levels of performance that
are maintained by well-trained normal animals, but they
were very good indeed for animals deprived of the largest single basic subcomponent of the telencephalon.
Notably, a similar paradigm was used by Barrett et al.
(2) in an experiment with rats of a strain whose members are normally poor avoidance learners, and their
findings for those subjects were essentially the same
as our findings for decorticated subjects.

We believe that these studies are clearly supportive
of the notion that engrams, once they are established,
are exceptionally hard to get rid of. We believe, in

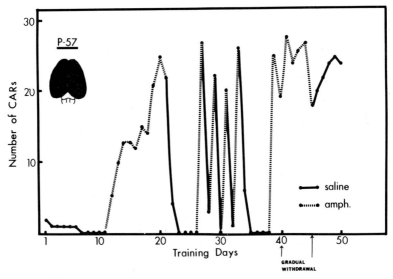

FIG. 6. Number of conditioned avoidance responses (CARs) exhibited by an extensively decorticated rat that was given initial training with saline injections, then trained under d-amphetamine, then trained under a schedule of alternating saline and amphetamine injections. Gradual withdrawal via daily reductions in amphetamine from 1 mg/kg to the saline vehicle alone resulted in maintained performance during the final saline test days.

addition, that they show that engrams can form and then be latent in subjects that exhibit almost no progress in the mastery of the task in question. However, it is nonetheless possible to think that the traces with which we were concerned in these studies were not necessarily exemplary of engrams in general. They were stable, but there also were traces that were formed over several days and many trials of training, and hence many students of memory would regard them as having no bearing on a second and more fundamental issue. That issue has to do with whether new memories have comparatively labile traces, and whether such traces are preliminary to the establishment of durable engrams.

It is widely believed, and the width of the belief is manifest in many different ways, that short-term memories are in that respect completely different from long-term memories. Hebb (14) first proposed the most attractive concept that they are, and his two-stage theory is frequently presented in conjunction with the view that the hippocampus is involved in the transcription of the substrates of memories from one form to the other form. While these two ideas can be dissociated, they have not been by many students of memory who employ interventional procedures. Thus it has become the

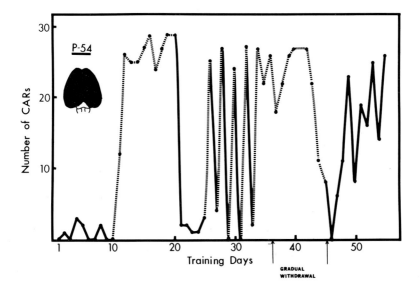

FIG. 7. A second example of the effects of alternation of saline and amphetamine conditions, and of subsequent withdrawal of amphetamine, upon maintenance of CARs by a rat prepared with a bilateral dorsal pallial ablation. Solid lines represent saline conditions, dashed lines represent amphetamine conditions. (The *d*-amphetamine employed in these investigations was graciously supplied to us by Smith, Kline, & French.)

contemporary custom for treatments to be given rapidly, and for methods to be used which will ensure that the agents will have effects upon the hippocampus.

First we shall consider the concept that hippocampal processes are crucially involved in the establishment of long-term memories. One of its bases are the findings of Scoville and Milner (40) and of Milner (30, 31) with respect to the deficits produced in man by basal bitemporal ablations. However, these findings, although they are unquestionably real, impressive, and important, are largely inconsistent with predictions from the findings as to what we might observe in animals subjected to bilateral hippocampal extirpations. Thus it has been found that monkeys subjected to Scoville's procedure, and by Scoville himself, are capable of long-term memory (6, 7, 8). The same thing is true of rats with hippocampal lesions (18), and also rats subjected to bilateral hippocampal spreading depression (39). This is not to say that there are no costs whatever of damage to the hippocampus, but the bulk of the evidence at hand is not in keeping with the thesis that long-term memory formation depends upon hippocampal functions.

We need nonetheless to comment upon a finding of
Kesner and Conner (21), who studied the effects of hippocampal stimulation upon the short-term and long-term
retention by rats of passive avoidance habits which
were formed five sec before the interventions were performed. Kesner and Conner observed that the habits
were well-retained when tests were conducted 55 sec later, but were not well-retained when the tests were
conducted one day later. That result was taken by Kesner (20) to mean that hippocampal stimulation interferes with long-term storage. However, the findings of
Kesner and Conner were not a proof of that contention
because, as we have noted, an engram can form and yet
go undetected unless special methods are used to demonstrate its existence.

Next, we shall discuss the concept that short-term
memories have labile substrates. To look at that idea,
we have no need to know what the routes are into the
memory banks of the brain provided that we have a means
of intervention that ought to play havoc with extra-
hippocampal as well as with hippocampal functions.
Grand mal seizures would seem to qualify, at least as a
first approximation. Moreover, such seizures have effects upon retentions of habits that may or may not be
memorial, and hence inductions of them have been widely employed as a technique for examining the two-stage
theory.

We have known since the classical experiment of
Duncan (11) that ECS treatments, if given very shortly
after a habit has been learned, have greater effects
upon retention of the habit than the same treatments
given later on. Results such as those which Duncan
first obtained are facts about ECS treatments, and they
also are consistent with the theory of Hebb that short-
term memories are labile. However, it has always been
possible to think that the time-dependent actions of
ECS treatments were due to their effects upon retrieval, or to keep an open mind on the question and suppose
that ECS treatments have effects upon memories as well
as upon retrievals of them.

The phenomenon of time dependence posed the question
as to whether the relation was obligatory, as it clearly had to be if the results of quick treatments were to
be interpreted as evidently due to effects upon consol-
idating traces. However, many studies have shown very
clearly that it isn't. The particular details of some
of these studies have been recently reviewed by Lewis
(27), whose own work has also made a fundamental contribution to our knowledge of memory. To illustrate,
he showed with Misanin and Miller (32) that a habit
which is learned in one training trial is subject to
suppression by an ECS treatment that is given 24 hours

after training if the rats are then given a "reminding" stimulus. Although explanations which seem to us contorted have been advanced to reconcile that finding with the two-stage theory, it nonetheless is highly suggestive that the age of a habit has relatively little to do with whether it can be suppressed with ECS treatments or not.

Here we will remark that the proof that old habits are sometimes suppressible by ECS treatments has come as no surprise to clinicians. ECS treatments have been used for many years in the treatment of mental disorders, and the treatments have commonly resulted in impairments of memorially-related functions. The impairments are typically severest with respect to recently-acquired information, although it must be stressed that clinicians will describe amnesias as impairments of recent memories if the habits in question had been learned, say, within a week or so. Also, the impairments, while they usually can be predicted from the ages of the habits, are sometimes spotty in the sense that recent happenings will be better-remembered than old ones (23, 42, 43).

Losses of the latter kinds are interesting because the time-dependent nature of clinical amnesias has also been construed as supportive of the view that memories are constantly changing. Again, we will stress that the time-frames to which this notion is applied are very much longer than the time-frames that have been examined in experiments related to the two-stage theory. However, experiments by Robbins and Meyer (38) Howard and Meyer (17), Thompson and Grossman (41), and Howard et al. (16) have examined this concept, and the findings contradict the notion that the ages of well-established habits are determinants of whether such habits are suppressible by ECS treatments.

In the Robbins-Meyer paradigms, groups of rats were trained in a Krechevsky maze (K-maze) on a series of two-choice visual discrimination habits. Each subject learned three habits, and the habits were established through the use of two different incentives. Thus a given rat might learn its first habit to avoid mild shocks to its feet, its second habit to obtain food placed within a goalbox, and its third habit to avoid mild shocks to its feet. Six groups of rats were employed, and each of the members of a given group was trained on its series of three successive habits through the use of a particular serial order of shock-avoidance or food-approach conditions. Thus, for some subjects, the first two habits were learned for food reward and the third was learned for shock-avoidance. For others, the first two habits were learned for shock avoidance and the third for food rewards. Other groups

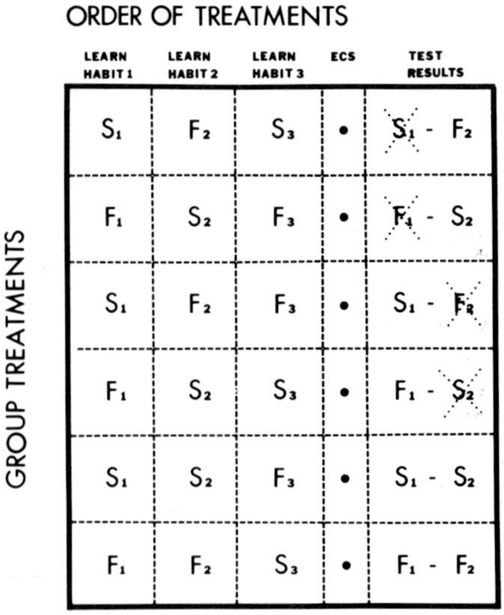

ORDER OF TREATMENTS

	LEARN HABIT 1	LEARN HABIT 2	LEARN HABIT 3	ECS	TEST RESULTS
GROUP TREATMENTS	S_1	F_2	S_3	•	S_1 - F_2
	F_1	S_2	F_3	•	F_1 - S_2
	S_1	F_2	F_3	•	S_1 - F_3
	F_1	S_2	S_3	•	F_1 - S_2
	S_1	S_2	F_3	•	S_1 - S_2
	F_1	F_2	S_3	•	F_1 - F_2

FIG. 8. The Robbins-Meyer paradigm. F refers to food-approach habits and S to shock-avoidance habits. Numerical subscripts indicate the order in which habits were learned. The habits which were found to be susceptible to ECS-induced suppressions of retention are crossed out in the "test results" column.

were trained with alternations of the two kinds of incentives, or else with one incentive for the first habit and the other for the second and third habits.

Typically, it took the rats about two weeks to learn their three successive habits. Then, as each subject reached criterion on its third discrimination, it was given a single ECS treatment. Thereafter, it was tested for retention of either the first or the second of the habits that it previously had learned. Robbins then observed that if the habit that was learned just prior to treatment was a footshock habit, the subject exhibited a loss of retention for an older habit if, and only if, that habit had also been established through the use of footshock. Conversely, if the third and last habit in the series has been learned under food-approach conditions, then the subject exhibited a loss of retention if, and only if, that habit had also been established through the use of food rewards. Thus older habits, regardless of whether they were first or second in the series, were well retained if they had been established with incentives which were different from the ones that were employed for establishing the final habits (Fig. 8).

Notably, the habits which were poorly retained were so poorly retained that one could readily believe that the treatments had completely obliterated memories for those habits. However, as Thompson and Grossman (41) demonstrated, the observed effects were not memorial. Thus they confirmed the fact that rats, if given training on a shock-related habit, then a food-related habit, and finally, another shock-related habit, the ani-

mals will show no retention of the first of these habits if given an ECS treatment. In addition, they observed that if, before the rats were tested for retention on the following day, they were given another ECS
treatment, the subjects exhibited excellent retention
of the first shock-related habit. Hence the observations served to show once again that failures of performance of a habit are much more likely to be due to
failures of retrieval than to losses of memory.

In summation, we believe that the aggregate of findings we have thus far presented are relevant to many
contemporary concepts of the nature of memorial encoding. We shall next briefly summarize, in terms of
three statements, what we think can be concluded from
studies of memory that involve interventional procedures. First, interventions which will readily produce
impairments of retentions of habits are grossly unlikely to have had their effects because they affected memories. Second, it is possible for memories to form
during times when a subject is showing no signs of progress in the learning of a task, and the memories thus
formed will then be usable if methods are employed
which will serve to facilitate retrieval of the memories. Third, if we exclude very-short-term memories,
that is, iconic memories, it is highly unlikely that
memories and their substrates undergo significant
changes as a function of time.

Next we shall consider a few implications of the
first of these general conclusions. One is that we
need to be extremely wary of characterizations of losses of retentions of habits as memorial deficits. To
illustrate, workers who have studied the effects of
antibiotics as interventive agents initially supposed
that these agents, when effective, had had their effects by blocking the syntheses of engrams. However,
as is clear from the admirable review of the status of
molecular memorial research that Barraco and Stettner
(1) have presented, the effects of antibiotics upon retentions of habits are usually reversible by pharmacological or behavioral procedures. This is as expected from our first conclusion, which suggests that memorial impairments are the last, and not the first
things that one should think of.

The first conclusion is also consistent with findings that have been obtained by Rigter and his colleagues (36, 37). These investigators have shown that
ACTH, ACTH 4-10, MSH, and an orally-active ACTH 4-9
analog (Organon 2766) will readily reverse CO_2-induced
amnesia. These effects are produced if the compounds
are given prior to the test for retrieval, but not if
the compounds are given prior to the time that the animals are trained. Moreover, at least some of the pep-

tides will serve to reverse, when given in this manner, amnesias for habits which are brought about by ECS treatments. Not very long ago, ECS-induced and CO_2-induced amnesias were, as the phrase went, generally accepted to be due to interferences with short-term labile memory traces. They obviously are not, for agents that facilitate retrievals must have something to retrieve, and hence these experiments are most impressive proofs that durable memories are formed very quickly.

To us, these results are highly reminiscent of our findings that treatments with amphetamine facilitate retrievals of habits by rats prepared with cerebral ablations. Hence, in some respects at least, as Dornbush et al. (10) have suggested, the actions of amphetamines and some of the peptides appear to be similar, although we are amazed by the differences between their potencies. Here we will note that our interest in amphetamine stemmed from our interest in the problem of recovery from stroke, and particularly in whether the so-called memorial impairments which are seen in victims of stroke are, in fact, memorial in nature. Our work has been primarily intended to show that it is reasonable to hope that such impairments will yield to pharmacological treatments, which of course would be impossible in principle if strokes of the kinds that men survive are destructive of the engrams of habits. Our findings have suggested that this is unlikely if the strokes are cerebral cortical strokes although, as we have noted, the impairments of performance can be so grave as to prompt a very different conclusion. Accordingly, our thinking has been very similar to the thinking of Rigter and his colleagues, and we salute their proposal that Organon 2766 should be tried as a therapeutic agent for patients with so-called memorial disorders.

We also have an interest in hyperkinesis and its treatment with amphetamine. Our second conclusion could well have a bearing on the problems that children with this so-called syndrome exhibit. They are typically described as being over-active and as having learning disabilities, but we think it is likely that the latter problems have been incorrectly characterized. Although it would be difficult to make a case for the presumption that amphetamine has no effects whatever upon learning, it does seem that students of the question have observed that it is not exactly easy to show that amphetamines have widespread and positive effects upon initial learning of habits. Hence we entertain an unproved suspicion that treatments with amphetamine, when given to children with hyperkinetic difficulties, have positive effects to the extent that they permit the children to retrieve the information

that they learned before the treatments were commenced
(28). We also suspect that at doses which produce po-
tentially desirable results, the drug is of either no
help at all or is a hindrance to subsequent learning.
The dilemma this produces, if our thoughts are correct,
suggests that other treatments should be sought and,
in our opinion, a good place to look for them would be
in the properties of peptides.

We suspect that our third conclusion will be viewed
as the most disturbing of the lot, and also as by far
the least likely to be worth consideration. However,
the argument that interventions which have time-dependent actions upon newly-formed habits produce their effects because they interfere with labile traces has
been tested, and found wanting. The argument that interventions which produce complete and lasting impairment of retention must therefore have interfered with
memory formation is not now, nor has it been for almost
a decade, worthy of serious belief. The argument that
time-dependent clinical amnesias imply that long-term
memories are in flux has been examined, and disproved.
Hence there is nothing to compel us to believe that
stable memories are not formed with great rapidity, or
to think that their substrates, whatever they may be,
are continuously changing as they age.

We contrast our conclusions with many of the notions
which we find in molar theories of memory, which include such terms as transfer, transformation, stages,
re-encoding, and the like. Although many workers will
think, at first glance, that our viewpoint is altogether novel, it is not, for it is virtually identical to
Penfield's (34) theory of memorial encoding. Penfield
derived his concept of memory from his finding that
stimulation of the temporal lobes of human beings will
sometimes elicit incredibly complex and veridical past
experiences. That fact prompted him to argue that the
substrates of memory, once they have been formed, undergo very few if any alterations as a function of the
passage of time. Although our own data base is different from his, we have come to the very same conclusion,
and we cheerfully acknowledge the fact that our pro-
posals are revivals instead of new departures.

ACKNOWLEDGMENTS

A number of the studies described in this report
were supported by United States Public Health Service
Grants MH-02035 and MH-06211.

Michael S. Beattie, United States Public Health Ser-
vice Predoctoral Fellow, was supported by Training
Grant MH-06748 to The Ohio State University, Columbus,
Ohio.

REFERENCES

1. Barraco, R. A. and Stettner, L. J. Antibiotics and memory. (1976): *Psychol. Bull.*, 83:242-302.
2. Barrett, R. J., Leith, N. J. and Ray, O. S. (1972): Permanent facilitation of avoidance behavior by *d*-amphetamine and scopolamine. *Psychopharmacologia* (Berlin), 25:321-333.
3. Beattie, M. S., Gray, T. S., Rosenfield, J. R., Meyer, P. M. and Meyer, D. R. (1976): *d*-amphetamine facilitation of conditioned avoidance response performance in rats with isocortical ablations. *(In preparation.)*
4. Braun, J. J., Meyer, P. M. and Meyer, D. R. (1966): Sparing of a brightness habit in rats following visual decortication. *J. Comp. Physiol. Psychol.*, 61:79-82.
5. Cicala, G. A., Ulm, R. R. and Drews, D. R. (1971): The effects of chlorpromazine and d-amphetamine on the acquisition and performance of a conditioned escape response in rats. *Psychol. Rec.*, 21:165-169.
6. Correll, R. E. and Scoville, W. B. (1965): Effects of medial temporal lesions on visual discrimination performance. *J. Comp. Physiol. Psychol.*, 60:175-181.
7. Correll, R. E. and Scoville, W. B. (1965): Performance on a delayed match following lesions of medial temporal lobe structures. *J. Comp. Physiol. Psychol.*, 60:360-367.
8. Correll, R. E. and Scoville, W. B. (1967): Significance of delay in performance of monkeys with medial temporal lobe resections. *Exp. Brain Res.*, 4:85-96.
9. Descartes, R. Traite de l'homme, 1664. *Treatise of Man.* French text and English translation by T. S. Hall, pp. 87-90. Harvard University Press, Cambridge, Massachusetts.
10. Dornbush, R. L. and Nikolovski, O. (1976): ACTH 4-10 and short term memory. *Pharmacol. Biochem. Behav. (Suppl.)*, 5:69-72.
11. Duncan, C. P. (1949): The retroactive effects of shock on learning. *J. Comp. Physiol. Psychol.*, 42:32-34.
12. Glendenning, R. L. (1972): Effects of training between two unilateral lesions of visual cortex upon ultimate retention of black-white habits by rats. *J. Comp. Physiol. Psychol.*, 80:216-229.
13. Hearst, E. and Whalen, R. E. (1963): Facilitating effects of d-Amphetamine upon discrimination avoidance performance. *J. Comp. Physiol. Psychol.*, 56:124-128.
14. Hebb, D. O. (1949): *The Organization of Behavior*, John Wiley, New York.
15. Horel, J. A., Bettinger, L. A., Royce, G. J. and Meyer, D. R. (1966): Role of neocortex in the learning and relearning of two visual habits by the rat. *J. Comp. Physiol. Psychol.*, 61:66-78.
16. Howard, R. L., Glendenning, R. L. and Meyer, D. R. (1974): Motivational control of retrograde amnesia: further explorations and effects. *J. Comp. Physiol. Psychol.*, 86:187-192.
17. Howard, R. L. and Meyer, D. R. (1971): Motivational control

of retrograde amnesia in rats: a replication and extension. *J. Comp. Physiol. Psychol.*, 74:37-40.

18. Isaacson, R. L., Douglas, R. J. and Moore, R. Y. (1961): The effect of radical hippocampal ablations on acquisition of avoidance response. *J. Comp. Physiol. Psychol.*, 54:625-628.

19. Jonason, K. R., Lauber, S. M., Robbins, M. J., Meyer, P. M. and Meyer, D. R. (1970): Effects of amphetamine upon relearning pattern and black-white discriminations following neocortical lesions in rats. *J. Comp. Physiol. Psychol.*, 73: 47-55.

20. Kesner, R. (1973): A neural system analysis of memory storage and retrieval. *Psych. Bull.*, 80:177-203.

21. Kesner, R. and Conner, H. S. (1972): Independence of short and long term memory: a neural system analysis. *Science*, 176: 432-434.

22. King, F. A. and Meyer, P. M. (1958): Effects of amygdaloid lesions upon septal hyperemotionality in the rat. *Science*, 128:655-656.

23. Landis, C. (1964): *Varieties of psychopathological experience*. Holt, Rinehart and Winston, New York.

24. Lashley, K. S. (1935): The mechanism of vision: XII. Nervous structures concerned in habits based on reactions to light. *Comp. Psychol.*, 11:43-79.

25. Lashley, K. S. (1950): In search of the engram. *Symposium of the Society for Experimental Biology*, pp. 454-482. Cambridge University Press, New York.

26. LeVere, T. E. and Morlock, G. M. (1973): The nature of visual recovery following posterior neodecortication in the hooded rat. *J. Comp. Physiol. Psychol.*, 83:62-67.

27. Lewis, D. J. (1976): A cognitive approach to experimental amnesia. *Am. J. Psychol.*, 89:51-80.

28. Meyer, D. R. (1972): Access to engrams. *Am. Psychologist*, 27:124-133.

29. Meyer, P. M., Johnson, D. A., and Baughn, D. W. (1970): The consequences of septal and neocortical ablations upon learning a two way conditioned avoidance response. *Brain Res.*, 22:113-120.

30. Milner, B. (1968): Disorders of memory after brain lesions in man. *Neuropsychologia*, 6:175-179.

31. Milner, B. (1970): Memory and the medial temporal regions of the brain. In: *The Biology of Memory*, edited by K. H. Pribram and D. E. Broadbent, pp. 29-50. Academic Press, New York.

32. Misanin, J. R., Miller, R. R. and Lewis, D. J. (1968): Retrograde amnesia produced by electroconvulsive shock after reactivation of a consolidated memory trace. *Science*, 160:554-555.

33. Pavlov, I. P. (1927): *Conditioned reflexes: An Investigation of the Physiological Activity of the Cerebral Cortex*. Translated by G. V. Anrep. Oxford University Press, London.

34. Penfield, W. (1958): *The Excitable Cortex in Conscious Man*, pp. 34-35. Liverpool University Press, Liverpool.

35. Rech, R. H. (1966): Amphetamine effects on poor performance

of rats in a shuttle-box.   *Psychopharmacologia,* (Berlin), 9:
110-117.

36. Rigter, H., Janssens-Elbertse, R. and van Riezen, H.   (1976):
Reversal of amnesia by an orally active ACTH analog (Org 2766).
Pharmacol. Biochem. Behav. (Suppl.), 5:53-58.

37. Rigter, H. and van Riezen, H.   (1975):   Anti-amnesic effect
of ACTH 4-10: Its independence of the nature of the anmesic
agent and the behavioral test.   *Physiol. Behav.,* 14:563-566.

38. Robbins, M. J. and Meyer, D. R.   (1970):   Motivational control of retrograde amnesia.   *J. Exp. Psychol.,* 84:220-225.

39. Schneider, A. M.   (1973):   Spreading depression: a behavioral
analysis.   In: *The Physiological Basis of Memory,* edited by
J. A. Deutsch.   Academic Press, New York.

40. Scoville, W. B. and Milner, B.   (1957):   Loss of recent memory after bilateral hippocampal lesions.   *J. Neurol. Neuro-
surg. Psychiatry,* 20:11.

41. Thompson, C. I. and Grossman, L. B.   (1972):   Loss and recovery of long-term memories after ECS in rats: evidence for
state-dependent recall.   *J. Comp. Physiol. Psychol.,* 78:248-
254.

42. Whitty, C. W. M. and Zangwill, O. L.   (1966):   Traumatic amnesia.   In: *Amnesia,* edited by C. W. M. Whitty and O. L.
Zangwill.   Spottiswoode, Ballantyne, London.

43. Yacorzynski, G. K.   (1965):   Organic mental disorders.   In:
Handbook of Clinical Psychology, edited by B. B. Wolman,
McGraw-Hill, New York.

*Neuropeptide Influences on the Brain
and Behavior,* edited by L.H. Miller,
C.A. Sandman, and A.J. Kastin.
Raven Press, New York © 1977.

Pituitary-Adrenal Hormones and Learned Taste Aversion

Seymour Levine, William P. Smotherman, and John W. Hennessy

*Department of Psychiatry and Behavioral Sciences, Stanford University,
Stanford, California 94305*

INTRODUCTION

Evidence accumulated during the past decade clearly indicates that a number of peptide hormones directly influence behavior in both animals and humans. Many peptides, both natural and synthetic, have been studied on a variety of behaviors. Although the large body of evidence has been concerned with behaviors that have been under aversive control, there are a number of studies which indicate that the effects of these peptides can indeed influence a variety of other behavioral processes, including extinction of an approach behavior (6), modulation of reversal learning of a complex brightness discrimination task (32, 33, 34, 37), facilitation of memory retrieval (31), and facilitation of sexually motivated behavior (3).

Since there now exist a number of excellent review papers and books (14) that have catalogued many of the effects of the pituitary peptides on behavior, it seems of little value to present in this chapter another extensive review of the variety of studies which have been concerned with this general problem. However, when one examines, in detail, the many studies that have been concerned with the role of the pituitary-adrenal system and peptides related to ACTH and ACTH analogues, there are very few studies which have dealt extensively with the relationship of these compounds to passive avoidance. In 1965 Levine and Jones reported that the administration of ACTH in a passive avoidance situation which involved shocking animals after they had stabilized on a bar press for water, significantly affected the passive avoidance behavior. Animals given ACTH failed to return to bar pressing after the administration of two shocks in contrast to control animals which, after a brief period of response inhibition, subsequently began to bar press for water. These results were difficult to interpret since it was impossible to discriminate between whether an animal was better at learning the passive avoidance response or whether the animal was indeed showing a failure to extinguish.

In subsequent studies that looked at the effects of ACTH on passive avoidance it was demonstrated that ACTH could have an effect on both processes and it appears as though ACTH can affect both the acquisition and the retention of a passive avoidance response (17). There has, however, been remarkably little research on the role of the analogues of ACTH and other pituitary peptides on passive avoidance behavior. Lissak and Bohus (25) have reported that there was an enhancement of passive avoidance retention when Pitressin, lysine[8] vasopressin, or ACTH was given prior to learning. In contrast, hypophysectomy led to an interference of passive avoidance retention. Although these data do indicate a possible role of pituitary peptides in passive avoidance performance, the traditional shock-induced passive avoidance does have at least one serious methodological problem for studying the influence of the pituitary-adrenal system in relationship to learning and extinction. It has recently been demonstrated by Rigter (29) that animals, once exposed to electric shock in passive avoidance, when subsequently placed in the apparatus without shock, show a conditioned elevation of corticoids, indicating an activation of the pituitary-adrenal system following a single exposure to shock. Thus, when attempting to study either learning or retention of passive avoidance, one is faced with the problem that the organism *already*, at the time of testing, has high endogenous levels of these compounds so that it is difficult to assess the effects of the endogenous hormones versus the exogenous administration of pituitary-adrenal hormones or any other peptide related to this system.

Over the past several years there has been a growing literature, using an aversion technique which is different in many of its characteristics from traditional shock-induced passive avoidance and yet, still appears capable of being subsumed under a passive avoidance model. This technique goes under a variety of names including flavor toxicosis, conditioned taste aversion and bait shyness (13, 28). This procedure involves presenting the animal with a preferred substance, normally a sweetened compound, and following the animal's exposure to this preferred substance, the animal is made ill by injection of toxins or x-radiation. What has been found consistently is that the animal, when

subsequently re-exposed to the preferred drinking substance, will then avoid this substance for a considerable period of time before it starts to drink it again.
Although this paradigm differs from the more traditional shock-induced passive avoidance, in the temporal aspects of the relationship between the conditioned stimulus, it clearly appears to have some of the same characteristics; namely, that the animal is exposed only
one time to a noxious, unconditioned stimulus and then
subsequently avoids the stimulus paired with that noxious event. It seems of interest to examine whether or
not this paradigm shows some of the same hormonal characteristics as passive avoidance, both in terms of the
steroid response to the preferred substance which has
been paired with illness, and in terms of whether hormones of the pituitary-adrenal system influence the
learning and retention of this type of passive avoidance performance.

The following series of studies, therefore, constitute an extensive investigation into both aspects of
the problem. Initially, we investigated the animal's
pituitary-adrenal response to lithium chloride (LiCl),
and to a variety of conditions when re-exposed to the
substance (in our case milk) following illness, and
finally to hormone manipulation, including pituitary
peptides which might influence the course of learning
and retention of learned taste aversions.

GENERAL METHODS AND SUBJECTS

In all experiments subjects were male Sprague-Dawley
rats (300 to 350 g). They were housed individually in
controlled temperature and humidity colony rooms on
regulated 12-hr-on/12-hr-off light cycles.

In the taste-aversion experiments, all subjects were
first trained to drink on cue in their home cage. A
sucrose solution (20%) was presented in 15 min sessions
for seven days. Thereafter, the sucrose solution and
sweetened milk were presented on alternate days until
each animal received five milk presentations. With the
exception of the first few sucrose presentations, the
subjects were maintained under *ad lib.* food and water
conditions. For toxicosis conditioning, the fifth milk
drinking session was followed 25 to 35 min later by an
i.p. injection of LiCl (0.40 M; 7.50 mg/kg). The subjects were allowed 72 hr to recover from the LiCl
treatment, and the remaining milk presentations can be
considered as extinction or recovery sessions. We have
found that recovery is reasonably complete in untreated
animals after 10 extinction sessions (sessions where
animals have *ad lib.* access to food and water). We will
refer to these as free extinction sessions. An alter-

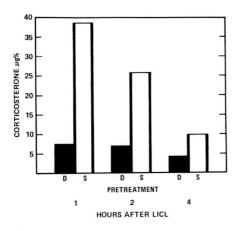

FIG. 1. Plasma corticosterone levels following an injection of LiCl in animals pretreated with dexamethasone (D) or saline (S).

nate procedure was used in some instances (forced extinction) where animals were food deprived for four days with water being withheld for the last two of these four. Unless otherwise stated, the extinction data were collected using the free extinction procedure.

When necessary, animals were quickly anesthetized with ether and blood samples (0.8 ml) were collected by cardiac puncture (4) in heparinized syringes. The blood was then centrifuged at 2,000 rpm for 10 min, the plasma extracted, and quickly frozen until a time at which it could be assayed for corticosterone levels. The micro-method of Glick, von Redlich and Levine (15) was used to determine plasma levels of corticosterone.

Pituitary-Adrenal Changes that Accompany Conditioned Taste Aversion

It has been well established that a variety of stimuli, including aversive-unconditioned stimuli (UCS) used in passive-avoidance situations, activate the pituitary-adrenal system (11, 12). Does the illness produced by LiCl injection act as an UCS in terms of the pituitary-adrenal system, as evidenced by increased levels of circulating glucocorticoids?

We found that injections of LiCl in a dosage and concentration (7.50 mg/kg of 0.40 M) sufficient to produce a learned taste aversion, resulted in sustained increases in plasma corticosterone levels which lasted from 2 to 4 hr (see Fig. 1). These data suggest that both ACTH and corticosterone are elevated at the time of taste-aversion learning. Further, they indicate that, like the UCS (footshock) used to produce passive-avoidance behavior, LiCl treatment used in producing a conditioned taste aversion activates the pituitary-adrenal system (18).

Other investigators (1, 29) have demonstrated in passive-avoidance paradigms that stimuli paired with shock, in the absence of that shock, lead to conditioned activation of the pituitary-adrenal system. Given that LiCl injections cause a sustained increase in plasma corticosterone, we asked whether changes in corticosterone levels could be conditioned. In other words, would animals show corticosterone elevations on the first day of extinction (recovery) when they were again presented with the substance that was, on the prior presentation, paired with the toxic aftereffects of LiCl?

To answer this question, individual groups of animals were conditioned to show a taste aversion to a sweetened milk solution. Following the fifth milk (CS) presentation they were treated with LiCl (conditioned group) or an equal volume of isotonic saline (control group), which did not produce a taste aversion. Three days after these injections, during which food and water were continuously available, the milk was again presented and animals in both groups had blood samples taken 20 min after the end of the drinking session for determination of plasma levels of corticosterone. Table 1 (upper panel) summarizes the effects. Clearly, the conditioned animals developed an aversion for the milk that was not evidenced by controls. On the other hand, this avoidance behavior (flavor aversion) was not accompanied by an elevation in plasma levels of corticosterone.

The milk had clearly become aversive as evidenced by the postconditioning suppression in drinking. As was evidenced by the fact that milk drinking was not completely suppressed, animals had been re-exposed to the CS. Some postconditioning sampling of the milk occurred. In a taste-aversion paradigm where subjects were re-exposed to the CS (the taste of milk) paired earlier with the malaise produced by LiCl injection, corticosterone levels remained low (35). Under these testing conditions the avoidance behavior was not accompanied by pituitary-adrenal activation.

At this point another experiment was designed which was intended to maximize the possibility that subjects would re-experience the CS. Following the taste-illness pairing and a free extinction session, subjects were placed on food deprivation for four days with water being withheld for the last two of these four days. With this procedure subjects were forced to consume either a neutral substance (tap water) or the aversive substance (milk). Subjects had blood samples taken to determine plasma corticosterone levels. These data are summarized in the bottom panel of Table 1.

TABLE 1. Conditioned plasma corticosterone elevations during recovery from LiCl-induced taste aversions

	Plasma corticosterone µg/100 ml	Milk consumption (g)	
	Free extinction	Pretoxicosis	Posttoxicosis
Conditioned animals N=13	4.5 ± 0.5	11.7	3.1
Control animals N=13	6.9 ± 0.8	11.6	11.6

	Plasma corticosterone µg/100 ml		Milk consumption (g)	
	Free extinction	Forced extinction	Free extinction	Forced extinction
Neutral solution (tap H$_2$O) N=9	16.1	16.0	–	–
Aversive solution (sweetened milk) N=9	15.0	28.5[a]	2.2	8.4

[a] $p<.01$ Newman-Keuls post hoc comparison following significant interaction effect

As with the first experiment, under the conditions of free extinction (*ad lib.* access to food and water), avoidance of the milk was not accompanied by elevations in corticosterone. However, following the deprivation procedure, which reversed to some extent the aversion, animals that drank the aversive substance had higher levels of corticosterone than animals drinking tap water (a neutral substance). With this procedure, conditioned elevations in plasma corticosterone were demonstrated. With both the free and forced extinction procedures, conditioned animals drank a substance paired with negative postingestive consequences produced by LiCl treatment. However, only under the conditions of forced extinction did a conditioned activation of the pituitary-adrenal system occur (35).

If the food and water deprivation procedure (forced extinction) motivates the animal, and the milk drinking data verify that it has, the animal is thus in a conflict situation, motivated to drink, and presented only with the aversive substance. It is only in this

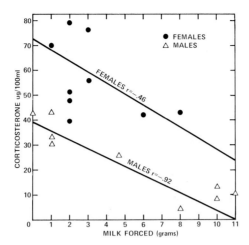

FIG. 2. A plot showing the correlation between the plasma corticosterone concentrations (determined after the forced extinction
session) and the amount of milk forced (forced extinction minus
free extinction milk consumption). A lower mile forced value
represents a greater aversion.

conflict situation that endogenous steroid levels elevate.

Dupont, Endröczi, and Fortier (7) and Endröczi and
Fekete (10) have reported a correlation between pituitary-adrenal activity and behavior in a passive-avoidance situation. Animals showing the largest steroid
elevations in response to the UCS (shock) subsequently
exhibited the greatest passive avoidance behavior. We
have seen (36) a similar corticosterone/behavior relationship using a conditioned aversion paradigm. Figure
2 shows this relationship. The magnitude of the aversion, as measured by the suppression of milk drinking
and plasma levels of corticosterone were related in a
linear fashion. In both males ($r = -.92$) and females
($r = -.46$) this relationship was such that the greater
the strength of the aversion (more suppression in milk
drinking) the greater were the steroid elevations.

These data suggest that changes in pituitary-adrenal
activity as measured by circulating levels of glucocorticoids reflec† the strength of conditioned taste
aversions. Again these data from a taste-aversion paradigm parallel those reported by Dupont et al. (7) for
a shock/fear motivated passive avoidance situation.

In summary, we have shown that LiCl in a dosage and
concentration that produces a conditioned taste aversion, like other aversive stimuli, activates the pituitary-adrenal system. When subjects have *ad lib.* access
to food and water (free extinction) and control the
amount of milk they consume, endogenous steroid levels

do not elevate. However, forcing the animal to consume
the aversive substance (forced extinction) results in
conditioned corticosterone elevations. In general the
steroid/behavior relationship in this taste-aversion
paradigm parallels closely that reported for more traditional passive-avoidance situations. The results
demonstrate the task generality of conditioned pituitary-adrenal changes that accompany avoidance conditioning.

Altered Endogenous Steroid Levels and Their Effects on Conditioned Taste-Aversion

As stated earlier, LiCl injections caused an activation of the pituitary-adrenal system. Given that
corticosterone, and presumably ACTH, levels are elevated at the time conditioning occurs, we studied the
effects of changes in pituitary-adrenal function upon
taste aversion acquisition and performance. As a first
step, to assess the effects of both dexamethasone (DEX)
pretreatment and LiCl injections upon pituitary-adrenal
activity, animals were assigned to one of six independent groups. Pretreatment injections were administered
2.5 hr prior to LiCl injection; one-half of the subjects received 400 μg of dexamethasone phosphate and
the remainder received an equivalent volume of isotonic
saline. Blood samples were taken either 1, 2, or 4 hr
after LiCl injection (.40 M solution; 7.50 mg/kg) for
these three groups of animals within a pretreatment
condition. Plasma corticosterone levels were determined and the results are shown in Fig. 1. For the
saline pretreated groups, plasma corticoid levels were
elevated for 2 to 4 hr following LiCl administration.
As was expected, dexamethasone pretreatment uniformly
suppressed these corticosterone elevations (18).

A factorial design was employed with four groups of
animals receiving DEX or saline 2 hr prior to drinking
on either the conditioning day, or throughout recovery,
or both. Thus, four independent groups were employed:
(1) those pretreated with DEX prior to both conditioning and during recovery (D-D); (2) those receiving DEX
prior to conditioning and saline during recovery (D-S);
(3) those receiving saline pretreatment for conditioning and DEX during recovery (S-D); and (4) those pretreated with saline throughout (S-S). The results
(Fig. 3) indicated that both groups pretreated with DEX
on the conditioning day (D-D and D-S) showed an attenuated
taste aversion relative to those treated with saline
(S-D and S-S). The effect was present on the first day
of testing and lasted throughout extinction.

In the same series of experiments, we investigated
the possibility that manipulation of the ACTH-steroid

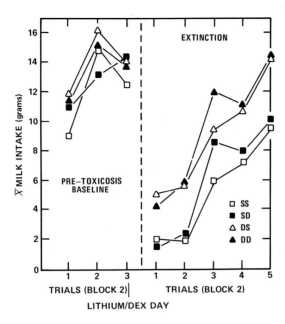

FIG. 3. The effects of DEX pretreatment during conditioning and/
or extinction on taste aversion to milk.

levels, via exogenous administration, might also affect
performance in this type of avoidance paradigm. Preliminary evidence (18) had shown that ACTH injections
administered prior to both conditioning and extinction
sessions tended to prolong recovery, i.e., ACTH-injected groups drank less milk during extinction. Again,
a factorial design was employed to measure the effects
of presession ACTH injections during either conditioning or recovery (19). It was found that ACTH injections, when given *prior to recovery sessions,* affected performance and prolonged the extinction process (Fig. 4).
It is interesting to note here that the group receiving
ACTH injections prior to the conditioning trial and
saline injections during recovery (AS) showed a trend
toward an attenuated aversion; a possible state-dependent phenomenon. Since ACTH injections produce elevations in both ACTH and corticosterone levels, the possibility exists that ACTH injections may exaggerate the
avoidance response by elevating corticoid levels. Rigter (29) has recently reported that the peptide ACTH 4-
10, which is virtually devoid of corticotropic activity, will also prolong the recovery of a learned taste
aversion. We have recently replicated this effect
(35a) and found that ACTH 4-10 injections produce recovery which is intermediate to that seen in ACTH and
saline treated subjects.

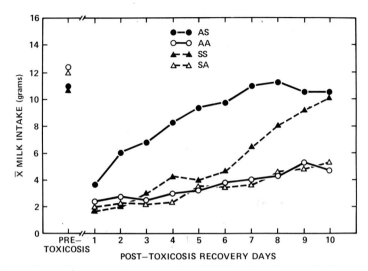

FIG. 4. The effects of presession ACTH injections during conditioning and/or extinction on taste aversion to milk.

The data reported here are generally in line with
the literature on passive avoidance. The effect of
DEX compares favorably, but not entirely, with other
effects of glucocorticoid administration (2, 24, 26).
The fact that ACTH prolongs recovery is consonant with
data from passive avoidance (17, 23) and active avoidance extinction (6), although the stage of training
when injections are effective may differ (*cf.*, 16, 17).
Also, it is interesting to note that the effectiveness
of both DEX and ACTH injections is consistent with our·
measures of pituitary-adrenal activity during the different phases of conditioning. DEX is effective at the
time of conditioning, when in untreated animals endogenous pituitary-adrenal activity is high. Since manipulation studies to date have used animals which had
free access to food and water (free extinction), endogenous activity during recovery is low. ACTH injections
are effective only when administered during recovery,
presumably by elevating hormonal levels at that time.
The data from studies of pituitary-adrenal manipulation have suggested that this system can affect both
the learning and performance in the taste-aversion paradigm. Our initial interpretation of these data focused on the importance of the elevated levels of ACTH
at the time of conditioning. Since a DEX block of ACTH
release during illness can reduce the degree of aversion, we concluded that ACTH participates, in some un-
specified manner, in learning that ingestion of some
substances may result in illness. This notion is cer-

tainly compatible with the reinforcement-memory function proposed by Pfaff (27). In a similar manner, the effects of ACTH injections can be related to the high levels of pituitary-adrenal activity at the time of conditioning. If high ACTH levels act as a salient component of the stimulus complex associated with illness, then treatment of the subjects with ACTH prior to recovery sessions may facilitate the retrieval of memories associated with the aversive event (20, 21, 22, 31).

More recently, we have investigated the hypothesis that the effect of DEX on the conditioning process was due to reduced ACTH levels (18a). Since intracranial implants of hydrocortisone block ACTH release (but also reduce peripheral steroid levels), the performance of implanted subjects was measured in a taste-aversion learning situation. It was found that, unlike DEX, hydrocortisone implants in the median eminence did not attenuate the aversion, although both procedures block ACTH release. The role of ACTH in the conditioning process must be questioned and the possibility that DEX is operating via an independent glucocorticoid effect seems more probable (5, 8, 38, 39).

SUMMARY AND CONCLUSIONS

1. Lithium chloride (LiCl), in these experiments, causes a marked and prolonged elevation of adrenal corticoids is significantly more prolonged than has been demonstrated for more acute stressful conditions. The time course of corticosterone elevations following exposure to a brief, intense electric shock or 1 min of ether normally shows a peak elevation roughly 15 to 30 min after the initial exposure, but by the end of 2 hr most values have returned to resting levels. It is possible, therefore, that prolonged ACTH secretion, which would be essential to maintain corticosteroid values elevated for a long period of time, could indeed be acting as a component of the unconditioned stimulus or response associated with LiCl injections.

2. The data indicate that under certain types of retention (forced extinction) pituitary-adrenal activity can be conditioned. Thus, when an animal is forced to drink following prolonged deprivation, exposure to the milk which had been associated with illness now causes a significant elevation of plasma corticosterone. Further, there is a negative correlation between the elevation of plasma corticosterone and the amount of milk consumed under forced extinction conditions. It is therefore possible that plasma levels of corticosterone may provide an alternate index for the strength of conditioned taste aversions.

3. The steroid elevations observed under the forced
extinction conditions give further evidence of the fact
that learned taste aversions can be subsumed under the
general category of passive avoidance. The elevations
of steroids seen under the forced extinction conditions
are similar to those observed in shock-induced passive
avoidance, when the animal is placed in the apparatus
and thus is exposed to those stimuli which have been
associated with shock.

4. Manipulating the hormones associated with the
pituitary-adrenal system also affects the degree of
learned taste aversion and influences recovery. Thus,
if one administers DEX prior to the administration of
LiCl, learned taste aversion is attenuated. It would,
however, appear that ACTH is not involved in the acquisition of learned taste aversion since a central
block of ACTH does not affect the magnitude of the
aversion. If ACTH is injected during recovery, animals tend to show a more prolonged suppression of
drinking. These data appear to be best explained using a memory-retrieval model.

5. The manipulations of hormones and their effects
on learned taste aversions appear to follow the effects
observed endogenously. Thus, ACTH administered to animals during the conditioning phase does not appear to
have any effect upon the learning of the aversion.
Since LiCl markedly elevates ACTH, as indicated by prolonged elevations of steroids, the additional ACTH
given exogenously at the time of conditioning does not
appear to add to the effects already attributable to
endogenous ACTH. Conversely, DEX given during recovery
appears to have no effect upon the recovery function.
Since ACTH is low during the free extinction procedure,
the further reduction of ACTH by DEX appears to have
no function upon recovery.

6. The effects of ACTH are in part due to a peptide
function. Thus, ACTH 4-10, which has no effect upon
the adrenal, does have an effect on recovery similar
to that of the parent peptide, ACTH. However, the effects are not as profound as those seen with the whole
ACTH molecule, although they do significantly prolong
the recovery of drinking.

7. Finally, it appears that the learned taste aversion may be especially well suited for the study of
peptides. During the free extinction procedure, in
which endogenous levels of ACTH and steroids are not
elevated, peptide influence upon the recovery of
learned taste aversions can be studied systematically
without the concern that endogenous hormone levels can
interfere and override the effects of these peptides.

ACKNOWLEDGMENTS

This study was supported by Research Grant NICH&HD-02881 from the National Institutes of Health (SL), Biosciences Training Grant MH-8304 (WPS), and a grant from the Foundations' Fund for Research in Psychiatry (JWH).
Dr. Levine is supported by USPHS Research Scientist Award K5-MH-19936 from the National Institute of Mental Health.

REFERENCES

1. Auerbach, P. and Carlton, P. L. (1971): Retention deficit correlated with a deficit in the corticoid response to stress. *Science,* 173:1148-1149.
2. Bohus, B. (1973): Pituitary-adrenal influences on avoidance and approach behavior of the rat. *Prog. Brain Res.,* 39:407-419.
3. Bohus, B., Hendrick, H. H. L., van Kolfschoten, A. A., and Krediet, T. G. (1975): Effects of corticotrophin-like neuropeptides on male sexual behaviour in the rat. *J. Endocrinol.,* 64:37P.
4. Davidson, J. M., Jones, L. E., and Levine, S. (1968): Feedback regulation of adrenocorticotropin secretion in "basal" and "stress" conditions: Acute and chronic effects of intrahypothalamic corticoid implantation. *Endocrinology,* 82:655-663.
5. de Wied, D. (1974): Pituitary-adrenal system hormones and behavior. In: *The Neurosciences, Third Study Program,* edited by F. O. Schmitt and F. G. Worden, pp. 653-666. M.I.T. Press, Cambridge.
6. de Wied, D., van Delft, A. M. L., Gispen, W. H., Weijnen, J. A. W. M., and van Wimersma Greidanus, Tj. B. (1972): The role of pituitary-adrenal system hormones in active avoidance conditioning. *Hormones and Behavior,* edited by S. Levine, pp. 136-171. Academic Press, New York.
7. Dupont, A., Endröczi, E., and Fortier, C. (1971): Influence of hormones on the nervous system. In: *Proceedings of the International Society of Psychoneuroendocrinology,* edited by D. H. Ford, pp. 451-462. Karger, Basel.
8. Endröczi, E. (1972a): Pavlovian conditioning and adaptive hormones. In: *Hormones and Behavior,* edited by S. Levine, pp. 173-207. Academic Press, New York.
9. Endröczi, E. (1972b): *Limbic System, Learning and Pituitary Adrenal Function.* Akademiai Kiado, Budapest.
10. Endröczi, E. and Fekete, T. (1973): Correlations between the pituitary-adrenal function and the exploratory activity, learning behavior and limbic functions. In: *Hormones and Brain Function,* edited by K. Lissak, pp. 399-408. International Society for Psychoneuroendocrinology, Budapest.
11. Friedman, S. B. and Ader, R. (1967): Adrenocortical response to novelty and noxious stimulation. *Neuroendocrinology,* 2:209-212.

12. Ganong, W. F. and Forsham, P. H. (1960): Adenohypophysis and adrenal cortex. *Annu. Rev. Physiol.*, 22:579-614.

13. Garcia, J., Hankins, W. G., and Rusiniak, K. W. (1974): Behavioral regulation of milieu interne in man and rat. *Science* 185:824-831.

14. Gispen, W. H., van Wimersma Greidanus, Tj. B., Bohus, B., and de Wied, D. (1975): (eds.) *Prog. Brain Res.*, 42.

15. Glick, D., von Redlich, D., and Levine, S. (1964): Fluorometric determination of corticosterone and cortisol in 0.02-0.05 milliliters of plasma or submilligram samples of adrenal tissue. *Endocrinology*, 74:653-655.

16. Gray, P. (1975): Effect of adrenocorticotropic hormone on conditioned avoidance in rats interpreted as state-dependent learning. *J. Comp. Physiol. Psychol.*, 88:281-284.

17. Guth, S., Seward, J. P., and Levine, S. (1971): Differential manipulation of passive avoidance by exogenous ACTH. *Horm. Behav.*, 2:127-138.

18. Hennessy, J. W., Smotherman, W. P., and Levine, S. (1976): Conditioned taste aversion and the pituitary-adrenal system. *Behav. Biol.*, 16:413-424.

18a. Hennessy, J. W., Smotherman, W. P., and Levine, S. (1977): Investigations of the nature of the dexamethasone and ACTH effects upon taste aversion. *Horm. Behav. (In press.)*

19. Kendler, K., Hennessy, J. W., Smotherman, W. P. and Levine, S. (1976): An ACTH effect on recovery from conditioned taste aversion. *Behav. Biol.*, 17:225-229.

20. Keyes, J. B. (1974): Effect of ACTH on ECS-produced amnesia of a passive avoidance task. *Physiol. Psychol.*, 2:307-309.

21. Klein, S. B. (1972): Adrenal-pituitary influence in reactivation of avoidance-learning memory in the rat after intermediate intervals. *J. Comp. Physiol. Psychol.*, 79:341-359.

22. Levine, S. and Brush, F. R. (1967): Adrenocortical activity and avoidance learning as a function of time after avoidance training. *Physiol. Behav.*, 2:385-388.

23. Levine, S. and Jones, L. E. (1965): Adrenocorticotropic hormone (ACTH) and passive avoidance learning. *J. Comp. Physiol. Psychol.*, 59:357-360.

24. Levine, S. and Levin, R. (1970): Pituitary-adrenal influences on passive avoidance in two inbred strains of mice. *Horm. Behav.*, 1:105-110.

25. Lissak, K. and Bohus, B. (1972): Pituitary hormones and avoidance behavior of the rat. *Int. J. Psychobiol.*, 2:103-115.

26. Pappas, B. A. and Gray, P. (1971): Cue value of dexamethasone for fear-motivated behavior. *Physiol. Behav.*, 6:127-130.

27. Pfaff, D. (1969): Parsimonious biological models of memory and reinforcement. *Psychol. Rev.*, 76:70-81.

28. Revusky, S. and Garcia, J. (1970): Learned associations over long delays. In: *The Psychology of Learning and Motivation: Advances in Research and Theory, Vol. 4,* edited by G. H. Bower, pp. 1-84. Academic Press, New York.

29. Rigter, H. (1975): Peptide hormones and the extinction of conditioned taste aversion. Paper presented at the meeting of the British Society of Pharmacology, September 1975, London, England.

30. Rigter, H. and van Riezen, H. (1975): Anti-amnesic effect of ACTH 4-10: Its independence of the nature of the amnesic agent and the behavioral test. *Physiol. Behav.,* 14:563-566.

31. Rigter, H., van Riezen, H., and de Wied, D. (1974): The effect of ACTH- and vasopressin-analogues on CO_2-induced retrograde amnesia in rats. *Physiol. Behav.,* 13:381-388.

32. Sandman, C. A., Miller, L. H., Kastin, A. J., and Schally, A. V. (1972): Neuroendocrine influence on attention and memory. *J. Comp. Physiol. Psychol.,* 80:54-58.

33. Sandman, C. A., Alexander, W. D., and Kastin, A. J. (1973): Neuroendocrine influences on visual discrimination and reversal learning in the albino and hooded rat. *Physiol. Behav.,* 11:613-617.

34. Sandman, C. A., George, J. M., Nolan, J. D., van Riezen, H., and Kastin, A. J. (1975): Enhancement of attention in man with ACTH/MSH 4-10. *Physiol. Behav.,* 15:427-431.

35. Smotherman, W. P., Hennessy, J. W., and Levine, S. (1976): Plasma corticosterone levels during recovery from LiCl produced taste aversions. *Behav. Biol.,* 16:401-412.

35a. Smotherman, W. P. and Levine, S. (1977): ACTH and ACTH 4-10 modification of neophobia and taste-aversion responses in the rat. *J. Comp. Physiol. Psychol. (In press.)*

36. Smotherman, W. P., Hennessy, J. W., and Levine, S. (1976): Plasma corticosterone levels as an index of the strength of illness-induced taste aversions. *Physiol. Behav.,* 17:903-908.

37. Stratton, L. O. and Kastin, A. J. (1973): Melanocyte stimulating hormone in learning and extinction of two problems. *Physiol. Behav.,* 10:689-692.

38. Weiss, J. M., McEwen, B. S., Silva, M. T. A., and Kalkut, M. F. (1969): Pituitary-adrenal influences on fear responding. *Science,* 163:197-199.

39. Weiss, J. M., McEwen, B. S., Silva, M. T. A., and Kalkut, M. F. (1970): Pituitary-adrenal alterations and fear responding. *Am. J. Physiol.,* 218:864-868.

*Neuropeptide Influences on the Brain
and Behavior,* edited by L.H. Miller,
C.A. Sandman, and A.J. Kastin.
Raven Press, New York © 1977.

Brain Mechanisms Involved in ACTH-Induced Changes of Exploratory Activity and Conditioned Avoidance Behavior

Elemér Endröczi

*Central Research Division, and Institute of Experimental and Clinical Laboratory
Investigations, Postgraduate Medical School, 1389 Budapest, Hungary*

In 1953, Mirsky et al. (12) and Murphy and Miller (13) reported that ACTH administration produced an extraadrenal action on conditioned avoidance behavior in monkeys and rats. Subsequent studies indicated that both ACTH fragments and analogues like α- and β-MSH, induce delayed extinction of avoidance responses, increase the retention of newly acquired responses, improve visual discrimination, and possess antiamnesic effects (1, 2, 8, 9, 15, 18). ACTH fragments such as ACTH 4-10 have proven to be effective in increasing both protein and RNA synthesis of brainstem tissue *in vitro* (5, 6, 14, 16). Among other actions on neurotransmitters, it has been found that both systemic and intraventricular injection of ACTH 4-10 results in an increased norepinephrine (NE) turnover in different brain regions (3, 10, 17). The possible role of NE neuronal transmission in ACTH-induced behavioral reactions has been suggested by several investigators (3, 11).

Recent studies support the view that a catecholaminergic neuronal system plays a role in ACTH-induced behavioral reactions, although the presence of specific peptidergic receptors involved in mediation of responses cannot be excluded.

Exploratory Activity

Male rats were used in the study and the adrenal glands were removed 2 weeks prior to the behavioral investigations. The exploration was tested in a 12-cell maze and it was scored by the number of gates crossed by the animal during the 10 min observation period.

179

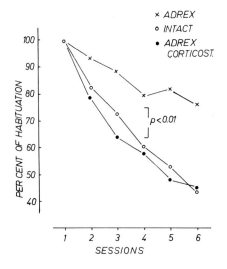

FIG. 1. Habituation of exploratory activity in consecutive sessions of 12 hr intervals in intact, adrenalectomized, and cortiocoste-
rone-treated male rats.

For studying the habituation of exploratory activity
the testing was repeated in 12 hr intervals. It was
found that adrenalectomy produced a greater resistance
to habituation of exploratory activity which could be
restored by administration of 100 μg/100 g corticosterone (i.p., for 3 days before testing). These observations led us to assume that an increase in endogenous ACTH secretion as a result of the adrenalectomy
delays the habituation of exploratory activity in a
novel situation (Fig. 1).

ACTH-Induced Changes in Brain NE Metabolism

The intraventricular injection of ACTH 1-24 and ACTH
4-10 with a tracer amount of ^{3}H-NE produced an increase
of the disappearance rate of the labeled pool from different brain regions. Earlier studies had revealed
that administration of Pargylin or alpha-methyltyrosine
(α-MT) did not prevent the ACTH-induced increase of the
NE turnover (3) (Figs. 2, 3, 4).

Local implantation of ACTH 4-10 in agarose gel into
the brainstem reticular formation, the medial forebrain
bundle in the niveau of the hypothalamic ventromedial
nucleus, and the subcommissural septal region was used
to study the possible site of the peptide action. The
implantation was performed 2 days prior to the intraventricular injection of the ^{3}H-NE and the animals were
killed in the 6th and 12th hrs following the injection.
Bilateral ACTH implants in the brainstem reticular formation (locus ceruleus region) produced a significant
increase of the disappearance rate of labeled NE pool.
In contrast to these observations the bilateral ACTH

HYPOTHALAMUS

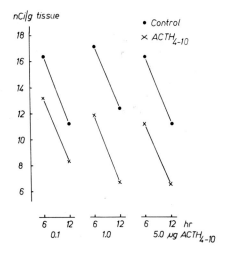

FIG. 2. Effect of intraventricular injection of ACTH 4-10 on the disappearance rate of labeled NE pool from the hypothalamus in male rats. The animals were sacrificed in the 6th and 12th hr after injection of the tracer with different amounts of the peptide. The means were calculated from 6 to 8 determinations.

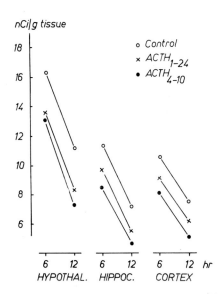

FIG. 3. Changes in the disappearance rate of the labeled NE pool from different brain regions after intraventricular injection of 0.5 µg ACTH 4-10 and 1.0 µg ACTH 1-24. The disappearance of labeled NE pool was significantly increased after ACTH peptide administration.

implants in the forebrain regions did not alter the NE metabolism (Fig. 5).

Correlations Between the Acquisition of Active Avoidance Response and Brain NE Metabolism

Male rats were trained in a shuttle-box by 50 associations of a buzzer as conditional signal with electrical footshocks in one session. The intraventricular

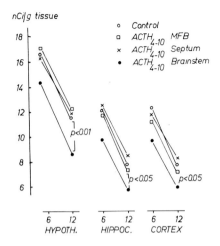

FIG. 4. Changes in the labeled NE pool after bilateral implantation of ACTH 4-10 into the brainstem reticular formation, medial forebrain bundle, and septal region.

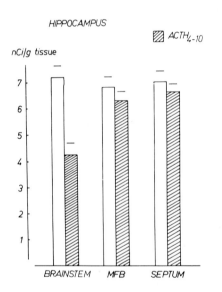

FIG. 5. Changes in the labeled NE pool of the hippocampus after bilateral implantation of ACTH 4-10 into the locus ceruleus, medial forebrain bundle, and septal area in male rats.

injection of ^{3}H-NE was performed 16 hr prior to the training period and the rats were killed immediately after the session. It was found that rats with high acquisition rate showed a greater disappearance of the labeled NE pool than those with poor performance level. In another experimental series the animals were trained in similar conditions to those mentioned before, but the intraventricular injection of the ^{3}H-NE was made 2 days later and the animals were killed without exposing them to the experimental situation. There

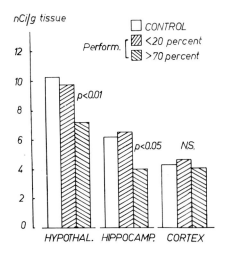

FIG. 6. Changes in the labeled NE pool in different brain regions of rats with low and high performance during 50 trials in two-way avoidance conditioning.

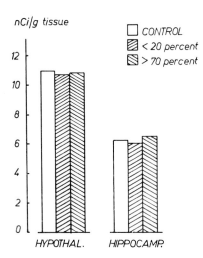

FIG. 7. The labeled NE pool of different brain regions in rats with low and high performance levels in two days after the training session in resting condition.

was no difference between the NE turnover of the "good" and "poor" performers which indicated that an increase of the NE turnover is closely related to the development of temporary linkage between the conditioned signal and goal-directed motor performance (Figs. 6, 7).

Correlations Between the Extinction of
Avoidance Response and the Brain NE Metabolism

Male rats were trained in a shuttle-box up to 90 percent criterion level. Twenty associations were presented in each daily session for 6 days. On the fourth day after the last training session ^{3}H-NE was injected

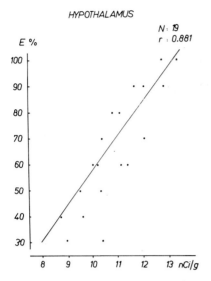

FIG. 8. Correlation between the extinction of avoidance response and the disappearance rate of labeled NE pool from the hypothalamus in male rats.

into the lateral ventricle and 16 hr later extinction was effected by the presentation of 30 nonreinforced trials. At the end of the extinction test the animals were killed immediately for measurement of plasma ACTH level by radioimmunoassay technique and the brain was removed for studying NE metabolism. The animals showed a high performance level and the presentation of 30 nonreinforced trials in 30 sec intervals resulted in a partial extinction of the avoidance response. It was found that both plasma ACTH concentration and NE turnover rate are in an inverse correlation to the extinction of avoidance response (Figs. 8, 9, 10).

The increased NE turnover in rats with high acquisition and retention of avoidance responding suggested that a NE neuronal system is involved in the integration of goal-directed motor patterns. On the other hand, the involvement of fear and punishment in activation of brain catecholaminergic system seems unlikely. These observations are in accord with the findings of Hanson (7) and Fuxe and Hanson (4) who reported increased NE turnover in telencephalic structures during acquisition of avoidance responses in rats.

CONCLUSIONS

A relatively long-term effect of the ACTH peptides on behavior has been confirmed by many investigators (2, 18). This property of the peptides with a short half-life in the extracellular space suggests the existence of peptidergic receptors in the central nervous system. Moreover, it seems to be very likely that

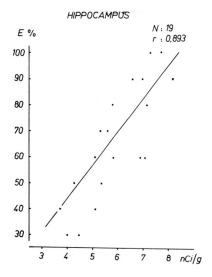

FIG. 9. Correlation between the extinction of avoidance response and the disappearance rate of labeled NE pool from the hippocampus in male rats.

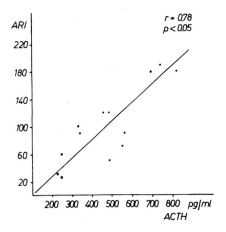

FIG. 10. Correlation between the extinction of avoidance response (ARI = avoidance response index) and the plasma ACTH response values in male rats.

ACTH peptides can activate ascending catecholaminergic pathways at the brainstem level, although a direct action on the nerve terminals in the telencephalon cannot be excluded.

The involvement of a NE neuronal system in learning behavior, and many similarities between the NE metabolism and behavioral reactions induced by ACTH peptides to those following administration of sympathomimetic drugs, do not exclude the possibility that ACTH peptides exert multiple influence on the brain functions. A similar conclusion was drawn by McGaugh et al. (11) who postulated NE transmission as a secondary messenger in the ACTH action.

The ACTH-induced increases in the retention of avoidance responses may be interpreted as a facilitatory influence of the peptide on development of temporary linkage between the conditional and the unconditional signal, on the one hand, and between the conditional signal and the motor pattern (or its withdrawal in a passive avoidance situation), on the other hand. The present findings indicate the involvement of a NE neuronal system in these events. This assumption is in accord with the relevant data from the literature that blocking of NE biosynthesis or β-adrenergic receptors results in a marked impairment of the acquisition and retention of avoidance behavior.

REFERENCES

1. Bohus, B. and de Wied, D. (1966): Inhibitory and facilitatory effect of two related peptides on extinction of avoidance behavior. *Science,* 153:318-320.
2. de Wied, D., Bohus, B., and Wimersma-Greidanus, van Tj. B. (1974): The hypothalamic-neurohypophyseal system and the preservation of conditioned avoidance behavior in rats. *Prog. Brain Res.,* 41:417-428.
3. Endröczi, E., Hraschek, A., Nyakas, Cs., and Szabo, G. (1975): Brain catecholamines and pituitary-adrenal function. In: *Cellular and Molecular Bases of Neuroendocrine Processes,* edited by E. Endroczi, pp. 607-618. Akademiai Kiado, Budapest.
4. Fuxe, K. and Hanson, L. C. F. (1967): Central catecholamine neurons and conditioned avoidance behavior. *Psychopharmacologia,* 11:439-447.
5. Gispen, W. H., de Wied, D., Schotman, P., and Jansz, H. S. (1970): Effects of hypophysectomy on RNA metabolism in rat brain stem. *J. Neurochem.,* 17:751-761.
6. Gispen, W. H., de Kloet, E. R., Reith, M. E., Wiegant, V. M., and Schotman, P. (1975): Pituitary peptides and brain function: some neurochemical aspects. *Brain Res.,* 66:368-369.
7. Hanson, L. C. F. (1965): The disruption of conditioned avoidance response following selective depletion of brain catecholamines. *Psychopharmacologia,* 6:100-109.
8. Kastin, A. J., Sandman, C. A., Stratton, O. L., Schally, A. V., and Miller, L. H. (1975): Behavioral and electrographic changes in rat and man after MSH. In: *Hormones, Homeostasis and the Brain,* edited by W. H. Gispen, Tj. B. van Wimersma-Greidanus, D. de Wied, and B. Bohus, *Prog. Brain Res.,* 42:143-151.
9. Koranyi, L. and Endröczi, E. (1967): The effect of ACTH on nervous processes. *Neuroendocrinology,* 1:144-157.
10. Leonard, B. E. (1974): The effect of two synthetic ACTH analogues on the metabolism of biogenic amines of the rat brain. *Arch. Int. Pharmacol. Therap.,* 207:242-253.

11. McGaugh, J. L., Gold, P. E., van Buskirk, R., and Haycock, J. (1975): Modulating influences of hormones and catecholamines on memory storage processes. *In:* Hormones, Homeostasis and the Brain, edited by W. H. Gispen, Tj. B. Wimersma-Greidanus, B. Bohus, and D. de Wied, *Prog. Brain Res.*, 42:151-162.
12. Mirsky, I., Miller, R., and Stein, M. (1953): Relation of adrenocortical activity and adaptive behavior. *Psychosom. Med.*, 15:574-584.
13. Murphy, J. V. and Miller, R. (1955): The effect of adrenocorticotrophic hormone (ACTH) on avoidance learning in the rat. *J. Comp. Physiol. Psychol.*, 48:47-49.
14. Reith, M. E. A., Schotman, P. and Gispen, W. H. (1975): Effect of behaviorally active ACTH analogues on brain protein metabolism. In: *Hormones, Homeostasis and the Brain,* edited by W. H. Gispen, Tj. B. van Wimersma-Greidanus, B. Bohus, and D. de Wied. *Prog. Brain Res.*, 42:195-201.
15. Rigter, H., Elbertse, R. and van Riezen, H. (1975): Time-dependent antiamnesic effect of ACTH 4-10 and desglycinamide-lysin-vasopressin. In: *Hormones, Homeostasis and the Brain,* edited by W. H. Gispen, Tj. B. van Wimersma-Greidanus, B. Bohus, and D. de Wied, *Prog. Brain Res.*, 42:163-173.
16. Schotman, P. and Gispen, W. H. (1974): Analogues of ACTH, conditioned avoidance behaviour and metabolism of macromolecules in the brain of rat. In: *Central Nervous System: Studies on Metabolic Regulation and Function,* edited by E. Genazzani and H. Herken, pp. 231-235. Springer-Verlag, Berlin.
17. Versteeg, D. H. G. (1973): The effect of two ACTH analogues on noradrenaline metabolism in rat brain. *Brain Res.,* 49:483-485.
18. van Wimersma Greidanus, Tj. B., Bohus, B. and de Wied, D. (1975): The role of vasopressin in memory processes. In: *Hormones, Homeostasis and the Brain,* edited by W. H. Gispen, Tj. B. van Wimersma-Greidanus, B. Bohus and D. de Wied. *Prog. Brain Res.*, 42:135-143.

Neuropeptide Influences on the Brain and Behavior, edited by L.H. Miller, C.A. Sandman, and A.J. Kastin. Raven Press, New York © 1977.

Is Learning Involved in Neuropeptide Effects on Behavior?

Gregory A. Kimble

Department of Psychology, The University of Colorado, Boulder, Colorado 80309

ALTERNATIVES TO LEARNING

In this chapter I will answer the question: Is learning involved in the effects of the neuropeptides on behavior? Then I will turn to some other questions that came to mind as I read some of the chapters in this volume. This second set of questions defines certain areas of research that appear quite promising. The answer to the first part will probably seem simple and straightforward to some and complex and uncertain to others. It will all depend in individual cases on what the social psychologists call your "tolerance for ambiguity." What you are about to find me saying is that effects on learning probably have not been established. Even if they have, the influences of the neuropeptides are surely broader than that.

It is too much to hope that all the neuropeptides will have exactly the same behavioral effects. In order to keep this discussion in bounds I have concentrated on the reported effects of ACTH- and MSH-related peptides. It is almost certain that the conclusions I reach will not hold for vasopressin, growth hormone, and the other peptides. In fact, several chapters in this volume suggest that even the D- and L-isomers of the same neuropeptide fraction may have different (possibly opposite) effects. On the other hand, I shall try now to raise certain questions that should be asked about these other hormones. Perhaps this will point the way to a more complete discussion.

Learned Versus Unlearned

Although the distinction between learned and unlearned behavior has blurred in recent years it still retains some utility. Reflex reactions, released re-

189

sponses and what is called instinctive behavior seem
quite clearly to differ from foresightful behavior,
concept formation, and complex problem solving. The
literature contains persuasive evidence that the neuropeptides have an effect upon behavior in the first
category, that is upon unlearned behavior.

Dunn and his colleagues (3) report that the injection of ACTH fractions produce significant increases
in grooming, stretching, and yawning in mice as well
as an insignificant decrease in eating behavior. Gispen et al. (5) report the same effect on grooming after injection of the complete ACTH molecule and also
mention a heightened level of sexual excitement. Champney et al. (1) refer to "a significant enhancement of
gregariousness," resulting from neonatal intraperitoneal injections of MSH. All of these influences seem to
be on behaviors that are unlearned rather than learned.

Champney also adds a dimension of complexity to the
picture. He reports that the effects of ACTH 4-9 interact with sex. For example, hormone-treated female
rats showed a decrement in passive avoidance responding; males showed an increase. At least the interaction, if not the separate effects, is hard to conceptu-
alize in terms of learning and seems instead to be related to inborn sexual differences.

Learning Versus Performance

In the traditional theories of learning it was standard practice to look at behavior as the joint product
of two different sets of variables called learning variables and performance variables. In that tradition,
learning was usually defined as a relatively permanent
change in behavior. The most important determining
variables were experience (practice) in some defini-
tions and experience plus reinforcement in others. The
translation of this permanent capacity into action de-
pended on the more temporary performance variables.
Motivation, fatigue, anxiety, stress, and arousal are
examples. I have listed these particular ones because
they are mentioned time and time again in this volume
as effects of the neuropeptides. This strongly suggests that a major part of the influence is on performance rather than learning.

In the late 1940s or early 1950s Clifford T. Morgan
proposed that the effects of food deprivation were
mediated physiologically by what he called a "hunger
hormone." Norman Guttman and I conceived the idea that
this hunger hormone might be ACTH. We coopted the assistance of a friend in the department of endocrinology
at Duke University Medical School, who supplied a tech-
nician and the necessary substances. Guttman and I

trained about eight rats to press the bar in a Skinner
box to obtain pellets of food. Then when the animals
were not very hungry we injected them with ACTH, naive-
ly hoping for a subsequent flurry of bar pressing. All
that happened was that the animals stopped doing anything for hours. Even the normal slow rate of bar
pressing disappeared. Had I been asked for a theoretical account of this result, I would have said that the
rats were sick. The experiment lasted for two nights
of investigation.

The main point that I want to make with the aid of
this example is that this suppression of behavior was
an effect on performance rather than learning. The
animals still had the bar-pressing habit as they were
able to demonstrate the next day. The second point is
that it is possible that Guttman and I were on a productive track in this work and that we aborted the
study prematurely. I say this because of the fairly
frequent observation in the research reported here that
the dose-response curve for the neuropeptides is nonmonotonic. Perhaps if we had lowered the dosage the
expected enhancement of performance would have appeared.
If it had, we would then have had to face the question
of whether the influence was on learning or performance.
The weight of the evidence seems to suggest an effect
on performance.

It is interesting to consider the results reported
by Strand and her colleagues (17). These investigators
report that several ACTH-like peptides increase the
amplitude of muscle action potentials and reduce fatigue. Elsewhere Dunn and his co-workers (3) report
that the administration of lysine vasopressin "resulted
in dramatic behavior in which the mice frantically and
unceasingly moved about the cage, often foraging
through the wood-shavings and occasionally eating or
grooming." It seems probable that Endröczi's (4) observation of ACTH-induced increases in exploratory activity is the same phenomenon.

The most immediate significance of these influences
is that they alone could account for the most dependable behavioral consequences of the administration of
the neuropeptides—the delayed extinction of conditioned
avoidance responses. The explanation would be that the
peptide-injected animals are just "revved up" and they
continue to perform the avoidance response because they
have to do something.

Several authors have noted that such an explanation
will not account for all of the behavioral effects of
the neuropeptides. For example it would predict the
opposite of what actually occurs in experiments involving shifted discriminations. Subjects should persist
in their original behavior and be slow to acquire the

new discrimination. It appears, however, that the usual result is that an intradimensional shift occurs more quickly in ACTH-injected subjects than in normals. This aspect will be discussed further.

Behavior Versus Stimulation

The arguments presented so far on the question of the locus of neuropeptide effects can be summarized quickly. These influences appear not to be effects on learning but rather to result from an influence on responses. There is an alternative to the second part of this interpretation that needs to be explored. It is that the effects of the neuropeptides might be due to changes in sensitivity, particularly to noxious stimuli. Gray and Garrud (7) come close to making this point and I would offer two observations in support of taking it seriously. The first is that some of the cleanest demonstrations of neuropeptide effects involve aversive stimuli as motivators. These include avoidance conditioning and the experiments involving intradimensional shifts. Then from Gispen et al. (5) we learn that certain ACTH analogs interfere with the analgesic action of morphine. If this effect is through some influence on a gating mechanism, it could be that the neuropeptides increase the effective intensity of painful and other unpleasant stimuli and exert some of their influence in that way.

Obviously, if this idea is to be applied to the results of several of the studies reported, it will have to be generalized considerably—to enhanced nauseous effects of lithium chloride (LiCl) injections studied by Levine and his associates (9), and to increases in fear or anxiety which presumably motivate the performance of avoidance responses. Since studies of the extinction of these reactions usually involve administration of peptides after the response had been learned, shock does not occur at the point in the experiment where the peptides are having their effect. Thus the effect must be on some residue of the previous experience, fear being the most attractive candidate.

A final, possibly more important, relevance of this point is to performance in reversed discriminations. For example, if we hypothesize that Marx (11) is exactly accurate in her description of this work in *Science:* Rats were trained "to run to a *lighted* door in one arm of a Y-shaped maze in order to escape an electric shock. Then they made the *dark* door the escape route from the shock. Rats treated with MSH learned this reversal faster than those receiving the control solution" (p. 368, emphasis added). Such data have been taken as one line of evidence for an effect of neuropeptides on attention.

But consider this result in the light of the fact
mentioned by Panksepp and his associates (13) that MSH
increases the well-known dark preferences of rats. The
quicker mastery of the reversed problem by rats injected with MSH could be an expression of this preference
rather than anything directly related to attention. In
studies where there has been an attempt to control for
the effects of brightness, the variable still remains
as a complicating problem. Obviously the test apparatus employed has to be some *color*, and treatment with a
neuropeptide seems likely to alter the animal's preference for this color. Just how such an increased or decreased preference will affect learning the discrimination is something that I do not know. Until the nature
of such influences is clearer I remain unconvinced that
the data on discrimination reversal support any particular interpretation of the influence of the neuropeptides, including the interpretation in terms of attention.

Learning Versus Attention

There are two substantial reports of research with
human subjects that seem to suggest that the conclusion
I have just reached should not be applied across the
board. These are the reports of Miller et al. (12)
and Sandman et al. (15). These investigators present
several results that concur with our findings when they
are considered as resulting from improved attention
produced by the administration of MSH/ACTH 4-10. These
results would be taken as evidence for an influence on
mechanisms other than those we call learning when
viewed in terms of the somewhat old-fashioned theoretical perspective I have been using up to now. A newer
point of view which reorganizes the field and posits
stages of information processing tends to diminish the
importance of the concept of learning. In these terms
it seems advisable to argue that these data show that
an important part of the neuropeptide influence is on
stages early in the sequence of processing.

Learning Versus (?) Memory Formation

I have mentioned the information-processing point of
view because I will rely on it in the final portion of
this section which deals with neuropeptide influences
on memory. The information processing theory concerns
itself with the "fate" of information presented to an
organism. The general idea is that such information
undergoes a series of stages of processing during which

some of it is lost and some ends up permanently stored in long-term memory. The number of stages of processing involved is a matter of modest controversy. The usual postulated number is three—immediate, short-term and long-term memory—but some theorists have argued for four, adding a stage of intermediate memory. I will make my point in terms of three stages, chiefly in the interest of space.

Immediate memory. The first of these stages (immediate memory) is one in which incoming materials remain briefly in the sensory-neural registers of the organism. The duration of this stage is only 1 or 2 sec but a great deal happens during that brief time. Images are formed. Materials are identified for what they are. Somehow this involves contact with long-term memory which must be consulted if the organism is to recognize the materials as things he has experienced before. The evidence reported by Miller et al. (12) strongly suggests an influence of the neuropeptides on this stage of processing. We are considering here the improved visual memory that the peptides seem to produce. This could come about as a result of stronger initial registration.

Short-term memory. Most of the inputs to immediate memory are lost at that stage. Only those to which the organism attends are subject to further processing. As I have mentioned there is evidence for an effect of the peptides on attention suggesting an additional influence of these substances at the interface between immediate and short-term memory.

Information that finds its way from immediate memory to short-term memory stays in the latter stage for another 15 to 30 sec. During this period there is evidence in human beings that verbal materials are represented in a form that is largely acoustic and highly susceptible to interference. These ideas constitute part of the research reported by Dornbush (2). Although this study shows neuropeptide effects possibly on attention but more likely on arousal there were no effects on short-term memory itself. I am inclined to postpone judgment on the question of whether such effects exist. Dornbush's strategy was only one of many possible approaches—not a sufficient basis for giving up the possibility.

Long-term memory. The circumstances required to transfer information from short-term to long-term memory are no doubt complex. A part of it must be some means of keeping the materials "alive" beyond the brief duration of short-term memory itself. The best candidate appears to be a behavioral one, specifically rehearsal. But rehearsal is only part of what goes on. Clinical and experimental literature has been accumulating for years indicating that a fairly long-term process (15 to 20 min)—sometimes called memory formation, sometimes consolidation—is also involved. Consolidation almost has to be an automatic neurochemical process. Certainly it cannot be continued rehearsal. Imagine the utter inefficiency of an organism that had to rehearse an experience for 15 to 20 min in order to learn it.

In this case we have evidence in the report of Gold and McGaugh (6) that the neuropeptides may promote consolidation or interfere with it. The argument for an hormonal effect on this aspect of information processing is a strong one.

Interim Summary

Do neuropeptides have an influence on learning or not? In the terms that are usually implicit in the asking of this question the answer appears to be "no." There are effects on instinctive behavior, on performance variables, on sensitivity, and on attention, but no effects that I would assign directly to learning unless one wished to argue that consolidation and learning are the same thing. But recent theoretical developments in psychology begin to suggest that the original question may not be based on the most productive way to organize an answer. When we look at neuropeptide effects in terms of an information-processing model, these effects appear in most of the theoretical stages.

CONCLUDING COMMENTS

As discussed previously, the first and possibly most important issue concerns an overall view of the field of neuropeptide research. When such research is directed at behavioral effects, it seems to me that it should include attention to the following issues: (a) the effect of environmental conditions and behavior upon the level of naturally occurring peptides; and (b) the behavioral consequences of these levels both in intact organisms and in organisms without the target organ of the peptide.

Comments on these problems seem to be missing from the literature. I do not see how it is possible to arrive at a complete picture of influence of the neuropeptides in the absence of such information. Now I realize that an investigator with mainly applied motives might be concerned with the therapeutic effectiveness of these hormones and with some justification look at their value for the alleviation of clinical symptoms. Some authors do take that point of view. In general, however, the findings are not impressive. It seems to me that using injections of neuropeptides in these works was just a *shot in the dark*.

Having made this general point I would like to offer
some fairly specific suggestions of lines of research
that seem to be important.

Study Neuropeptide Effects on Learned Helplessness

As most of you know, rats or dogs that are subjected
to unavoidable and inescapable shock are unable, later
on, to learn to avoid shock when avoidance becomes possible. The best reference on the topic is the 1976 paper by Maier and Seligman (10). This phenomenon has
several features to recommend it. (a) The administration of unavoidable shock is highly stressful and
should affect the neuropeptide levels. (b) The later
inability to cope with avoidable shock (learned helplessness) is dramatic, often an all-or-none phenomenon.
(c) These effects are of great current theoretical interest and of obvious potential relevance to real life
situations.

Find Out More About the Conditionability of Peptide Release

Levine and his associates (9) offer some evidence
that the release of the neuropeptides is a condition-
able response. If this is a dependable effect, the
conditioned reaction surely must have something to do
with the results of peptide administration. Moreover,
the extent of this conditioning probably varies from
one procedure to another and might help explain contradictory results. If I were in this field, one of the
first studies I would undertake would involve a neuropeptide assay following three conditioning procedures:
unsignalled unavoidable shock, signalled unavoidable
shock (classical conditioning), and signalled avoidable shock (operant conditioning). I selected these
three procedures for two reasons: (a) they are known
to be differentially stressful in terms of the production of stomach ulcers, and (b) properly controlled
they are the essential experimental conditions for the
study of learned helplessness. This offers an attractive opportunity to bring an important degree of integration to the field. At the same time, however, the
effects of conditioning with unconditioned stimuli other than shock should be investigated.

Do Simpler Experiments

The authors of this volume are in agreement that the
neuropeptides have profound influences on fundamental
behavioral mechanisms. In lower animals these include
effects on instinctive behavior and sensitivity to en-

vironmental events. It seems to me that understanding
of more complex processes might be hastened by the accumulation of more detailed data on such matters.

It is interesting that none of the authors has com-
mented on the effects of neuropeptides on experience as
might be revealed by clinical-type interviews. Even
psychologists are no longer nervous about the use of
introspective methods. If such information has not
yet been collected, it seems to me that it should be.
If nothing else, these data might narrow the range of
psychological processes that come under neuropeptide
influence.

Determine Dose/Response Curves More Completely

The chapters in this volume reveal that the field of
neuropeptide research is one of great complexity. Where
relevant data are reported they often suggest that the
dose/response curve is nonmonotonic for several behavioral indices. Moreover the conditions against which
the effects of these hormones are assessed (e.g.,
stress) also have nonmonotonic relationships to behavior. Baseline data in both areas appear to be necessary if progress is to occur in the area.

Standardize Measurement

The recommendation to standardize measurement first
came to mind when I noted that one of the studies reported used a 0.25-mA shock in the conditioning portion
of the experiment. There is a great deal of evidence
to suggest that this shock is too weak to obtain good
avoidance learning. I suspect the notorious impreci-
sion of shock values provided by the settings on shock
generators.

If I am wrong in this diagnosis, there is a different point to make. In the rat a 0.25-mA shock is nearly optimal for the elicitation of a class of responses
that I (8) once called "flinch" responses. Stronger
shocks produce jumping and a high level of activity.
It could be that the avoidant behavior produced by weak
shocks is quite different from that obtained with
stronger unconditioned stimuli. One of the "simpler
experiments" that ought to be done is a psychophysical
study of shock sensitivity in animals injected with
neuropeptides.

Take Advantage of the Power Inherent in the Psychophysics of Signal Detectability

In some studies presented in support of an effect of
the neuropeptides on attention [e.g., Miller et al.

(12)], the measures are the probability that a signal
will be detected. This probability, however, depends
in part on the bias of the observer or the criterion he
sets for making a positive response. A high level of
hits *can* result from a tendency to respond positively
to almost anything rather than increased sensitivity.
Measures provided by the theory of signal detectability
make it possible to obtain separate indices of sensitivity and bias. Although the results of Miller et al.
seem to suggest that the influence is on sensitivity,
the matter should be pursued. Altered levels of motivation, relaxed criteria, or a psychological state of
"impulsiveness" might also be involved. Incidentally
these same indices can be obtained for performance in
certain types of memory experiments.

*Look at Neuropeptide Effects in Several of the Information-Pro-
cessing Paradigms*

The past two decades have produced a set of powerful methods for determining what occurs in that critical 1 or 2 sec following the presentation of materials
to an observer. Since this determines what remains
available for more elaborate processing, it seems important to ask whether there are hormonal effects at
this stage.

The Sperling paradigm. In 1960 Sperling (16) reported
an experiment in which he first presented a tachisto-
scopic array of 12 symbols. Then, at intervals ranging up to about 2 sec, he gave a signal that asked the
observer to report particular subsets of the array.
Sperling's results showed that, immediately after presentation, essentially all of the symbols were available for this partial report. With time they quickly
disappeared. If the neuropeptides have an effect at
this level they might hasten or postpone the decay.

The Posner paradigm. Somewhat later Posner (see ref. 14)
showed that letters presented for identification exist
in consciousness first as a physical entity, then with
a name (for example "a") attached, then as a member of
a category, for example a vowel. It would be interesting to know whether the neuropeptides affect this series.

The Sternberg paradigm. In 1966, Sternberg (18) did the
following experiment: First, observers memorized a set
of one to six numbers. Then Sternberg presented a
probe number which sometimes was and sometimes was not
a member of the set in memory. All the observer had to
do was to report as quickly as possible whether the
probe was or was not one of the numbers in memory. The
somewhat startling result was that the time required to
make the report was an increasing linear function of

the size of the set in memory and had the same slope
for "yes" and "no" responses. Although Sternberg's
interpretation has been questioned, he concluded that
observers processed serially and exhaustively in this
experiment. It would be interesting to know whether
peptide-injected observers perform in the same way.
Exact interpretations would be less important than the
nature of the effect.

REFERENCES

1. Champney, T. F., Sahley, T. L., and Sandman, C. A. (1976):
   Effects of neonatal cerebral ventricular injection of ACTH 4-
   9 and subsequent adult injections on learning in male and female albino rats. *Pharmacol. Biochem. Behav. (Suppl.)*, 5:3-
   10.
2. Dornbush, R. L. and Nikolovski, O. (1976): ACTH 4-10 and
   Short-term Memory. *Pharmacol. Biochem. Behav.* (Suppl.), 5:
   69-72.
3. Dunn, A. J., Rees, H. D., and Iuvone, P. M. (1976): Behavioral and biochemical responses of mice to the intraventricular administration of ACTH peptides and Lysine vasopressin.
   Pharmacol. Biochem. Behav. (Suppl.), 5:139-146.
4. Endröczi, E. (1976): Brain mechanisms involved in ACTH-induced changes of exploratory activity and conditioned avoidance behavior. *(This volume.)*
5. Gispen, W. H., Reith, M. E. A., Schotman, P., Wiegant, V. M.,
   Zwiers, H., and de Wied, D. (1976): The CNS and ACTH-like
   peptides: Neurochemical response and interaction with opiates.
   (This volume.)
6. Gold, P. E. and McGaugh, J. L. (1977): Hormones and memory.
   (This volume.)
7. Gray, J. A. and Garrud, P. (1977): Adrenopituitary hormones
   and frustrative nonreward. *(This volume.)*
8. Kimble, G. A. (1955): Shock intensity and avoidance learning. *J. Comp. Physiol. Psychol.*, 48:281-284.
9. Levine, S., Smotherman, W. P., and Hennessy, J. W. (1976):
   Pituitary-adrenal hormones and learned taste aversion. *(This
   volume.)*
10. Maier, S. F. and Seligman, M. E. P. (1976): Learned helpless-
    ness: Theory and evidence. *J. Exp. Gen. Psychol.*, 105:3-46.
11. Marx, J. L. (1975): Learning and behavior (I): Effects of
    pituitary hormones. *Science*, 190:367-370.
12. Miller, L. H., Harris, L. C., Kastin, A. J. and van Riezen, H.
    (1976): A neuropeptide influence on attention and memory in
    man. *Pharmacol. Biochem. Behav.* (Suppl.), 5:17-22.
13. Panksepp, J., Reilly, P., Bishop, P., Meeker, R. B., Vilberg,
    T. R., and Kastin, A. J. (1976): Effects of α-MSH on moti-
    vation, vigilance and brain respiration. *Pharmacol. Biochem.
    Behav.* (Suppl.), 5:59-64.
14. Posner, M. I. and Warren, R. E. (1972): Traces, concepts and
    conscious constructions: In: *Coding Processes in Human Memory*,

edited by A. W. Melton and R. Martin. Wiley, New York.

15. Sandman, C. A., George, J., Walker, B., Nolan, J. D., and Kastin, A. J. (1976): The heptapeptide MSH/ACTH 4-10 enhances attention in the mentally retarded. *Pharmacol. Biochem. Behav.* (Suppl.), 5:23-28.

16. Sperling, G. (1960): The information available in brief visual presentations. *Psychol. Monogr.,* 74:498.

17. Strand, F. L., Cayer, A., Gonzalez E., and Stoboy, H. (1976): Peptide enhancement of neuromuscular function: Animal and clinical studies. *Pharmacol. Biochem. Behav.,* (Suppl.), 5: 179-188.

18. Sternberg, S. (1966): High-speed scanning in human memory. *Science,* 153:652-654.

Neuropeptide Influences on the Brain and Behavior, edited by L.H. Miller, C.A. Sandman, and A.J. Kastin. Raven Press, New York © 1977.

Adrenopituitary Hormones and Frustrative Nonreward

Jeffrey A. Gray and Paul Garrud

Department of Experimental Psychology, Oxford University, Oxford OX1 3UD England

Our first venture into the study of the hormones of the adrenopituitary system was in test of a prediction that was disproved at once. Since then this field has continued to provide a ready grave for promising hypotheses. Over the last few years we have collected a number of observations of the behavioral effects of the adrenopituitary hormones, and of some of the peptide fragments of the full molecule of adrenocorticotropic hormone (ACTH), which will need to be incorporated into any complete account of the action of these compounds.

The prediction which we first disproved (21, 25) was that ACTH would increase the behavioral effects of what Amsel (2) has called 'frustrative nonreward', i.e., the omission of reward which has previously followed an instrumental response. This prediction was based upon a general hypothesis that the behavioral effects of frustrative nonreward and those of punishment are functionally, and perhaps physiologically, identical (20, 22, 33, 36, 37) coupled with the finding (32) that exogenous ACTH increased passive avoidance behavior. The argument presented was as follows: Any treatment that increases the behavioral effects of punishment (as in a passive avoidance situation) should increase the behavioral effects of frustrative nonreward; ACTH does the former, therefore it should do the latter as well. We tested this prediction by administering the hormone to rats during extinction of an appetitively motivated running response, previously acquired under continuous food reinforcement (CR). We expected that ACTH would, by boosting the effects of nonreward, cause extinction to take place more quickly. To our surprise, the reverse happened: extinction was significantly retarded (21). ACTH, in other words, acted as though it reduced the behavioral effects of nonreward.

201

To test this possibility, we investigated the effects of ACTH in a partial reinforcement (PR) situation. It is well known that, if a rat is rewarded in the straight alley on only a proportion of trials chosen at random (PR schedule), it subsequently displays much greater resistance to extinction than control rats run for an equal number of trials but rewarded on every one of them (CR schedule). This is known as the 'partial reinforcement extinction effect' (PREE). A second phenomenon which is observed in partial reinforcement experiments occurs during acquisition: as originally described by Goodrich (19) and Haggard (29) PR animals run faster than CR animals, especially in early segments of the alley and late in training. However, the Goodrich-Haggard effect is not so robust as the PREE, and the conditions under which it occurs are still obscure. If the retardation of extinction produced by ACTH in Gray's (21) study was due to an attenuation of the behavioral effects of nonreward, we would expect that this hormone, injected during acquisition, would reduce the partial reinforcement effects. Exactly this outcome was obtained by Gray, Mayes, and Wilson (25), who were able to block both the Goodrich-Haggard effect and the PREE with ACTH administered during acquisition only. Furthermore, the pattern of change produced by the hormone in this study was consistent with the hypothesis of altered reactivity to nonreward: the influence of ACTH was limited to the group of rats exposed to the PR schedule (whose behavior came to resemble more closely that of the CR group), CR animals being unaffected by the hormone.

These experiments suggested that, far from increasing the behavioral effects of nonreward, as we had predicted from Levine and Jones' (32) experiment on passive avoidance, ACTH had the reverse effect. A possible explanation of the failure to confirm the original hypothesis was that behavioral responses to nonreward were affected by both ACTH and by ACTH-occasioned release of corticosterone, but in opposite directions, and that the outcome in any particular experiment would depend on the balance between these two effects. Such a situation has been shown to exist in another behavioral test by de Wied and his collaborators: the extinction of active avoidance in the shuttle-box is retarded by ACTH but enhanced by corticosterone (8). We determined to find out whether the effect of ACTH on resistance to extinction of appetitive responses was due to an action of this hormone itself, or to an action of the adrenal steroids released by it.

The first experiment of this type used extinction in the straight alley after continuous food reinforcement as in Gray (21), the various compounds studied being

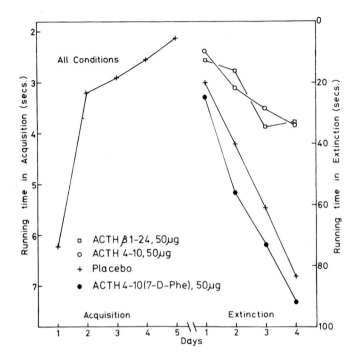

FIG. 1. Effects of ACTH 1-24, ACTH 4-10, and ACTH 4-10 (7-*d*-phe) on mean daily alley times in extinction, after continuous reinforcement in acquisition. The peptides were injected in extinction only.

injected during extinction only (17). We used ACTH 4-10, a fragment of the full ACTH molecule which has been shown to have no steroid-releasing effect but considerable behavioral potency (5, 26). As shown in Fig. 1, this had the same effect as the full ACTH molecule, i.e., it retarded extinction. Corticosterone was found to enhance extinction in the same situation (17). Thus in this situation as in shuttle-box avoidance (8), ACTH and corticosterone exert opposite influences on resistance to extinction. A further similarity between the results obtained by de Wied's group in the shuttle-box and our results emerged when we investigated the effects of ACTH 4-10 (7- *d* -phe), a compound in which the naturally occurring L-isomer of the phenylalanine at position number seven in the ACTH chain is substituted by the D-isomer. In shuttle-box avoidance this compound has been shown to produce the opposite behavioral effect to ACTH 4-10, enhancing extinction (9). We obtained analogous results when ACTH 4-10 (7- *d* -phe) was injected during extinction of the alley-running response (Fig. 1).

Two previous experiments failed to find an effect of ACTH on resistance to extinction of appetitive behavior (28, 30). In both of these experiments the hormone was administered during both acquisition and extinction. It is possible, therefore, that our results are due, not to a true effect of the hormone on extinction, but to some form of state dependency (34). This is unlikely, however, since the usual state dependency effect in positive reinforcement experiments is for resistance to extinction to be decreased. There are two possible alternative explanations of the negative findings reported by Guth, Levine, and Seward (28) and Hennessy, Cohen, and Rosen (30). First, antigenic activity may have been promoted by ACTH which differed in structure from rodent ACTH; this possibility is supported by the finding (21) that the effect of ACTH administered during extinction is blocked by one previous injection of the hormone at the start of acquisition. Second, repeated injections of ACTH in acquisition may have produced adrenal hypertrophy, and consequently an increased corticosterone secretion in response to later ACTH injection (9).

We recently followed up these findings using the partial reinforcement situation and hormone administration during acquisition only (18). The general method for the experiments was as follows: male Wistar rats were food-deprived and then trained to run in the straight alley for food reward. The training consisted of a period of pretraining (2 to 4 days) during which animals were allowed to explore the alley with food available in the goal-box. This was followed by acquisition training, consisting of eight trials a day for each animal. These trials were rewarded on a random 50% basis for the PR animals and on every trial for the CR animals. Acquisition continued until the animals were running at asymptotic speed (7 to 8 days). Extinction was then begun, except that in the two experiments using corticosterone there was a period of several days (seven in the first experiment, and three in the second) between acquisition and extinction, during which injections ceased, in order to allow the animals to recover from ill effects of continuous treatment with the propylene glycol vehicle. Extinction consisted of six nonrewarded trials a day for each animal, and was continued until half the placebo treated animals had stopped running (6 to 8 days). The various drugs tested were: 80 µg ACTH 4-10, 80 µg ACTH 4-10 (7-*d* - phe), both dissolved in saline; 1 mg corticosterone, 2.5 mg corticosterone, both made up in propylene glycol.

The drugs were given to the animals subcutaneously prior to each session of pretraining and acquisition

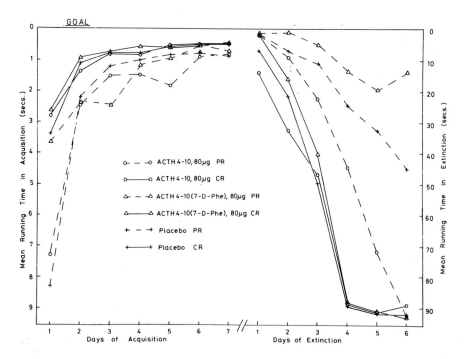

FIG. 2. Effects of ACTH 4-10 and ACTH 4-10 (7-*d*-phe) on mean daily alley times in acquisition and extinction, after continuous or partial reinforcement in acquisition. The peptides were injected in acquisition only.

(1 hr before running for the ACTH peptides; 2 hr before running for corticosterone), but no drug was given during extinction or on days between acquisition and extinction.

There were six groups in the first experiment, three CR groups and three PR groups. One CR and one PR group received ACTH 4-10, the second CR and PR groups received ACTH 4-10 (7-*d*-phe), and the third PR and CR groups received placebo (vehicle only), throughout acquisition. All the animals were injected with placebo in extinction. The results of this experiment are shown in Fig. 2. Analysis of variance showed that there was a significant interaction ($p < 0.01$) between the drug treatments, the reinforcement conditions, and days of extinction. There was virtually no effect of the two peptides on the extinction of the CR groups, but ACTH 4-10 increased the rate of extinction of PR animals and ACTH 4-10(7-*d*-phe) retarded the extinction of the PR animals. It can be seen from Fig. 2, that the placebo PR animals extinguished much more slowly than the CR placebo animals (the usual PREE), and so the effects of these two peptides can be interpreted as

ACTH 4-10 attenuating the PREE and ACTH 4-10(7-*d*-phe) enhancing it.

In the second experiment the effect of 1 mg corticosterone was examined. There were four groups of animals: corticosterone-treated CR and PR groups, and placebo-treated PR and CR groups. The substances were injected daily throughout pretraining and acquisition only, and no injections were given at all in extinction. The results of this experiment were negative. Although the placebo PR animals showed the normal slower extinction than the placebo CR animals (PREE), there was no effect of the treatment with corticosterone on the performance of either CR or PR animals.

In the third experiment, the effects of a much larger dose (2.5 mg) of corticosterone were investigated. There were four groups of animals exactly as in the second experiment. The results of this experiment again showed no effect on the PREE of the administration of corticosterone during acquisition.

This set of results gives support to the hypothesis that ACTH 4-10 attenuates the effects of frustrative nonreward, and, since no effect of corticosterone was found in these experiments, suggests that the previous finding of ACTH 1-39 blocking the PREE (25) was due to the extra-adrenal action of ACTH 4-10 and not to any increased secretion of corticosterone. The absence of any effect of corticosterone in the partial reinforcement experiments renders it unlikely that this hormone has any general effect on behavioral responses to nonreward. It is possible that the effect reported by Garrud et al. (17), namely that corticosterone administered during extinction enhanced the rate of extinction, was due, not to any specific effect of the hormone, but to the extra change in stimulus conditions between acquisition and extinction occasioned by its injection.

In these experiments ACTH 4-10(7-*d*-phe) was again found to have the opposite effect to ACTH and ACTH 4-10, enhancing the PREE. Combined with the earlier experiments on extinction after CR (17), it is reasonable to propose that this substance has the action of increasing the effects of frustrative nonreward.

It is clear from these experiments that the attenuation of the behavioral effects of nonreward originally described for ACTH 1-39 by Gray (21) and Gray et al. (25) were due to the extra-adrenal effects of this hormone. If this attenuation were part of a general reduction in sensitivity to aversive events, both frustrating and punishing, one might expect then that the increased passive avoidance found by Levine and Jones (32) with ACTH 1-39 was not due to such an extra-adrenal effect, but rather to the release of corticosterone.

This, however, is certainly not the case. Anderson et al. (3) obtained the same effect as Levine and Jones (32) in hypophysectomized animals. Furthermore, subsequent experiments have shown that passive avoidance and other punishment effects are increased by ACTH 4-10 (10, 15, 16, 25) while adrenal glucocorticosteroids have inconsistent effects (7, 14). The two sets of extra-adrenal ACTH effects present a pattern which, as far as we know, is unique. There are a considerable number of treatments that alter reactions to nonreward and punishment in the same direction, among them minor tranquilizing drugs (24), septal lesions (11, 33) and hippocampal lesions (1, 12). In contrast ACTH 4-10 appears to reduce the effects of the one, and to increase the effects of the other. This contrast caused us to re-examine the influence of both ACTH 4-10 and corticosterone on a further effect of nonreward.

We used a situation in which we could investigate responses to change of reward in favorable as well as unfavorable directions. A technique that meets this requirement has been developed by Baltzer and Weiskrantz (4); it has the advantage that adaptation to both favorable and unfavorable changes can be measured in the same individual concurrently and repeatedly. Baltzer and Weiskrantz trained rats on a variable interval schedule, for which small and large reward values were alternated from day to day, with stimulus conditions associated with each value also alternating appropriately. Within each daily session, there were two brief intrusions of the contrasting reward condition, together with its associated stimulus. They found that the response rates within each session were highly sensitive to reward value, animals responding faster in the high value sessions than in the low value sessions, and that the response rates in the intrusion periods altered according to the direction of change in reward value (increase for high value intrusions and decrease for low value intrusions). Indeed, the rates of responding in the intrusion periods were actually higher or lower than the corresponding rates of responding in the high value or low value baseline sessions. They termed these overadjustments of responding in the intrusion periods 'elation' and 'depression' effects, respectively. The present experiment differed from Baltzer and Weiskrantz's in the use of frequency rather than magnitude of reinforcement as the two reward values.

Four mildly food-deprived male Lister rats were trained in a Skinner box on variable interval (VI) 2 min (the Lo reward value) and VI 30 sec (the Hi reward value) in alternate half-hour sessions, with illumination of houselight or stimulus light respectively as

the discriminative stimuli. In each baseline session
there was one 4-min intrusion of the contrasting VI
schedule with its discriminative stimulus, during
which responding was rewarded on that schedule. After
the intrusion, the baseline condition and associated
stimulus were reinstated for the remainder of the session. There were two sessions every day. The animals
were trained until they showed a reliable and stable
difference in response rate on the two baseline schedules, and then the effects of 80 µg ACTH 4-10 and 1 mg
corticosterone were examined by chronic administration
of the drugs for ten days each, with an equal number of
placebo days prior to each drug treatment. Route and
time of injection were the same as in the alley experiments.

All animals showed a significant difference between
the two baseline response rates, and also a significant
difference between the rates of response in the baseline and in the intrusion period within each session.
When a comparison was made between rates in the Hi intrusion and Hi baseline periods of the two sessions on
the same day, it was clear that there was no overshoot
or 'elation effect' in the Hi intrusion period, response rate being very similar in both Hi intrusion and
baseline. A similar comparison between rates in the Lo
intrusion and the Lo baseline periods of the same day's
sessions showed, however, that there was a significant
undershoot or 'depression effect' in the Lo intrusion
period, response rate being much lower in the Lo intrusion than the baseline. These comparisons are called
in 'between-session intrusion effects.' Figure 3 shows
the results of treatment with ACTH 4-10 and corticosterone on these between-session intrusion effects.

The principal effect of ACTH 4-10 was to reduce the
between-session intrusion effect for both the Hi and Lo
intrusions; i.e., ACTH 4-10 interfered with the alteration in response rate that the subjects normally showed
when reward conditions changed within a session. ACTH
4-10 treatment also increased the difference between
the baseline response rates on the Hi and Lo baselines.
Treatment with corticosterone did not have such striking effects on the behavioral reactions shown in the
intrusion periods. No change was produced by this
treatment in the between-session Hi intrusion effect,
and although there was an overall increase in the between-session Lo intrusion effect, it was not consistent between subjects, one subject showing a slight decrease and the other three subjects an increase in the
effect. Corticosterone treatment did, however, reduce
the difference in response rate between the two baseline reward conditions, the opposite effect to ACTH 4-
10.

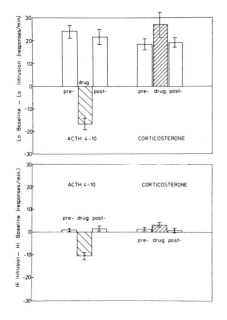

FIG. 3. Effects of 80 µg ACTH 4-10 and 1 mg corticosterone on between-session intrusion effects. Hi intrusion effect is measured as *Hi intrusion response rate - Hi baseline response rate*; Lo intrusion effect is measured as *Lo baseline response rate - Lo intrusion response rate*. *Upper panel, Lo intrusion effect. Lower panel, Hi intrusion effect.*

This final experiment shows once again that ACTH 4-10 impairs the behavioral reaction to reduction in reward, a reduction this time to a non-zero value. Furthermore, this impairment is not due to a failure to discriminate either the reinforcement schedules or the discriminative stimuli which were associated with them, since the peptide actually enhanced the difference between the two baseline response rates. However, ACTH 4-10 also impaired the behavioral response to increase in reward. Thus these results raise the possibility that the effects of this peptide on reactions to non-reward are part of a more general change in the ability of an animal to alter its behavior in response to unpredictable changes in reinforcement contingencies. Other data suggest that unpredictability of reinforcement conditions is a necessary condition for the occurrence of such ACTH-produced impairments (6, 13, 16).

It should be noted that the changes we found in the Baltzer and Weiskrantz (4) situation are clearly performance, not learning, effects. Thus, although ACTH 4-10 may affect retention (31, 35), it also has other effects.

Although, as we have pointed out, the effects of ACTH 4-10 on behavioral responses to nonreward may not be specific to this event, it remains true that the series of experiments we have described indicate that this peptide rather consistently reduces such responses. Given the evidence (10, 16, 27) that ACTH 4-10 also enhances behavioral responses to punishment, our findings are incompatible with the hypothesis of a functional identity between punishment and nonreward (23). Indeed, in our view the behavioral effects of ACTH 4-10 constitute the most severe obstacle which this otherwise promising hypothesis has so far encountered.

ACKNOWLEDGMENTS

We would like to thank the UK Medical Research Council for financial help in carrying out this research, and the Mental Health Foundation, who supported one of us (P.G.) with a Leverhulme Research Fellowship.

The synthetic ACTH 1-24, ACTH 4-10 (Org OI 63) and ACTH 4-10 (7-*d*-phe) (Org OI 64) were generously supplied by N. V. Organon, Oss, The Netherlands.

REFERENCES

1. Altman, J., Brunner, R. L., and Bayer, S. A.   (1973):   The hippocampus and behavioral maturation. *Behav. Biol.*, 8:557-596.
2. Amsel, A.   (1962):   Frustrative nonreward in learning: Some recent history and a theoretical extension. *Psychol. Rev.*, 69:306-328.
3. Anderson, D. C., Winn, W., and Tam, T.   (1968):   Adrenocorticotrophic hormone and acquisition of a passive avoidance response: A replication and extension. *J. Comp. Physiol. Psychol.*, 66:497-499.
4. Baltzer, V., and Weiskrantz, L.   (1970):   Negative and positive behavioral contrast in the same animals. *Nature*, 228:581-582.
5. Bohus, B., and de Wied, D.   (1966):   Inhibitory and facilitatory effect of two related peptides on extinction of avoidance behavior. *Science*, 153:318-320.
6. Bohus, B., de Wied, D., and Lissak, K.   (1971):   Heart rate changes during fear extinction in rats treated with pituitary peptides or corticosteroids.   In: Proceedings of the 25th International Congress of the International Union for Physiological Science, Vol. IX, p. 72.
7. Bohus, B., Grubits, J., Kovacs, G., and Lissak, K.   (1970):   Effect of corticosteroids on passive avoidance behavior of rats. *Acta Physiol. Acad. Sci. Hung.*, 38:381-391.
8. de Wied, D.   (1966):   Opposite effects of ACTH and glucocorticosteroids on extinction of conditioned avoidance behavior. *Excerpta Medica*, 132:945-951.
9. de Wied, D.   (1969):   Effects of peptide hormones on behavior. In: *Frontiers in Neuroendocrinology*, edited by W. F. Ganong and L. Martini, pp. 97-140.   Oxford University Press, New York.
10. de Wied, D.   (1974):   Pituitary-adrenal system hormones and behavior. In: *The Neurosciences, Third Study Program*, edited by F. O. Schmitt and F. G. Worden, pp. 653-666.   MIT Press,

Cambridge, Massachusetts.

11. Dickinson, A. (1974): Response suppression and facilitation by aversive stimuli following septal lesions in rats: a review and model. *Physiol. Psychol.*, 2:444-456.

12. Douglas, R. J. (1967): The hippocampus and behavior. *Psychol. Bull.*, 67:416-442.

13. Dupont, A., Endröczi, E., and Fortier, C. (1971): Relationship of pituitary-thyroid and pituitary-adrenocortical activities to conditioned behavior in the rat. In: *Influence of Hormones on the Nervous System, Proceedings of the International Society of Psychoneuroendocrinology*, edited by D. H. Ford, pp. 19-28. S. Karger, Basel.

14. Endröczi, E. (1972): *Limbic System, Learning and Pituitary-Adrenal Function*. Akademiai Kiado, Budapest.

15. Garrud, P. (1975): Effects of lysine-8-vasopressin on punishment-induced suppression of a lever-holding response. In: *Progress in Brain Research,* Vol. 42, *Hormones, Homeostasis and the Brain,* edited by W. H. Gispen, Tj. B. van Wimersma-Greidanus, B. Bohus and D. de Wied, pp. 173-186. Elsevier, Amsterdam.

16. Garrud, P. (1976): *A Behavioral Analysis of the Effects of Pituitary-Adrenal Hormones*. Unpublished D. Phil. Thesis, Oxford University.

17. Garrud, P., Gray, J. A., and de Wied, D. (1974): Pituitary-adrenal hormones and extinction of rewarded behavior in the rat. *Physiol. Behav.*, 12:109-119.

18. Garrud, P., Gray, J. A., Rickwood, L. and Coen, C. (1977): Pituitary-adrenal hormones and effects of partial reinforcement on appetitive behaviour in the rat. *Physiol. Behav.*, 18:1-6.

19. Goodrich, K. P. (1959): Performance in different segments of an instrumental response chain as a function of reinforcement schedule. *J. Exp. Psychol.*, 57:57-63.

20. Gray, J. A. (1967): Disappointment and drugs in the rat. *Adv. Sci.*, 23:595-605.

21. Gray, J. A. (1971a): Effect of ACTH on extinction of rewarded behaviour is blocked by previous administration of ACTH. *Nature*, 229:52-54.

22. Gray, J. A. (1971b): *The Psychology of Fear and Stress,* Weidenfeld and Nicolson, London.

23. Gray, J. A. (1975): *Elements of a Two-Process Theory of Learning,* Academic Press, London.

24. Gray, J. A. (1977): Drug effects on fear and frustration: possible limbic site of action of minor tranquilizers. In: *Handbook of Psychopharmacology,* Vol. 8 edited by L. L. Iversen, S. D. Iversen and S. H. Snyder. Plenum, New York.

25. Gray, J. A., Mayes, A. R. and Wilson, M. (1971): A barbiturate-like effect of adrenocorticotrophic hormone on the partial reinforcement acquisition and extinction effects. *Neuropharmacology*, 10:223-230.

26. Greven, H. M. and de Wied, D. (1967): The active sequence in the ACTH molecule responsible for inhibition of the extinc-

tion of conditioned avoidance behavior in rats. *Eur. J. Pharmacol.*, 2:14-16.

27. Greven, H. M. and de Wied, D. (1973): The influence of peptides derived from corticotrophin (ACTH) on performance. In: *Drug Effects on Neuroendocrine Regulation, Progress in Brain Research,* Vol. 39, edited by E. Zimmerman, W. H. Gispen, B. H. Marks and D. de Wied, pp. 429-444. Elsevier, Amsterdam.

28. Guth, S., Levine, S., and Seward, J. P. (1971): Appetitive acquisition and extinction effects with exogenous ACTH. *Physiol. Behav.*, 7:195-200.

29. Haggard, D. F. (1959): Acquisition of a simple running response as a function of partial and continuous schedules of reinforcement. *Psycholog. Rep.*, 9:11-18.

30. Hennessy, J. W., Cohen, M. E., and Rosen, A. J. (1973): Adrenocortical influences upon the extinction of an appetitive runway response. *Physiol. Behav.*, 11:767-770.

31. Keyes, J. B. (1974): Effect of ACTH on ECS-produced amnesia of a passive avoidance task. *Physiol. Psychol.*, 2:307-309.

32. Levine, S., and Jones, L. E. (1965): Adrenocorticotropic hormone (ACTH) and passive avoidance learning. *J. Comp. Physiol. Psychol.*, 59:357-360.

33. McCleary, R. A. (1966): Response-modulating functions of the limbic system: initiation and suppression. In: *Progress in Physiological Psychology,* Vol. 1, edited by E. Stellar and J. M. Sprague, pp. 209-272. Academic Press, New York.

34. Overton, D. A. (1966): State-dependent learning produced by depressant and atropine-like drugs. *Psychopharmacologia*, 10:6-31.

35. Rigter, H., Elbertse, R., and van Riezen, H. (1975): Time-dependent anti-amnesic effect of ACTH 4-10 and desglycinamide-lysine vasopressin. In: *Hormones, Homeostasis and the Brain, Progress in Brain Research,* Vol. 42, edited by W. H. Gispen, Tj. B. van Wimersma Greidanus, B. Bohus and D. de Wied, pp. 163-171. Elsevier, Amsterdam.

36. Wagner, A. R. (1966): Frustration and punishment. In: *Current Research on Motivation,* edited by R. M. Haber, pp. 229-239. Holt, Rinehart and Winston, New York.

37. Wagner, A. R. (1969): Frustrative nonreward: A variety of punishment? In: *Punishment and Aversive Behavior,* edited by B. A. Campbell and R. M. Church, pp. 157-181. Appleton-Century-Crofts, New York.

Neuropeptide Influences on the Brain and Behavior, edited by L.H. Miller, C.A. Sandman, and A.J. Kastin. Raven Press, New York © 1977.

Peptides and Protocritic Processes

Karl H. Pribram

Department of Psychology, Stanford University, Stanford, California 94305

INTRODUCTION

The organizers approached this conference with a unique proposal. They have asked some of us who are ignorant of the wealth of research findings on the role of brain peptides in behavior to comment on that wealth. I seized this opportunity to learn and find out just what is known. After reviewing the chapters I experienced an unusual postprandial satisfaction. Part of this satisfaction is due to a decision reached in the reading. Two modes of review were open to me: One, to have tried to organize the material to be reviewed on its own merits, or two, to try to integrate the peptide results into the frame of theory already developed on the basis of other data, especially those from my own laboratory. I chose the integrative approach as being the richer, but realized the difficulties of exposition which then had to be faced. For it must be made clear that I did not approach the peptide data with any view toward forcing them to the frame. Rather, the data evoked their own clear organization, an organization which paralleled that obtained from the other research data.

The frame of the theory regards what I have called protocritic processes. The term is derived from Head (35) who, on the basis of experiments in which he severed his own peripheral nerves and studied his sensations as regeneration occurred, discerned two modes of feeling: an epicritic and a protopathic. Epicritic sensations carried local sign i.e., they allowed the stimulus to be referred to a point in space-time. By contrast, protopathic feelings, which occurred while the nerves were regenerating and before they had reestablished their normal spectrum of fiber-sizes, globally reflected the intensive dimension of the stimulus.

213

In Head's experiments these protopathic sensations were clearly linked to pathology-the cut nerves. Subsequent research, however, showed that two classes of nerve fibers, distinguishable by their fiber size were responsible for the two types of sensation: a large diameter system with a fast conduction rate mediates epicritic processes, while a set of small fibers is responsible for protopathic sensations (26).

Much of this research has dealt with pain and discomfort. Recently, the relationship between epicritic and protopathic processes has been viewed as somewhat more complex than just two parallel systems. Melzak and Wall (53) have proposed that epicritic processes act as a "gate" on the protopathic-i.e., when there is sufficient organization of input in space-time, protopathic sensations are eliminated.

Once the gate theory had been forwarded a further complication became apparent. In tracing the ventral spinothalamic tract-the severing of which abolished pain (85)-cephalad, only about one-third of the fibers reached the ventrobasal thalamus and parietal cortex. The other two-thirds of the fibers disappeared along the way, many of them ending in core brainstem structures such as the periaqueductal gray and medial thalamus (44).

These anatomical data were supplemented by the results of psychosurgical procedures undertaken to assuage pain and distress. Parietal cortex resections helped little while frontal leukotomies did (93) and frontal cortex received its input from the medial thalamus (67, 69). What then, might be the relationship at the thalamic level between epicritic and protopathic processes? Could a ventrobasal-parietal (or, as Mountcastle suggested some years ago [54], a closely related posterior thalamic-posterior parietal system) act as a gate on the more medially placed corebrain-frontal system? And perhaps vice versa?

PAIN AND TEMPERATURE

These questions would remain unanswered as long as we knew little about the corebrain-frontal mechanism involved in the protopathic process. However, to study pain in the animal experimental laboratory is difficult. Threshold studies can of course be done readily, but the organism's behavioral response to aversive stimulation is primarily one of escape and avoidance-and these measures entail such other factors as level of activity, memory, conflict, etc., which, as the reports presented at this conference make clear, pose problems of analysis for the experimenter.

In order to circumvent some of these problems, I
searched for another sensory modality closely related
to pain, that would not bring with it these disadvan-
tages.

In the spinal cord, the pathways for pain and temperature appear to be inseparable. The temperature
sense thus suggested itself as an obvious candidate for
exploration. Further, just as in the case of pain, parietal lobe excisions had failed to influence temperature discrimination in a host of studies (17). Perhaps
the cortical involvement in temperature, as in pain, is
frontal rather than parietal.

An experiment was performed in which temperature
discrimination was disrupted by electrical stimulation
of the posterior orbital surface of the frontal lobe,
the amygdala and the stria terminalis (11). Parietal
lobe stimulations had no such effect. These results
suggest that a neural system based on the pain and temperature modalities may remain separate not only in the
spinal cord but through the brainstem and into the forebrain. The orbital locus of the rostral terminus of
the system is not far removed from the site of the temperature regulating mechanism in the anterior hypothalamus; it should not be altogether surprising to find
the regulatory and discriminative functions adjacent to
one another.

In the brainstem and diencephalon the sites from
which pain (aversive response) can be obtained are adjacent and often intermingled with those from which
positive reinforcement due to electrical self-stimula-
tion is elicited. Further, as is now well-known, electrical stimulation of many of these sites with low frequency (10 to 20 hz) currents produce analgesia (47,
48) and when such stimulations are performed in man
sensations of cooling accompany the analgesia (78).

These data suggest the hypothesis of a neural sys-
tem-or set of systems-based on the pain and temperature
senses-that deal with the hedonic dimension (distress-
comfort). As noted earlier, the term protocritic
(rather than protopathic since discrimination not pathology is critical) distinguishes these systems from
the epicritic which deal with organism-environment relationships in space-time (58, 63).

THE AMYGDALA

The central locus of the effect of electrical stimulation on temperature discrimination is the amygdala.
(The other two effective sites, the oribital cortex and
stria terminalis are respectively the source of a heavy
input to the amygdala and serve its output.) The amygdala, classically classified as a basal ganglion and

more recently as a part of the limbic forebrain, has
over the past 30 years received considerable attention
from the neuroscientific community (see 19). In addition to influencing temperature regulation (82) and
discrimination (11), the amygdala has been implicated
in a complex of behaviors initially brought together
under a rubic "the four F's"-Feeding, Fighting, Flee-
ing, and Sex (57, 59, 66, 75). The involvement of
amygdala function was then further extended to encom-
pass a variety of problem solving behaviors related to
reinforcement (83), stimulus equivalence (4, 36, 37,
84), delayed alternation (71), the orienting reaction
(1, 3), and classical conditioning (2).

These apparently disparate behaviors can be shown
by careful analysis to be influenced by a common mechanism (28, 60, 64, 72). It is worth summarizing the
highlight of this analysis because identifying a common mechanism operating on apparently disparate behaviors is a recurring problem in neuroscience as it is in
genetics (where it involves identifying genotype from
phenotypical behaviors).

With regard to feeding, the amygdala has been shown
to be a modulator of the satiety mechanism centered in
the ventromedial region of the hypothalamus. First,
it was noted that the increased feeding of amygdalectomized subjects was due to their failure to *stop* eating
as readily as their controls (24). Then, a very precise relationship was established between the amounts
of carbachol injected and amount of feeding (or drinking) once they had been initiated (33, 80).

This modulation of a *stop* mechanism was also shown
responsible for changes in fighting behavior. Fall in
a dominance hierarchy after amygdalectomy was, when it
occurred, related to the amount of aggressive interaction between the dominant and submissive animals of the
group. After amygdalectomy such interactions were
overly prolonged leading to a reorganization of the
dominance hierarchy (81). It was as if the amygdalectomized monkeys approached each interaction as novel.
Prior experience which modulated the behavior of the
control subjects seemed to have little influence after
amygdalectomy. We shall have occasion to return to
this finding repeatedly.

Analyses of the effects of amygdalectomy and electrical stimulations of the amygdala on avoidance (flee-
ing) behavior have come to a similar conclusion. Escape behavior is unaffected (59, 75) and sensitivity to
shock is not diminished (5). Nor is there a change in
generalization gradient to aversive stimulation (36,
37). What appears to be affected primarily is the mne-
monic aspect of avoidance-the expectation that aversive
stimulation will occur unless the behavior is *stopped*.

Such expectations are ordinarily referred to as "fear" but it must be clearly kept in mind that what distinguishes fear from pain (i.e., avoidance from escape) is an expectancy that stops the behavior from occurring.

The theme recurs when the effects of amygdalectomy on sexual behavior are analyzed. Hypersexuality is found to be not so much a quantitative increase in sexual behavior but an increased territory and range of situations over which the behavior is manifest (25, 57). Ordinarily cats *stop* such behavior in unfamiliar territory.

The gap between the involvement of amygdala function on the Four F's and on problem solving behavior is clearly not as great as it initially seemed. A pertinent example that has been detailed is that of so called passive avoidance which sets up a conflict between approach and avoidance behavior. After amygdalectomy animals fail to *stop* their approach on the basis of an aversive experience. Such conflict is, however, not limited to situations that involve aversive reinforcement. Approach-approach conflicts such as occur in delayed alternation partake of the same sorts of processes. Therefore, we tested amygdalectomized subjects on various forms of alternation tasks and found the monkeys with lesions to be impaired (71). Once again, the function of the amygdala is not limited to the aversive domain but rather extends wherever immediately current behavior involves *stopping* prior ongoing behavior.

The finding that the amygdala is involved in *stopping* ongoing behavior led to a series of studies on its role in the orienting reaction. This series of studies clearly showed that the visceroautonomic components of orienting were markedly affected by amygdalectomy and that the habituation of orienting was dependent on the occurrence of these visceroautonomic responses. Behavioral habituation, the indicator of familiarity, occurs in part, therefore, as a result of visceroautonomic activity. What is oriented to the novel, is a function of the familiar, the expected, on the basis of prior experience. However, the prior episode must have included a visceroautonomic reaction to be effectively experienced.

It is, of course, clear from a host of other studies relating brain and behavior, that all memory processes do not critically depend on the occurrence of visceroautonomic responses. The learning of motor skills, perceptual differentiation, rote memorization, etc. are examples where the memory mechanism operates more on the basis of simple repetition (see 61, 62 for review). Still, it is equally clear that there are occasions when memory is dependent on a "booster" that

stops ongoing behavior and derives from the importance
(novel, intense, distressing, or hedonic) of the situation to the organism. It is this booster type of
memory process in which the amygdala is involved.

AROUSAL, ACTIVATION, THE HYPOTHALAMUS
AND BASAL GANGLIA

A precise operational definition of this involvement
can be given (72). This definition is based on the
studies of visceroautonomic indicators. Such studies
show that amygdalectomy influences the phasic components of the indicators rather than their tonic components. The term "arousal" is commonly used to describe
the organism's phasic, i.e., brief response to input as
in the orienting reaction, in alerting when expectations are disconfirmed etc.

The advantage of defining arousal precisely comes
when it is distinguished from other similar processes
with which it is ordinarily confounded. Confusion occurs most often when the phasic and tonic reactions of
organisms are lumped together. Elsewhere (72) we have
reviewed in detail the evidence that tonic visceroautonomic reactions are regulated by the brain mechanisms
that control the organism's readiness to respond, mechanisms which center on the basal ganglia (caudate nucleus and putamen) of the forebrain. We can therefore
clearly separate, both on the basis of peripheral indicators and the brain mechanisms involved, the process
of phasic arousal from that of tonic activation. Arousal is a function of a set of neural systems whose forebrain extension is the amygdala; activation is a function of a set of neural systems whose forebrain extensions are the basal ganglia.

The basal ganglia of the forebrain have, until recently, been thought of primarily as regulators of muscle tone. There is now a body of evidence which shows
that the basal ganglia also control sensory input (60,
61, 62). This finding is not altogether disparate to
the motor control functions of the basal ganglia since
these are to a large extent affected by changes in the
bias of muscle spindles, receptors that reflexly regulate muscle contraction by way of feedback.

We are now in a position to take up another experimental result which has posed explanatory difficulties
for decades. When lesions are made in the region of
the ventromedial nucleus of the hypothalamus, rats
overeat and become obese. As noted earlier, this finding led to a series of experimental results that indicated that the ventromedial hypothalamus is a critical
part of a "satiety" mechanism. Before these results
were available, however, it was also shown that these

same rats would eat less than their controls and might
even starve if an easily surmountable barrier were
placed between them and the food. The initiation of
behavior and its maintenance (stop mechanism) were
dissociated. Other experiments showed that the initiation of feeding was controlled by a mechanism centered
on the far-lateral region of the hypothalamus, a region
devoid of neurons but rich in fiber tracts (60, 90).
Recently, the far-lateral hypothalamic syndrome has
been replicated by administering drugs that inhibit the
formation of dopamine, the putative transmitter that
characterizes the nigrostriatal basal ganglia system.

Further, it was found that excitation of the ventromedial region of the hypothalamus not only stopped eating behavior but led to the stopping of other behavior.
Alerting, escape, and attack could be elicited depending on the strength of stimulation. These findings led
Grossman (34) to suggest that the ventromedial hypothalamus is involved in regulating "affect" not "appetite." Affect in this instance is defined on the basis
of phasic reactions to input and thus fits the definition of arousal already presented (60).

In summary, the experimental evidence falls into
place when it is grouped on the one hand, according to
a phasic, stop, satiety mechanism which regulates arousal; and, on the other, a tonic, start, appetitive readiness mechanism that regulates sensory and motor activation. Arousal is controlled by a neural system that
includes the ventromedial hypothalamus and amygdala.
Activation is controlled by the basal ganglia-in particular the nigrostriatal system whose pathways course
through the far-lateral hypothalamic region.

EFFORT AND THE HIPPOCAMPUS

In addition to phasic arousal and tonic activation,
a third process has been distinguished by psychophysiological analysis. This third process is also tonic but
differs from the activation of readiness in that the
visceroautonomic indicators are influenced in an opposite direction. Thus, during readiness heart rate de-
celerates while acceleration accompanies this third
process which we have called "effort." Other terms
that are used are chronic arousal, anxiety, and reaction to stress. Again, a detailed review and analysis
of the relevant neurobehavioral and psychophysiological
evidence has been performed (72) with the result that
the hippocampus has been shown central to the neural
systems involved in regulating "effort." In this review, effort was shown to be necessary to coordinate
phasic arousal and tonic readiness in situations that
invoke both processes—such as discrimination reversal

(70), alternation (76), problem-solving under distraction (18), and when reasoning depends on computable variations in the situation (14, 15, 87). A good deal is also known about how the hippocampus performs this coordinating function (70).

SOME NEUROCHEMICAL PRELIMINARIES

This has been a brief overview of the methods and results of some 30 years of neurobehavioral research. The relationship of the analysis to the problems of this conference is evident: Currently, a body of data has accumulated relating a variety of brain peptides, many of them derivatives of ACTH, to a variety of behaviors. Interestingly, the behaviors that have become involved in brain peptide research are to a large extent the same as those involved initially in amygdala research and then shown to be dependent on hypothalamic, basal ganglia, and hippocampal function as well. Thus the neural organization of the mechanisms of arousal, activation, and effort delineated by neurobehavioral and psychophysiological techniques may well be relevant to the analysis of the relationship between neurochemical and behavioral processes.

Perhaps the easiest place to start is the by now well established and dramatic finding of a dopaminergic nigrostriatal system (23, 91) which has already been discussed. The evidence has repeatedly been reviewed to the effect that dopamine is involved in the maintenance of postural readiness and motivational activation (50, 86). It is also known (e.g., King and Hoebel [43]) that assertive behavior such as predatory aggression depends on the activation of a cholinergic mechanism. Thus, it is likely that the dopamine fibers interdigitate a cholinergic matrix (25) to determine the activation level of the nervous system and the readiness of the organism.

Two other by now well known neurochemical systems are those involving serotonin and norepinephrine. A large amount of research (e.g., reviews by Jouvet [42]; Barchas et al. [6]) has related these substances to the phases of sleep-serotonin to ordinary (slow-wave) sleep and norepinephrine to paradoxical (rapid-eye-movement) sleep during which much dreaming occurs. The relationship between serotonergic and norepinephrinergic mechanisms and the amygdala, seems to be similar to that between acetylcholine (ACh) and dopamine, and the striatum of the basal ganglia. Serotonergic and norepinephrinergic systems of fibers densely innervate the amygdala, the norepinephrinergic interdigitating a serotonergic matrix (see Pribram and Isaacson [70] for review).

The regulation of sleep by the amygdala has not been quantitatively documented but sleep disturbances are commonplace immediately following amygdalectomy, the animals often falling into a torpor from which they are difficult to rouse for several days to several weeks.

However, norepinephrine has been related to a behavioral function in which the amygdala is thoroughly implicated-the effects of reinforcing events (88). Norepinephrine has also been related to orienting and affective agonistic reactions. Once again a phasic response to novelty-sensed against a background of familiarity—is norepinephrinergic, whereas "familiarity" in the guise of "territoriality" and "isolation" has been shown to some extent to be dependent on a serotonergic mechanism (see reviews by Reis [77]; and Goldstein [29]).

These data suggest that norepinephrine acts by modulating a serotonergic substrate (which is determining one or another basic condition of the organism) to produce paradoxical sleep, reinforcement, orienting to novelty and perhaps other behaviorally relevant neural events that interrupt an ongoing state. The data are not as clearly supportive of this suggestion as those that relate ACh to an assertive state that becomes modulated by the activity of dopamine to produce specific readinesses. Nonetheless, as a first approximation to the data at hand, let us hold these possible neurochemical relations in mind as a tentative model with which to analyze the mass of evidence on the behavioral neurochemistry of the polypeptides.

NEUROPEPTIDES AND THE EFFORT MECHANISM

The neurochemical evidence on ACTH related peptides leads directly to the hypothesis that they are involved in the hippocampal mechanism. To begin with, Bohus (7) and McEwen et al. (52) have shown that the hippocampal circuit (Hippocampus and septum) is the brain site most involved in the selective uptake of adrenal cortical steroids. As McEwen states:

> It is only quite recently that we have come to appreciate the role of the entire limbic brain, and not just the hypothalamus, in these endocrine-brain interactions.
> Our own involvement in this revelation arose from studies of the fate of injected radioactive adrenal steroids, particularly corticosterone, when they entered the brain from the blood. These studies were begun, under the impetus of recent advances in molecular biology of steroid hormone action, to look for intracellular hormone receptors in brain

tissue. We expected to find such putative receptors in the hypothalamus, where effects of adrenal
steroids on ACTH secretion have been demonstrated
(12, 32). Much to our surprise, the brain region
which binds the most corticosterone is not the hypothalamus but the hippocampus. (52)

Thus the receptors of adrenal cortical hormones can
set the neural state which becomes modulated by ACTH
related peptides. Evidence that such modulation of a
corticosterone determined state involves the hippocampus has been presented in this volume by van Wimersma
Greidanus and de Wied.

Second, as noted in the review by Pribram and Mc-
Guinness (72), the hippocampal circuit functions to coordinate arousal (phasic response to input) and activation (tonic readiness to respond). Thus, in any complex behavioral situation, coordination would be influenced by manipulations of this circuit-and a host of
apparently conflicting results might be obtained with
very slight changes in the conditions of the experiment. (The best known of such slight changes is the
one-way versus two-way conditioned avoidance task (see
Pribram et al. [71]; and van Wimersma Greidanus and de
Wied [92]).

Further, effects on phasic and tonic processes
(arousal and activation) as well as on their coordination (effort) would be expected. This expectation is
borne out in the catalogue of effects of manipulations
of ACTH related peptides: extinction of two-way but not
one-way avoidance (13) interference with passive avoidance (45), interference with learned taste avoidance
(the Garcia effect-Levine [46]), interference with discrimination reversal (81), facilitation of memory consolidation (92), facilitation of exploratory behavior
and conditioning (20).

Just as in the case of manipulations of hippocampal
activity, *ongoing* behavioral activity (memory consolidation, exploratory behavior) is facilitated while any
change in behavior (two-way shuttle, passive avoidance,
learned taste aversion, discrimination reversal) is
interfered with. This appears initially as tilting the
bias toward readiness. But as Pribram and Isaacson (70)
show for hippocampal function, and Sandman's group conclude in their various contributions to this conference,
such an interpretation does not hold up. In the case
of hippocampal research, the initial formulation stated
that after hippocampal resections, animals could not
inhibit their responses (51). This interpretation
foundered when such animals were shown to perform well
in go/no-go alternation tasks (49, 70) and that they
could withhold behavioral responses despite an increase

in reaction time when distractors were presented (16).
The most cogent analysis has been performed on discrimination reversals. Isaacson et al. (40) and Nonneman and Isaacson (56) have shown that reversal learning
encompasses three stages: Extinction of the previously
correct response, reversion to a position habit, and
acquisition of the currently correct response. Pribram,
Douglas, and Pribram (68) and Spevak and Pribram (87)
have shown that hippocampally lesioned monkeys are intact with regard to both the extinction and the new acquisition phases of the reversal training experience.
However, such monkeys seem to become "stuck" in the 50%
reinforcement phase or in position response patterns.
In short, the monkeys' behavior seems to be taken over
by a relatively low variable interval schedule of reinforcement and they fail to "make the effort" to "pay
attention" to the cues which would gain them a higher
rate of reward. Champney et al. (10) have shown ACTH
related peptides to operate on just this aspect of the
reversal experience-and, in fact, have shown interactions with sex differences.

Evidence such as this makes highly plausible the
hypothesis that ACTH related peptides operate on the
hippocampal circuit and therefore the "effort" process.
But there is more. Strand et al. (89) present direct
evidence that muscle fatigue is reduced by ACTH-related
neuropeptides and that this effect must be central.
Pribram and McGuinness (72) in their analysis review
the evidence for peripheral metabolic events that contribute to effort but could at the time show only indirect evidence for a central process devoid of peripheral concomitants (73). Strand et al.'s (89) current contribution is thus a most welcome addition.

THE PROTOCRITIC DIMENSION

The foregoing analysis and review of evidence indicates that systems of corebrain stem, basal ganglia,
and limbic forebrain structures can be discerned in
which neurochemical events determine to a large extent
the behavioral functions that are regulated by these
structures.

Regulation is in part effected by the establishment,
through central receptor sensitivities, of neural representations of peripheral endocrine processes, and by
direct influences on these representations of centrally
active neurochemical substances. Among the many relationships between endocrines and central sensitivities
some were singled out as providing sufficient evidence
that a systematization relevant to this volume might be
attempted. Others such as the possible central effect
of insulin, the special sensitivity of the amygdala to

sex hormones were not included although they cannot be
ignored in any future attempt at synthesis.

At the moment three classes of systems are discern-
ible. One class determines specific neuromuscular and
neurosensory readinesses. A second deals with the momentary cessations of ongoing behavior, cessations due
to interrupting distractors, the intervention of satiety or the recurrence of reinforcing events. The third
class of systems coordinates the readinesses of the
organism with the processes that lead to their momentary suspension.

The proposal was made that states of specific readiness were due to a cholinergic mechanism operated upon,
i.e., modulated by, dopaminergic systems. The basal
ganglia are the major gross forebrain embodiments of
readiness mechanism.

The gross forebrain locus upon which the systems
that deal with momentary cessation of behavior converge
is the amygdala. Neurochemically, these systems are
posited to be basically serotonergic with norepinephrinergic operators modulating the basic serotonergic
state.

Finally, a coordinating mechanism was discerned
whose forebrain extension lies within the hippocampal
circuit. The neurochemical constitution of this class
of systems is hormonal with neuropeptides operating on
the hormonally induced neural state to regulate behavior. Corticosteroids and ACTH related neuropeptides
are examples of the functions of this third class of
systems.

In conclusion, I would like to venture that the protocritic process-the brain organization of the pain-
temperature dimension of experience-is central to these
three classes of systems. As first proposed by Brobeck
(9) and reviewed in detail by Grossman (33) temperature
regulation anchors muscular tonicity, water metabolism,
and food intake. As reported by Feldberg and Myers (22)
and elaborated more recently by Myers (55), *two* recip-
rocal hypothalamic neurochemical mechanisms can be discerned as controlling these functions. One is a sero-
tonin-norepinephrine mechanism (serotonin elevates and
norepinephrine lowers temperature) and the other is an
ACh-dopamine mechanism (ACh elevates and dopamine lowers temperature). ACh also induces drinking and the
catechols induce feeding. Thus, once again, the "arousal" and "activation" systems can be separately identified. However, according to the proposal made here
norepinephrine should operate on the satiety mechanism
in the ventromedial hypothalamus. So far, the evidence
is not clear whether the increased food intake resulting from hypothalamically injected norepinephrine does
in fact result from such action. Amphetamines, usually

found to stimulate norepinephrine receptor sites in the brainstem (8) decrease appetite.

At a higher level of control are the coordinating (effort) mechanisms that utilize hormones and neuropeptides to organize behavior dependent on the smooth interaction of tonically activated sensory and motor readinesses and episodic (phasic) arousals to internal and external inputs.

The role of pain in these sets of hierarchies of controls is just beginning to be established. The discovery of a morphine-like neurosecretion (eukephalin) by Hughes (38, 39), makes it plausible to treat the regulation of pain (and itch) in homeostatic terms (see 58, 63). Further, the evidence presented by Gispen et al. (27), that ACTH and some of the related neuropeptides could serve as endogenous ligands on opiate receptors provides an initial suggestion that the pain-analgesia (effort-comfort) process may function at the coordinating (hippocampal) level of the hierarchy of controls.

POSTSCRIPT

As a postscript, I will summarize the relationship of neuropeptides to emotion. On earlier occasions I have identified emotional processes as rooted in the phasic arousal mechanisms discussed here (60, 65, 74, 94) and distinguished them from motivational processes rooted in the readiness mechanisms. The classification of arousal, activation, and effort mechanisms was developed in order to understand the effects of brain operations and recordings on attentional and intentional behavior (72). And the relationship of attention and intention to learning and remembering has been reviewed as well (58, 63). Thus the neurochemical analysis undertaken here is relevant to the topic assigned. The analysis would predict that neuropeptides would be only indirectly involved in the regulation of emotion (affect) and motivation. Only when emotional and motivational processes need be coordinated would neuropeptide manipulations show an effect. The reports presented at the conference bear out this prediction. Emotion and affect are found minimally influenced by ACTH related compounds in man (18). Conflict producing tasks such as passive avoidance (45), learned taste aversion (46), two-way shuttles (13, 92), and frustrative non-reward (31) are the instruments of choice for demonstrating the effects of neuropeptides. One-way shuttles and simple punishments show either no effect or a mild facilitation of the reinforcing process.

As in the case of emotion and motivation, the effects of neuropeptides on learning and memory consolidation appear to be secondary to their coordinating role. This is brought out most clearly in the myriad of neurochemical effects of neuropeptide manipulation described in the papers dealing with these topics in this volume.

My conclusion is, therefore, that brain peptides regulate those "protocritic" processes that serve primarily to coordinate phasic arousal and tonic activation. Emotional, motivational, learning and memory processes are influenced only secondarily by neuropeptides when coordination between phasic arousal and activation is demanded. The function of the neuropeptides appears to be primarily manifest in the behavioral processes of attention and intention (decision) and in brain systems whose forebrain extension is the hippocampal circuit.

REFERENCES

1. Bagshaw, M. H. and Benzies, S. (1968): Multiple measures of the orienting reaction and their dissociation after amygdalectomy in monkeys. *Exp. Neurol.*, 20:175-187.
2. Bagshaw, M. H. and Coppock, H. W. (1968): Galvanic skin response conditioning deficit in amygdalectomized monkeys. *Exp. Neurol.*, 20:188-196.
3. Bagshaw, M. H., Kimble, D. P., and Pribram, K. H. (1965): The GSR of monkeys during orienting and habituation and after ablation of the amygdala, hippocampus and inferotemporal cortex. *Neuropsychologia,* 3:11-119.
4. Bagshaw, M. H. and Pribram, K. H. (1965): Effect of amygdalectomy on transfer of training in monkeys. *J. Comp. Physiol. Psychol.*, 59:118-121.
5. Bagshaw, M. H. and Pribram, J. D. (1968): Effect of amygdalectomy on stimulus threshold of the monkey. *Exp. Neurol.*, 20:197-202.
6. Barchas, J. D., Ciaranello, R. D., Stolk, J. M., Brodie, H. H., and Hamburg, D. A. (1972): Biogenic amines and behavior. In: *Hormones and Behavior,* edited by S. Levine, pp. 235-329. Academic Press, New York.
7. Bohus, B. (1976): The hippocampus and the pituitary adrenal system hormones. In: *The Hippocampus,* edited by R. L. Isaacson and K. H. Pribram, pp. 323-353. Plenum Press, New York.
8. Bradley, P. B. (1968): Synaptic transmission in the central nervous system and its relevance for drug action. *Int. Rev. Neurobiol.*, 11:1.
9. Brobeck, J. R. (1948): Food intake as a mechanism of temperature regulation. *Yale J. Biol. Med.*, 20:545-552.
10. Champney, T. F., Sahley, T. L., and Sandman, C. A. (1976): Effects of neonatal cerebral ventricular injection of ACTH 4-9 and subsequent adult injections on learning in male and female albino rats. *Pharmacol. Biochem. Behav. (Suppl.),* 5:3-10.

11. Chin, J. H., Pribram, K. H., Drake, K. and Green, L. O. (1976): Disruption of temperature discrimination during limbic forebrain stimulation in monkeys. *Neuropsychologia,* 14: 293-310.
12. Davidson, J. M., Jones, L. E., and Levine, S. (1968): Feedback regulation of adrenocorticotropin secretion in "basal" and "stress" conditions: Acute and chronic effects of intrahypothalamic corticoid implantation. *Endocrinology,* 82:655-663.
13. de Wied, D. Pituitary-adrenal system hormones and behavior. (1974): In *The Neurosciences III,* edited by F. O. Schmitt and E. G. Worden, pp. 653-660. M.I.T. Press, Cambridge.
14. Douglas, R. J., Barrett, T. W., Pribram, K. H., and Cerny, M. C. (1969): Limbic lesions and error reduction. *J. Comp. Physiol. Psychol.,* 68:437-441.
15. Douglas, R. J. and Pribram, K. H. (1966): Learning and limbic lesions. *Neuropsychologia,* 4:197-220.
16. Douglas, R. J. and Pribram, K. H. (1969): Distraction and habituation in monkeys with limbic lesions. *J. Comp. Physiol. Psychol.,* 69:473-480.
17. Downer, J. and Zubeck, J. P. (1954): Role of the cerebral cortex in temperature discrimination in the rat. *J. Comp. Physiol. Psychol.,* 47:199-203.
18. Ehrensing, R. H. and Kastin, A. J. (1976): Clinical investigations for emotional effects of neuropeptide hormones. *Pharmacol. Biochem. Behav. (Suppl.),* 5:89-94.
19. Eleftheriou, B. E. (1972): The Neurobiology of the Amygdala, Plenum Press, New York.
20. Endröczi, E. (1976): Brain mechanisms involved in ACTH-induced changes of exploratory activity and conditioned avoidance behavior. *(This volume.)*
21. Endröczi, E. (1972): Pavlovian conditioning and adaptive hormones. In: *Hormones and Behavior,* edited by S. Levine, pp. 173-207. Academic Press, New York.
22. Feldberg, W. and Myers, R.D. (1963): A new concept of temperature regulation by amines in the hypothalamus. *Nature,* 200:1325.
23. Fibiger, H. C., Phillips, A. G., and Clouston, R. A. (1973): Regulatory deficits after unilateral electrolytic or 6-OHDA lesions of the substantia nigra. *Am. J. Physiol.,* 225: (6) 1282-1287.
24. Fuller, J. L., Rosvold, H. E., and Pribram, K. H. (1957): The effect on affective and cognitive behavior in the dog of lesions of the pyriform-amygdala-hippocampal complex. *J. Comp. Physiol. Psychol.,* 50:89-96.
25. Fuxe, E. (1977): The dopaminergic pathways. In: *Proceedings of the American Neuropathological Association. (In press.)*
26. Gasser, H. S. and Erlanger, J. (1922): *Am. J. Physiol.,* 62:496-524.
27. Gispen, W. H., Reith, M. E. A., Schotman, P., Wiegant, V. M., Zwiers, H., and de Wied, D. (1976): The CNS and ACTH-like peptides: neurochemical responses and interaction with opiates. *(This volume.)*

28. Goddard, G. V.   (1972):   Long term alteration following amygdaloid stimulation.   In: *The Neurobiology of the Amygdala*, pp.
581-596.
29. Goldstein, M.   (1974):   Brain research and violent behavior.
Arch. Neurol., 30:1-35.
30. Green, J. D., Clemente, C. D., and de Groot, J.   (1957):
Rinencephalic lesions and behavior in cats.   An analysis of
the Klüver-Bucy syndrome with particular reference to normal
and abnormal sexual behavior.   *J. Comp. Neurol.*, 108:505-545.
31. Gray, J. A. and Garrud, P.   (1977):   Adrenopituitary hormones
and frustrative nonreward.   *(This volume.)*
32. Grimm, Y. and Kendall, J. W.   (1968):   A study of feedback
suppression of ACTH secretion utilizing glucocorticoid implants in the hypothalamus: the comparative effects of cortisol, corticosterone and their 21 acetates.   *Neuroendocrinology*,
3:55-63.
33. Grossman, S. P.   (1967):   *A Textbook of Physiological Psychology*.   John Wiley & Sons, New York.
34. Grossman, S. P.   (1966):   The VMH: A center for affective reactions, satiety, or both?   *Physiol. Behav.*, 1:1-10.   Pergamon Press, London.
35. Head, H.   (1920):   *Studies in Neurology*, Vol. 2.   Oxford University Press, Oxford.
36. Hearst, E. and Pribram, K. H.   (1964a):   Facilitation of
avoidance behavior by unavoidable shocks in normal and amygdalectomized monkeys.   *Psychol. Rep.*, 14:39-42.
37. Hearst, E. and Pribram, K. H.   (1964b):   Appetitive and aversive generalization gradients in amygdalectomized monkeys.   *J.
Comp. Physiol. Psychol.*, 58:296-298.
38. Hughes, T.   (1975):   Isolation of an endogenous compound from
the brain with pharmacological properties similar to morphine.
Brain Res., 88:295-308.
39. Hughes, T., Smith, T. W., Kosterlitz, H. W., Fothergill, L.
A., Morgan, B. A., and Morris, H. R.   (1975):   Identification
of two related pentapeptides from the brain with potent opiate
activity.   *Nature*, 258:557-559.
40. Isaacson, R. L., Nonneman, A. J., and Schwartz, L. W.   (1968):
Behavioral and anatomical sequelae of the infant limbic system.   In: *The Neuropsychology of Development, A Symposium*.
John Wiley & Sons, New York.
41. Isaacson, R. L. and Pribram, K. H.   (1976):   Neurophysiology
and behavior.   *The Hippocampus*, Vol. II, edited by R. L.
Isaacson and K. H. Pribram.   Plenum Press, New York.
42. Jouvet, M.   (1974):   Monoaminergic regulation of the sleep-
waking cycle in the cat.   In: *The Neurosciences*, III, pp. 499-
508.
43. King, M. B. and Hoebel, B. G.   (1968):   Killing elicited by
brain stimulation in rats.   *Community Behav. Biol.*, (Part A),
2:173-177.
44. Kunc, Z.   (1966):   Significance of fresh anatomic data on spinal trigeminal tract for possibility of selective tractotomies.
In: *Pain. Henry Ford International Symposium*, edited by R. S.

Knight and P. R. Dumke, pp. 351-371. Churchill Livingstone, London.

45. Levine, S. and Jones, L. E. (1970): Adrenocorticotropic hormone (ACTH) and passive avoidance in two inbred strains of mice. *Horm. Behav.*, 1:105-110.

46. Levine, S., Smotherman, W. P., and Hennessy, J. W. (1976): Pituitary-adrenal hormones and learned taste aversion. *(This volume.)*

47. Liebeskind, J. C., Guilbaud, G., Benson, J. M., and Oliveras, J. L. (1973): Analgesia from electrical stimulation of the periaqueductal gray matter in the cat: behavioral observations and inhibitory effects on spinal cord interneurons. *Brain Res.*, 50:441-446.

48. Liebeskind, J. C., Mayer, D. J., and Akil, H. (1974): Central mechanisms of pain inhibition: Studies of analgesia from focal brain stimulation. In: *Advances in Neurology, Vol. 4, Pain,* edited by J. J. Bonica. Raven Press, New York.

49. Mahut, H. (1971): Spatial and object reversal learning in monkeys with partial temporal lobe ablations. *Neuropsychologia,* 9:409-424.

50. Matthysse, S. (1974): Schizophrenia: Relationship to dopamine transmission, motor control, and feature extraction. In: *The Neurosciences III,* pp. 733-737.

51. McCleary, R. A. (1961): Response specificity in the behavioral effects of limbic system lesions in the cat. *J. Comp. Physiol. Psychol.,* 54:605-613.

52. McEwen, B. S., Gerlach, J. L., and Micco, D. J. (1976): Putative glucocorticoid receptors in hippocampus and other regions of the rat brain. In: *The Hippocampus,* edited by R. L. Isaacson and K. H. Pribram, pp. 285-322. Plenum Press, New York.

53. Melzack, R. and Wall, P. D. (1965): Pain mechanisms: A new theory. *Science,* 50:971-979.

54. Mountcastle, V. B., Poggio, G. F., and Werner, G. (1963): The relation of thalamic cell response to peripheral stimuli varied over an intensive continuum. *J. Neurophysiol.,* 26:807-834.

55. Myers, R. D. (1969): Temperature regulation: Neurochemical systems in the hypothalamus. In: *The Hypothalamus,* edited by W. Haymaker, E. Anderson, and W. J. H. Nauta, pp. 506-523. Charles C. Thomas, Springfield, Illinois.

56. Nonneman, A. J. and Isaacson, R. L. (1973): Task dependent recovery after early brain damage. *Behav. Biol.,* 8:143-172.

57. Pribram, K. H. (1960): A review of theory in physiological psychology. In: *Annual Review of Psychology,* Palo Alto Annual Reviews, Inc., pp. 1-40.

58. Pribram, K. H. (1976): Closing remarks on mind it does matter. In *Philosophical Dimensions of the Neuro-Medical Sciences,* edited by S. F. Spicker and H. T. Engelhardt, Jr., pp. 246-252.

59. Pribram, K. H. (1954): Concerning three rhinencephalic systems. *EEG Clin. Neurophysiol.,* 6:708-709.

60. Pribram, K. H. (1971): *Languages of the Brain: Experimental*

Paradoxes and Principles in Neuropsychology. Prentice-Hall, Englewood Cliffs, New Jersey.

61. Pribram, K. H. (1977): Modes of central processing in human learning. In: *Brain and Learning,* edited by Timothy Teyler, Greylock. *(In press.)*

62. Pribram, K. H. (1977): New dimensions in the functions of the basal ganglia. *Proc. Am. Psychopathol. Assoc. (In press.)*

63. Pribram, K. H. (1976): Self-consciousness and intentionality. In: *Consciousness and Self-Regulation: Advances in Research.* Plenum Press, New York.

64. Pribram, K. H. (1969): The neurobehavioral analysis of limbic forebrain mechanisms: Revision and progress report. In: *Advances in the Study of Behavior,* edited by D. S. Lehrman, R. A. Hinde, and E. Shaw, pp. 297-332. Academic Press, New York.

65. Pribram, K. H. (1967): The new neurology and the biology of emotion: A structural approach. *Am. Psychol.* 22:(No. 10), 830-838.

66. Pribram, K. H. and Bagshaw, M. H. (1953): Further analysis of the temporal lobe syndrome utilizing frontotemporal ablations in monkeys. *J. Comp. Neurol.,* 99:347-375.

67. Pribram, K. H., Chow, K. L., and Semmes, J. (1953): Limit and organization of the cortical projection from the medial thalamic nucleus in monkeys. *J. Comp. Neurol.,* 98:433-448.

68. Pribram, K. H., Douglas, R., and Pribram, B. J. (1969): The nature of non-limbic learning. *J. Comp. Physiol. Psychol.,* 69:765-772.

69. Pribram, K. H. and Fulton, J. F. (1954): An experimental critique of the effects of anterior cingulate ablations in monkeys. *Brain,* 77, (No. 1):34-44.

70. Pribram, K. H. and Isaacson, R. L. (1976): *The Hippocampus Vol. II,* edited by R. L. Isaacson, and K. H. Pribram, pp. 429-441. Plenum Press, New York.

71. Pribram, K. H., Lim, H., Poppen, R., and Bagshaw, M. H. (1966): Limbic lesions and the temporal structure of redundancy. *J. Comp. Physiol. Psychol.,* 61:365-373.

72. Pribram, K. H. and McGuinness, D. (1975a): Arousal, Activation and Effort in the control of attention. *Psychol. Rev.,* 82:(2):116-149.

73. Pribram, K. H. and McGuinness, D. (1975b): Arousal, activation and effort. Separate neural systems. In: *Brain Work, Alfred Benzon Symposium VIII.* Munksgaard, pp. 428-451.

74. Pribram, K. H. and Melges, F. T. (1969): Emotion: The search for control. In: *Handbook of Clinical Neurology,* edited by P. J. Vinken and G. W. Bruyn, pp. 316-342. North Holland Publishing Co., Amsterdam.

75. Pribram, K. H. and Weiskrantz, L. (1957): A comparison of the effects of medial and lateral cerebral resections on conditioned avoidance behavior of monkeys. *J. Comp. Physiol. Psychol.,* 50:74-80.

76. Pribram, K. H., Wilson, W. A., and Connors, J. (1962): The

effects of lesions of the medial forebrain on alternation behavior of rhesus monkeys. *Exp. Neurol.*, 6:36-47.
77. Reis, D. J.   (1974):   The chemical coding of aggression in
brain.   In: *Neurohumeral Coding of Brain Function,* edited by
R. D. Myers and R. R. Drucker-Colin, pp. 125-150.
78. Richardson, D. E. and Akil, H.   (1974):   Chronic self-admin-
istration of brain stimulation for pain relief in human patients.   *Proceedings American Association of Neurological
Surgeons.*   St. Louis, Missouri.
79. Rosvold, H. E., Mirsky, A. F., and Pribram, K. H.   (1954):
Influence of amygdalectomy on social interaction in a monkey
group. *J. Comp. Physiol. Psychol.*, 47:173-178.
80. Russell, R. W., Singer, G., Flanagan, F., Stone, M., and
Russell, J. W.   (1968):   Quantitative relations in amygdala
modulation of drinking.   *Physiol. Behav.*, 3:871-875.
81. Sandman, C. A., George, J., Walker, B., Nolan, J. D., and
Kastin, A. J.   (1976):   Neuropeptide MSH/ACTH 4-10 enhances
attention in the mentally retarded.   *Pharmacol. Biochem. Behav.* (Suppl.), 5:23-28.
82. Satinoff, E.   (1974):   Neural control of thermoregulatory responses.   In: *Limbic and Autonomic Nervous System Research,*
edited by Leo V. DiCara, pp. 41-83.   Plenum Press, New York.
83. Schwartzbaum, J. S.   (1960):   Changes in reinforcing properties of stimuli following ablation of the amygdaloid complex
in monkeys. *J. Comp. Physiol. Psychol.*, 53:388-395.
84. Schwartzbaum, J. S. and Pribram, K. H.   (1960):   The effects
of amygdalectomy in monkeys on transposition along a brightness continuum. *J. Comp. Physiol. Psychol.*, 53:396-399.
85. Sjoqvist, L.   (1938):   Studies on pain conduction in the trigeminal nerve.   A contribution to the surgical treatment of
facial pain.   *Acta Psychiatr. Neurol. Scand.*, (Suppl.) 17:1-
139.
86. Snyder, S. H.   (1974):   Catecholamines as mediators of drug
effects in schizophrenia.   In: *The Neurosciences III,* 721-732.
87. Spevack, A. and Pribram, K. H.   (1973):   A decisional analysis
of the effects of limbic lesions in monkeys. *J. Comp. Physiol.
Psychol.*, 82(2):211-226.
88. Stein, L.   (1968):   Chemistry of reward and punishment.   In:
Psychopharmacology.   A Review of Progress 1957-1967, edited
by E. H. Effron, pp. 105-135.   U. S. Government Printing Office, Pub. Ser. Publ. No. 1836, Washington, D. C.
89. Strand, F. L., Cayer, A., Gonzalez, E., and Stoboy, H. (1976):
Peptide enhancement of neuromuscular function: animal and
clinical studies.   *Pharmacol. Biochem. Behav.* (Suppl.), 5:179-
188.
90. Teitelbaum, P.   (1955):   Sensory control of hypothalamic hy-
perphagia. *J. Comp. Physiol. Psychol.*, 48:156-163.
91. Ungerstedt, U.   (1974):   Brain dopamine neurons and behavior.
In: *The Neurosciences Third Study Program, III.*   pp. 695-704.
M.I.T. Press, Cambridge, Massachusetts.
92. van Wimersma Greidanus, Tj. B. and de Wied, D.   (1976):   The

dorsal hippocampus: a site of action of neuropeptides on avoidance behavior? *Pharmacol. Biochem. Behav.* (Suppl.),5: 29-34.

93. White, J. C. and Sweet, W. H.   (1969): *Pain and the Neurosurgeon. A forty year experience.* Charles C. Thomas, Springfield, Illinois.

94. Young, P. T.   (1973): *Emotion in Man and Animal: Its Nature and Dynamic Basis,* p. 479. Robert E. Krieger Publishing Company, Huntington, New York.

Neuropeptide Influences on the Brain and Behavior, edited by L.H. Miller, C.A. Sandman, and A.J. Kastin. Raven Press, New York ©1977.

Attention

Allan F. Mirsky and Merle M. Orren

Boston University School of Medicine, Laboratory of Neuropsychology, Division of Psychiatry, Boston, Massachusetts 02118

The assertion has been made in several publications (34, 35, 59) that improvement in visual attention follows administration of neuropeptides. It would therefore be useful to discuss this assertion in the context of a review of investigations from our laboratory, since the neuropsychology of attention (i.e., measurement of behavioral, electrophysiological, and anatomical factors in visual attention) has been our primary concern for approximately 20 years.

The study of attention in neuropsychology is concerned with the question of the way in which the organism makes contact with its environment; i.e., what anatomical systems, physiological, and neurophysiological events participate in the lawful and orderly regulation of behavior with respect to the multitude of stimuli present in the environment. As such, the study of attention shares a common interest with other fields of investigation, such as studies of sleep, consciousness, vigilance, and arousal (see Fig. 1). To a large extent, the distinctions implied by the numerous terms are somewhat artificial. It should not be assumed that each construct represents an independent function referable to a different part of the brain or regulated by a separate process. All such constructs are merely semantic abstractions which bridge the gap between stimulus inputs to the organism and behavioral outputs from the organism. The use of different constructs is useful however since it calls attention to the various methods by which different investigators approach the study of organism-environment interactions.

In investigations of orientation and habituation, the primary interest is in behavioral (and neurophysiological) responses to novel and repeated stimuli, respectively. Orientation and habituation are thereby distinguished from studies of attention which require a

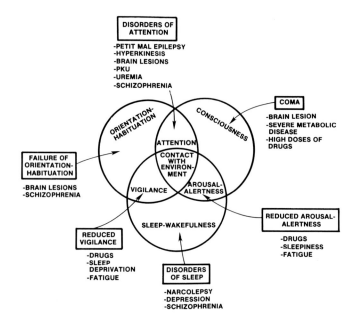

FIG. 1.   Conceptual diagram showing relationship among areas of research concerned with organism-environment interaction.

learned or verbally instructed response to a designated stimulus (that is not strictly speaking novel) which is part of a stimulus series (that is not strictly repetitive). Similarly, studies of both orientation-habituation and attention can be distinguished from studies of vigilance where the method of experimentation tests the organism's ability to detect the presence or absence of a given stimulus.

A second dimension differentiating the various constructs involves the responsiveness of the organism to stimuli of a given intensity, or conversely, the intensity of a stimulus needed to evoke a given response. For example, although sleep, wakefulness, and arousal may be distinguished on the basis of EEG patterns and physiological indicators (such as respiratory and pulse rate, etc.), it is also true that in the progression from sleep through relaxed wakefulness to alertness, stimuli of progressively diminishing intensity are necessary to evoke a behavioral response.

Finally, the several constructs applied to organism-environment interactions may also be considered to be independent by examining their disorders. For example, a failure to respond to critical or meaningful stimuli would indicate one type of dysfunction in the organism's contact with its environment. This deficit might occur as the result of cerebral events or neurological conditions (such as certain types of epilepsy) which may have no effect on the response to novel or repeated stimuli. Similarly, sleep-wake cycles may be affected by some disorders (such as schizophrenia) which do not produce a total loss of consciousness i.e., coma).

To discuss the different areas of investigation represented in Fig. 1 would go well beyond the scope of a single chapter. Instead it is our intent to describe the study of attention in certain patient populations which are of interest because they demonstrate either periodic or more chronic alterations in their response to environmental events. Where possible we have attempted to analyze attention deficits shown by such patients in terms of sensory or motor components. In addition, many studies are described in which animal models have been developed in order to study more directly the neural systems involved in attentive behavior.

Our studies have leaned heavily on a single method of studying attention; as such, they are neither exhaustive nor necessarily definitive. However, they do represent a systematic attempt to study attention as it might be measured or tested in a clinical setting. Moreover, the animal models which have been developed permit study of neurological variables under conditions of behavioral testing similar to those which have been used in man. The work to be described should therefore be considered an integrated, if somewhat circumscribed attempt to understand attention deficits as manifest in neurological and/or psychological disorders.

STUDIES OF THE SYMPTOM OF IMPAIRED ATTENTION IN PETIT MAL EPILEPSY

Periodic attention defects are perhaps best exemplified in certain epileptic disorders. Probably the most interesting and least well understood are the "generalized" epilepsies including petit mal and certain types of grand mal seizures. In contrast to the "focal" epilepsies (52) the seizure manifestations in these disorders cannot usually be related to the presence of a restricted or relatively restricted lesion which serves as a focus for the initiation of the abnormal discharge of neurons.

From the point of view of the neuropsychologist, the interest in petit mal stems largely from the behavioral symptom associated with this disorder: the staring spell or "absence" attack. The term "absence" is descriptive of the extent to which the patient periodically loses contact with the environment. Typically, the "absence" attack interrupts ongoing activity and

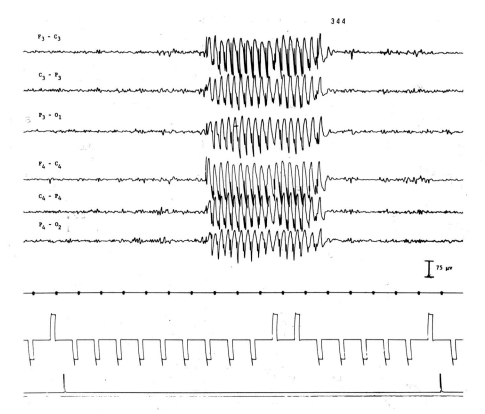

FIG. 2. The relation between a burst of spike and wave activity
and CPT performance in a patient suffering from petit mal epilepsy.
The top six channels in the tracing represent a standard anteroposterior EEG run, with electrode placements determined by the
"10-20" system (52). The seventh channel below this is a one sec
time mark. Below this in channel 8 are represented the stimuli
(duration = 0.2 sec) shown to the patient; those requiring a response (the letter X) are seen as deflections above the baseline;
other letter stimuli appear as deflections below the baseline.
The patient's response appears on channel 9 as an upward deflection. In this sample, the patient responded correctly to X's presented before and after the spike and wave burst but failed to
respond to the two occurring within the burst. (From Mirsky and
Tecce, ref. 42.)

the patient may stare into space as though distracted
by a thought.
     An example of a petit mal seizure, as recorded in
the EEG from scalp electrodes appears in Fig. 2. The
"absence" attack is indicated by the patient's failure
to respond to critical task stimuli which were presented during the high amplitude burst of spike-wave activity.

Behavioral studies of patients with petit mal or centrencephalic (we are using the terms interchangeably) epilepsy have been undertaken in order to quantify disease-related deficits by measuring performance on various stimulus-response or cognitive tasks. A method of studying sustained attention used in our investigations has been the Continuous Performance Test or CPT originally developed by Rosvold et al. (57) for study of brain damaged patients. The test makes use of a visual display in which single letters, colors, or numbers (.2 sec stimulus duration) are presented successively (1.0 sec between stimuli). The subject is instructed to press a response key whenever a previously designed critical stimulus appears such as the letter "X," (i.e., the "X" task). A more difficult version requires a key press for "X" only if it follows the letter "A" (i.e., the "AX" task). Critical stimuli appear randomly approximately 25% of the time. Subjects are required to perform this task for periods of 10 min and the analysis of performance looks specifically for two types of errors: errors of omission, or failure to press the response key for critical stimuli; and errors of commission, or pressing the response key for noncritical stimuli. The usual error made by patients with petit mal epilepsy is that of omission.

By way of summary of the behavioral studies using the CPT to test epileptic patients, Fig. 3 presents scores from the X and AX tasks for three groups of adult patients with centrencephalic and four with focal epilepsy. In addition, the AX task data from a study of epileptic children by Fedio and Mirsky (11) are included for comparison.

The significance levels listed above the grouped columns indicate where a statistically reliable separation among groups was found in a particular study: the means were corrected, if necessary, for differences in age or IQ, and occasionally for other variables such as duration of illness, seizure frequency, and degree of EEG abnormality. In only one case is there a reliable separation among groups with the X task, although the AX task discriminated successfully in three of four studies. Generally, there was greater variability of performance within the centrencephalic than the focal groups. This often took the form of a bimodal distribution of scores, with some centrencephalic cases performing as well as focal patients whereas others performed considerably more poorly. Variation in performance between centrencephalic groups tested in the different studies is also evident in Fig. 3. For example, among the adult groups of patients with focal epilepsy, the mean scores range between 90 and 96% correct and between 80 and 86% correct on the X and AX tasks re-

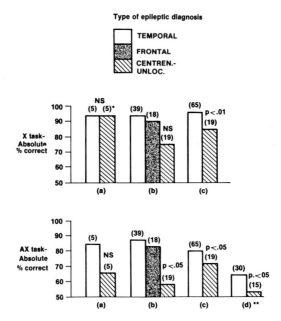

FIG. 3. Summary of mean CPT scores from focal and centrencephalic epileptic patients, including the data of three studies. The absolute % correct measure is the number of correct divided by the total number of critical stimuli. (a) (ref. 41); pilot study data; (b) (ref. 41); main study data; (c) (ref. 31); (d) (ref. 11); * = No. of subjects in study; ** = Children, average age 10.6.

spectively. For the adult centrencephalic groups, on the other hand, the X task means range between 75 and 94%; the AX task means, between 57 and 72%.

How do we interpret the numerous errors of omission made by patients with epilepsy of the centrencephalic type? Do they occur in conjunction with bursts of spike-wave activity? Or is erroneous performance on the CPT and similar tasks a static characteristic of persons with this illness, whether or not the EEG is displaying paroxysmal activity? To obtain information regarding the relation between errors and burst activity requires that the EEG be recorded during task performance. Mirsky and Van Buren (43) have provided data bearing on this question, some of which is presented in Table 1. The upper range of control scores as well as the mean, is somewhat inflated since the standard task parameters were eased for some subjects. It was thought that by providing for high levels of baseline performance during non-burst periods, the effects of spike-wave activity, especially if they were minimal, could be more easily assessed. As the results show, however,

TABLE 1. *Combined CPT % correct scores (X, AX tasks)*
visual and auditory versions; during spike-wave
bursts as compared with control periods

	DURING BURSTS	CONTROL PERIODS
Mean	24.1%	84.8%
Range	0 - 81.8%	64.7 - 99.4%

during the occurrence of spike-wave bursts, correct responding on the CPT is drastically reduced. Lengthening the inter-stimulus interval and increasing the stimulus duration did not improve performance during seizures.

In addition to demonstrating that bursts of spike-wave account for much of the impaired performance on the CPT, Mirsky and Van Buren found that specific characteristics of the EEG discharge are related to the degree of impairment. Thus, the variability in performance of the patients with centrencephalic epilepsy seen in the earlier described studies in which EEGs were not recorded may have been due to factors related to the type and number of bursts occurring.

Although much of the impairment of CPT performance shown by petit mal patients can be attributed to the occurrence of spike-wave activity, such patients still perform more poorly than those with other types of epilepsy even when seizure discharge is not occurring in the EEG. As shown in Fig. 3, the scores of adult focal epileptic patients on the X task ranged between 90 to 96% correct, and on the AX task between 80 to 86% correct. An analysis of the performance of one group of petit mal patients studied by Mirsky and Van Buren on a first testing session with the CPT (using standard parameters) showed average scores of only 75 to 80% correct on X or AX tasks, even when periods of spike-wave activity were eliminated. In some cases, scores as low as 17 to 20% were obtained from patients when there was no evidence of spike-wave activity in the EEG.

Mirsky and Van Buren (43) also attempted to explicate further the mechanisms of attention deficit in petit mal epilepsy by breaking down this complex concept into its component parts. Tasks which emphasized either sensory or the motor components of CPT were administered to some of the subjects. The sensory task or DID (delayed identification) consisted of presenting letters to the patient in either the visual or auditory modality before and during spike-wave bursts and requesting the patient to identify the stimulus only after the seizure ended. No motor response was required during the seizure period. It is recognized that this

TABLE 2. *Comparison of percentages
of impairment produced by spike-wave bursts
on DID, SMR and CPT tasks (N = 8 patients)*

CPT	82.8%
DID	58.0%
SMR	47.1%

is not a "pure" sensory task, since it involves memory which is also influenced by burst activity (14). Colored lights were sometimes used in an effort to simplify the cognitive aspect of the task. The motor task or SMR (simple motor response) required the patient to perform the same response (key pressing) as the CPT, but in a continuously repetitive fashion without reference to designated external stimulus events. The effects of the burst on this key-pressing response were evaluated and then compared with the DID and CPT data. Table 2 compares scores for the 8 patients who were administered all three tasks.

Performance on the CPT was significantly more impaired by burst activity ($p < .02$) than on either the DID or SMR tasks. The latter two tasks did not differ significantly from one another. The trend suggested by the data, however, is that the motor task performance is less affected by burst activity than is performance on the sensory task. This is borne out by considering some individual patient's scores, including some that are not represented in Table 2. Figure 4 shows the differential effect of spike-wave bursts on the CPT and SMR performance of one patient. Of 13 patients who performed the SMR task 5 never showed any arrest of key pressing during bursts. In contrast, every one of the eight cases on whom DID information was obtained showed some impairment, ranging from 12.5 to 100%. Orren (48) has recently obtained data similar to these.

We found more direct evidence of seizure effects on sensory events by study of visual evoked potentials during spike-wave activity. Orren found that for 3 of 4 patients this measure of sensory processing was indeed substantially altered during spike-wave discharge. The results of the evoked visual potential analysis from 3 of the patients appears in Fig. 5. In each case, the two topmost tracings within a subject's summary represent averages obtained from non-spike-wave (NSW) periods preceding and adjacent to spike-wave (SW) periods. Immediately below these is the average obtained during spike-wave (SW) burst activity. For subjects TS and DD there is no recognizable component during the first 150 msec of the 425 msec tracing depicted.

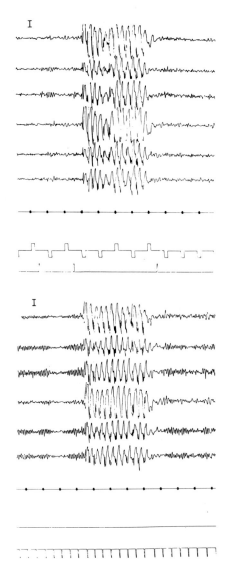

FIG. 4. Differential effect
of spike-wave activity on CPT
and SMR performance. Each
tracing shows six channels of
EEG, a one sec timer (channel
7), CPT stimuli (channel 8),
responses (channel 9). Calibration marks represent 50µV.
Top tracing: patient fails to
respond to a critical stimulus
(upward deflection) of the CPT
presented during a 4.0 sec
burst of spike-wave activity,
although correctly responding
before and after the burst.
Bottom tracing: when the identical response (key press) was
not contingent on CPT stimuli,
the same patient was able to
execute the response at a reg-
ular rate (SMR task) throughout another 4.0 sec burst.

For the subject CF, the spike-wave average is degraded
or distorted throughout the entire sweep (48).

The evoked potentials were recorded to flash-strobe
stimuli, and not to those of the CPT. When tested behaviorally using the flash as the stimulus, these patients showed impaired responding during spike-wave
bursts similar in degree to the impairment in their CPT
performance. Thus, the reduced amplitude evoked potential curves are consistent with the behavioral unrespon-

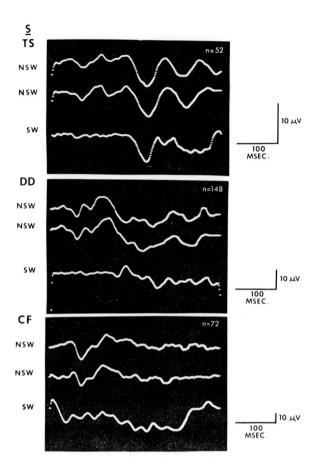

FIG. 5. Average evoked potentials during non-spike-wave (NSW) and
spike-wave (SW) activity; Subjects TS, DD, and CF. The averages
were obtained from parietal-occipital recordings (P_3-O_1 or P_4-O_2).
An upward deflection indicates positivity at the occipital relative to the parietal electrode. (From Orren, ref. 48.)

siveness seen when either flash or CPT stimuli were
used.

Since direct intracerebral exploration of patients
with petit mal epilepsy is rarely, if ever, justified
on therapeutic grounds, information as to the nature
and locus of neural events responsible for the various
behavioral and electrographic features of this disorder
will probably be forthcoming only from animal studies.
A number of investigators, beginning as early as 1947
with the study of Jasper and Droogleever-Fortuyn (21),
have used animal models to test various hypotheses of
the nature of the pathophysiological processes in epi-

lepsy. Much of this research was reviewed by Ajmone Marsan (1) and is detailed in the edited volumes by Jasper et al. (22) and Purpura et al. (53). The majority of these investigations carried out on either immobilized or anesthetized animals, were intended primarily to simulate the bilateral symmetrical and synchronous spike-wave discharges which are the EEG signature of petit mal epilepsy. We shall consider here primarily those studies aimed at simulating in alert and behaving monkeys the behavioral symptoms of petit mal, as defined by the human studies discussed above, and those attempting to account for these behavioral symptoms in terms of stimulus processing.

Simulating Behavioral Symptoms

Monkeys can be trained for either shock avoidance or water reinforcement to perform a simple version of the CPT (i.e., press for the red light, do not press for green or blue). The performance of monkeys on this task is influenced by the same variables that affect human performance on the CPT. As is the case with humans (28, 38), performance of the monkey on this task is differentially sensitive to the effects of chlorpromazine and sleep loss, as compared with secobarbital (37). The modification of the CPT for animal subjects has also provided the opportunity to study one type of behavior which seems to be impaired in human petit mal epilepsy. Two kinds of intracerebral manipulation found to affect this behavior have been performed. One involved the implantation of aluminum hydroxide cream via cannula into subcortical regions thought to be critical for petit mal symptoms; the other involved electrical stimulation of the brain.

Aluminum cream implantation procedure has been used by a number of workers (24, 25, 26) primarily as a way of simulating discharging cortical foci. Mirsky and Oshima (40) injected the substance into either midline thalamic nuclei or into upper brainstem structures, two of the anatomical candidates for the theoretical "centrencephalic" focus in petit mal epilepsy as proposed by Penfield and Jasper (52). The experimental effort in this case attempted to reproduce the effects of a subcortical "discharging" (i.e., epileptogenically active) lesion. The results indicated that destruction of even substantial amounts of medial thalamic tissue was without appreciable behavioral or electrographic effects; animals with such lesions could perform the CPT at high levels for months after the implantation procedure. By contrast, animals with brainstem lesions all showed either permanent or temporary performance impairment on the task, coupled in most cases with

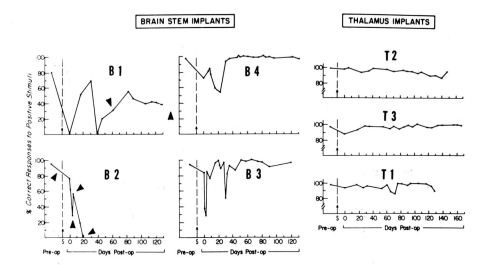

FIG. 6. Percentage of correct responses to positive stimuli for
animals with brainstem (B 1-4) and thalamic (T 1-3) implants.
The arrow indicated by "S" on the abscissa represents the time of
the surgical implant. The numbers along the abscissa refer to
days after the resumption of postoperative testing. The solid
triangles indicate days when EEG samples were obtained in B1 and
B2. (From Mirsky and Oshima, ref. 40.)

pathological (high voltage slow waves) EEG signs. Figure 6 presents the behavioral data, and Fig. 7 a re-
construction of the anatomical results of that investigation.

The histology verified that destruction of portions
of the mesencephalic reticular formation was common to
all the brainstem implanted animals. This suggests
that, to the extent that the monkey data model the human disease, mesencephalic rather than midline or in-
tralaminar thalamic structures are critical for "ab-
sence-like" symptoms. This same area may play a role
in the electrographic manifestations of petit mal; the
spike-wave pattern can be reproduced by high frequency
electrical stimulation of the mesencephalic "reticular
core" (73).

The aluminum cream study was followed by a detailed
and extensive stimulation study by Bakay Pragay et al.
(3). Five monkeys working on a shock-avoidance version
of the CPT were studied very extensively using moveable,
rather than fixed, stimulating electrodes. The electrode could be advanced into the brain millimeter by
millimeter, through small, stainless steel guides fixed
in the skull and resting on the dura. It was thus possible to describe in rather precise detail the locus of
effective points in each animal. The effects of stimu-

BRAIN STEM IMPLANTS

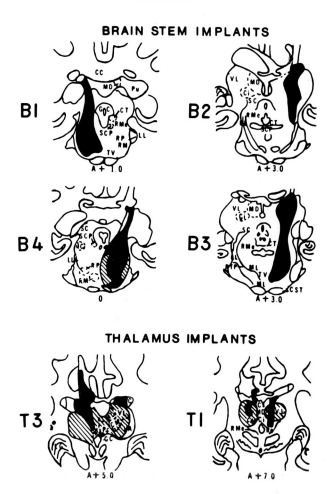

THALAMUS IMPLANTS

FIG. 7. Detail of section in each animal showing estimated maximal lesion. Abbreviations used are as follows: n = nucleus; r = reticularis; VA = n. ventralis anterior; VL = n. ventralis lateralis; MD = n. medialis dorsalis; C = n. caudatus; CM = n. centrum medianum; Re = n. reuniens; CS = n. centralis superior; Ci = n. centralis inferior; pc = n. parafascicularis; RMe = n. r. mesencephali; RP = n. r. pars parvocellularis; RM = n.r. pars magnocellularis; RTP = n. r. tegmenti pons; Pu = n. pulvinaris; TV = n. tegmenti ventralis; LG = n. geniculatis lateralis; CC = corpus callosum; CG = griseum centrale; CT = central tegmental tract; SC = superior colliculus; IC = inferior colliculus; SCP = superior cerebellar peduncle; LL = lateral lemiscus; ML = medial lemniscus; CTS = corticospinal tract. (From Mirsky and Oshima, ref. 40.)

lation on CPT performance and on the general behavior of the monkey outside the task situation were observed. In addition, stimulation at locations and parameters

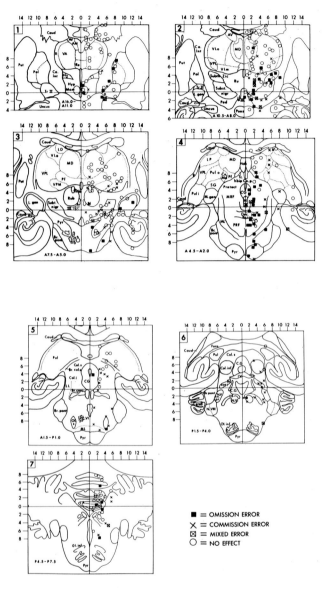

FIG. 8. Coronal sections through macaque brain showing locus of
stimulation induced effects on CPT. Effects were achieved with
exploring electrodes lowered into the brain through fixed guides.
(From Bakay Pragay et al., ref. 3.)

which produced alterations in behavior was repeated in
order to assess effects on the visual evoked potential.
Some portions of the results of that investigation are
presented in Figs. 8 through 10.

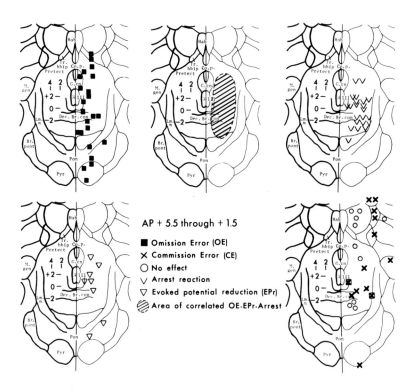

FIG. 9. Area of brainstem in macaque yielding stimulation-induced behavioral and evoked potential effects similar to those seen in human petit mal epilepsy. Upper left = omission error effects on CPT; lower left = reduced visual evoked potentials; upper right = "arrest" reaction. Central panel shows area of overlap of these effects. (From Bakay Pragay and Mirsky, ref. 36a.)

Figure 8 is a series of seven coronal sections through the macaque brain depicting the locus of 318 cerebral locations stimulated in this investigation. Not shown are the loci of the cortical points also stimulated, which were usually without significant effects on CPT performance (especially at the parameters which were effective in subcortical locations). As was the case of the aluminum cream study described above, the thalamus appears generally not to be involved in the maintenance of CPT behavior; of 88 locations stimulated within the thalamus only six (fewer than 7%) yielded omission or other errors, whereas 69 were without effect. This is clearly seen in sections 1 to 4 in Fig. 8. As was demonstrated in previous work, the region for eliciting errors is more ventral and caudal in

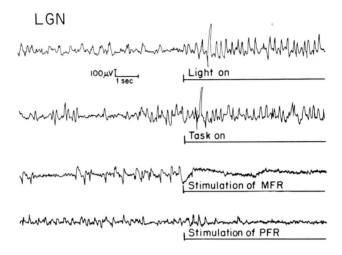

FIG. 10. Eye movement spike potentials recorded under various experimental conditions in lateral geniculate nucleus (LGN) of macaque. Top two traces show increase in spikes with visual stimulation. Bottom two traces show reduced spiking with electrical stimulation of mesencephalic (MFR) and pontine (PFR) reticular formation. (From Bakay Pragay and Mirsky, ref. 36a.)

location; thus for the midbrain, pons and medulla, where a total of 132 points were stimulated, 90 of these (more than 68%) produced either omission errors alone (33 points or 25% of the points) or other forms of erroneous behavior (57 points, or 42% of the points). This is most clearly seen in sections 2 to 4 in Fig. 8. Considering omission errors alone, behaviorally effective points are clustered in the mesencephalic and pontine reticular formations, pretectal area, pons, and red nucleus.

From the point of view of modeling petit mal epilepsy, an area of considerable interest was localized in the region of the junction zone between the mesencephalic and pontine reticular formation, represented schematically in Fig. 9. Stimulation of this region, which extends roughly 3 mm in anterior-posterior extent, produced a number of effects analagous to those seen in human petit mal seizures: errors of omission on the CPT task; arrest of ongoing behavior, including eye movements; and reduction in the amplitude of visual evoked responses recorded from occipital cortex. The reduction in eye movements, as reflected centrally, is seen in Fig. 10. The figure shows sharp, spike-like potentials recorded in the lateral geniculate nucleus under various experimental conditions. Potentials similar to these have been demonstrated to be associated with rap-

id eye movements (12) and can also be observed in the
pons and occipital cortex (7, 8).

The sharp lateral geniculate potentials are seen in
Fig. 10 to be absent during stimulation of either the
mesencephalic or pontine reticular formation (third and
fourth tracings). Such effects are possibly analagous
to the alteration or arrest in muscular activity which
in human petit mal epilepsy is referred to as a "staring spell". The final stimulation effect seen, i.e.,
reduced visual evoked potentials, is exemplified in
Fig. 11. The figure shows visual evoked potentials,
recorded from both the occipital cortex and the lateral
geniculate nucleus while the animal was being stimulated at points which elicited errors of omission on the
CPT. The reduction in visual evoked potentials is reminiscent of the findings of Orren (48) from patients
with petit mal epilepsy (see Fig. 5).

Collectively, then, these monkey studies, one with
aluminum cream implants, and one using intracerebral
stimulation, have provided evidence suggesting that the
brainstem, and in particular, the area of the mesencephalic and pontine reticular formation may be critical
for some of the behavioral (and electrographic) symptoms of human petit mal epilepsy and for the maintenance
of sustained visual attention.

Other Clinical Entities with
Impairment of Sustained Attention

The human and animal studies discussed to this point
have dealt almost exclusively with the "absence" phenomenon in petit mal epilepsy as the central problem in
the neuropsychology of attention. Are there other
groups of clinical entities which are also characterized by poor sustained attention? And, are there some
communalities, derived from either empirical or theoretical understanding, which link these in some way?
There have indeed been a number of clinical studies, in
addition to those dealing with epileptic disorders,
that have used the CPT to examine sustained attention
in a systematic way. Table 3 summarizes some of this
experimental work, and it is clear that the collection
of clinical entities is rather heterogeneous. The
studies have been organized into three general categories: those dealing with schizophrenia (A to D);
those dealing with social-educational problems (E to
I); and those concerned with toxic states, drug or metabolic (J to M). Some comments are in order on each of
the categories. However, it should be noted all the
studies in Table 3 included control groups and/or tests
in addition to the CPT that did not reveal deficit.

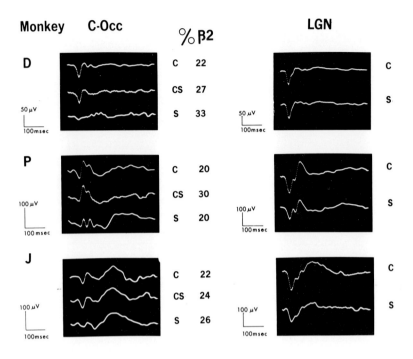

FIG. 11.   Reduction in visual evoked potentials from stimulation
in mesencephalic or pontine reticular formation (cross-hatched area
in center panel of Fig. 9) as seen in three monkey subjects D, P,
and J.   The set of tracings at the left are recorded from a cen-
tral-occipital cortex placement; those at the right are from the
lateral geniculate nucleus (LGN).   Within each tracing set the
topmost curve ("C") represents the control response to 2 Hz photic
stimulation; "S" at the bottom, represents the response to photic
stimulation during reticular formation stimulation; "CS" indicates
the response seen during stimulation of a control structure, usually located several mm from the behaviorally-effective point.
The numerical values to the right of the "C," "CS," or "S" desig-
nations indicate the percentage of β 2 activity (27 - 40 Hz) determined from a baseline-crossing frequency analysis of the EEG at
the time of the combined photic and reticular stimulation.   The
reduction in cortical VEP's during stimulation of behaviorally-effective points is clearly seen.   The effects are much less striking at LGN, and neither change is clearly related to any change in
"activation" as measured by the amount of β activity in the EEG.
The sweeps in each case are based on the average of 50 to 60 photic
stimulus presentations.   (From Bakay Pragay and Mirsky, ref. 36a.)

TABLE 3. *Summary of studies investigating sustained attention defect as a symptom of some clinical disorder/entity*

Clinical disorder or entity	Investigators	CPT impairment described	Comment on empirical or theoretical considerations
Schizophrenia	49, 50	Yes, in 40% of cases	
Schizophrenia	62	Yes, but with distraction only	Theoretical implication of reticular formation involvement "hyperarousal": (29, 36)
Remitted schizophrenia	77	Yes, but with distraction only	
Mother with schizophrenia "high risk" children	18	Yes, but only in 5-year olds, not 6-year-olds	Genetic disorder? (55)
Hyperkinetic children	65	Yes	Brain damage suspected in some children; heterogeneous disorder
Hyperkinetic behavior	66	Yes, but reversible with stimulants	
Mental retardation	57	Yes, MR + BD worse than MR alone	Diffuse and/or heterogenous brain damage
Mental retardation and brain damage	9	Yes, MR + BD worse than MR alone	
Learning disability	54	Yes, in 2nd grade children	Developmental delay suspected; brain damage uncertain
Chronic alcoholism	49	No	Damage to brain is cortical and/or subcortical but may spare reticular systems
Korsakoff's syndrome	16	No	
Uremia	44	Yes, reversible with dialysis in some cases	Clear evidence of reticular formation damage in severe cases (47), "petit mal"

Table 3 continued

Clinical disorder or entity	Investigators	CPT impairment described	Comment on empirical or theoretical considerations
			like EEG (20)
Phenylketonuria	2	Yes	"Petit mal-like" EEG (13)

Schizophrenia

A complete discussion of the nature of the evidence of attentive deficit in schizophrenia is beyond the scope of the present discussion. Mirsky (36) and Kornetsky and Mirsky (29) have reviewed this evidence, and have suggested that a disorder of the reticular formation of the brain, leading to a state of chronic hyperarousal, would account for this schizophrenic deficit. Orzack and Kornetsky (50) have had some success in showing differences in familial history and other variables between "good attenders" and "poor attenders" (the latter referring to the 40% of the schizophrenic population who show impairment of the CPT). It will be noted also that in two of the studies (62, 77) the deficit by schizophrenics on the CPT was revealed only under conditions of sensory distraction; this condition has little effect on the performance of children with petit mal epilepsy (11). The data provided by Grunebaum et al., (18) for children at risk for schizophrenia (by virtue of having a schizophrenic mother) are problematic. Poor CPT performance and other attentional deficits were seen only in 5- but not 6-year-olds. Moreover, it is not known how many, if any, of the children will eventually develop schizophrenic symptoms. Nevertheless, certain electrophysiological differences, reflected in the visual evoked potential, suggestive of developmentally less mature modes of stimulus or information processing, have been described in a sample of these high-risk children (19). These data suggest a possible physiological component to the putative genetic defect in schizophrenia (55) but a link to disordered brainstem mechanisms is not established at this time.

Social-educational Problems

Hyperactive children have shown poor CPT performance (65, 66) which is remediable, as is their general behavior with stimulant medication (66). The test thus

appears as a useful monitor of the hyperactive state.
There is no evidence clearly linking either this attention deficit or its remediation to brain mechanisms.
It is unlikely furthermore, that such evidence will be
easily forthcoming since hyperkinetic behavior is probably due to an enormously heterogeneous set of factors.
The same comment would appear to apply to mental retardation and learning disability as well. Judging from
the relative predominance of male subjects in studies
of hyperkinesis and learning disabilities (e.g., 23,
54) it seems that both of these syndromes affect many
more boys than girls. However, whether this is to be
attributed to greater vulnerability of the developing
male brain (17) to social-role factors, to both, or to
neither of these variables is impossible to say on the
basis of present knowledge.

Toxic States

Neither chronic alcoholics nor patients suffering
from Korsakoff's syndrome show deficits involving sustained attention. This latter group may shed some
light on the question of the neuropathological insult
necessary for attention defect in man. The brain structures damaged (mammillary bodies and medial dorsal nuclei of the thalamus) according to postmortem studies
of such patients (71) are probably *not* necessary for
sustained attention performance. Some positive evidence linking brain structures to attention may be provided by studies of persons suffering from severe uremic disorders. As in the case of petit mal patients,
difficulties with attention or concentration in uremic
patients are well documented (61, 67). However, the
resemblance to petit mal epilepsy is even more striking
as uremic individuals may show EEG patterns virtually
indistinguishable from those seen in petit mal epilepsy
(20). Although uremic patients perform poorly on the
CPT (44), it is not known whether errors of omission
are associated with slow wave discharges in the EEG.
It is known, however, from neuropathological studies of
persons who have died from uremic disease, that damage
to brainstem structures (particularly in reticular formation) is a common finding (47). The last toxic
state, that of phenylketonuria, has been shown to be
accompanied by significant impairment on a somewhat
simplified version of the CPT (2). This version, which
uses pictures rather than letter stimuli, was found to
be more suitable for the young patients afflicted with
this illness. The neuropathology of this defect is obscure, although some suggestion of "corticoreticular"
pathology is provided by the evidence of slow wave
burst and slow spike-wave activity in the EEGs of such
patients (13).

OTHER NEUROPSYCHOLOGICAL STUDIES
WITH ATTENTION DEFECT

The studies reviewed in this chapter have centered around the use of a particular technique for studying sustained attention-The Continuous Performance Test. Further, the primary clinical emphasis has been on the "absence" phenomenon shown by a particular subgroup of epileptic patients, those with petit mal epilepsy. There exists, however, a body of literature which is almost exclusively Russian that has described defects in behavioral and electrographic measures of attention in patients with extensive frontal lobe pathology. Such deficits can be demonstrated on tasks which prolong the orientation reflex by means of verbal instructions, as for example when the subjects must press a key in response to a signal.

> ...lesions of the frontal lobes make it impossible to evoke a state of activation in the cortex by means of verbal instruction. In other words, frontal lobe lesions violate the physiological basis underlying the regulation of the higher, specifically human, forms of attention.
>
> The above conclusion is particularly well supported by data from lesions of the polar, medial and probably mediobasal, parts of the frontal cortex, which, according to available data, are components of neural systems that insure the descending influences on the reticular formation and thus directly participate in the most complex forms of regulation of the states of neural activity (32).

The quotation suggests that tasks such as the CPT, which entail a verbal instruction to execute a given response (i.e., "press for X") should also be sensitive to lesions or pathology of the frontal lobes. However, several studies using the CPT to test patients with irritative or destructive lesions involving the frontal lobes have failed to reveal significant deficits in sustained attention. The data presented in Fig. 3 include 18 patients with epileptogenic foci localized in the frontal lobes. The CPT performance of these patients was not significantly different from that of persons with temporal lobe foci (41)-the latter group scoring as well as normal subjects of similar age and IQ (57).

Seizure foci, which are irritative and discharge periodically, may not be functionally equivalent in their behavioral effects to permanent damage and tissue

TABLE 4. *Comparison of CPT scores X-A%[a] and AX-A%, in controls and two groups of persons with prefrontal psychosurgical lesions*

		Lobotomy[b] (N=12)		Mixed psychosurgery[c] (N=11)	Controls (N=9)
	Mean	84.7	(92.5)	98.3	98.4
X-A%	SD	27.7	(7.9)	4.1	1.3
	Range	0-100	(77-100)	86-100	96-100
	Mean	80.1	(85.5)	—	93.3
AX-A%	SD	27.8	(21.4)	—	6.1
	Range	20-100	(33-100)	—	79-99
	Mean	40.7	(39.3)	46.9	39.0
AGE	Range	29-57	(29-57)	29-60	26-51
I.Q.	Mean	115.6	(115.1)	113.0	111.3

[a] X-A% and AX-A% refer, respectively, to absolute percentage of correct responses (no. correct/total positive stimuli) on the X and AX tasks.

[b] Includes one case with two prefrontal lobotomies; all others had one bilateral operation. Figures in brackets omit scores of one case who was unable to perform X task of CPT.

[c] Includes eight cases with bilateral medial orbital undercutting (one of whom had prior cingulotomy); two lobotomies and one transorbital lobotomy.

loss which are often the consequence of the lesions and tumors described by Luria. But more direct evidence concerning the possible role of the frontal lobes in mediating the type of attentive behavior measured by the CPT can be provided by patient populations undergoing surgical destruction of portions of the frontal lobes. Table 4 compares the CPT performance of two independently studied patient groups subjected to surgery involving the frontal lobes (39, 56) with the performance of normal subjects, similar in age and I.Q., who served as a control group in one of these studies (56).

The lobotomy group studied by Rosvold and Mirsky (56) consisted of 12 patients who underwent anterior prefrontal lobotomy (plus an additional, more posterior lobotomy in one case) for relief of schizophrenia. The CPT and IQ scores were obtained 5 years post-surgery. In the 11 cases comprising the mixed psychosurgery group (39) the primary diagnosis was depression or ob-

sessive-compulsive behavior, for which the surgical
treatment consisted of medial orbital undercutting or
lobotomy (including one transorbital lobotomy). This
latter group was also tested approximately 5 years after surgery.

Table 4 shows the CPT performance of the mixed psychosurgery group (tested only on the X task) to be virtually indistinguishable from that of the control subjects. Although the mean score of the lobotomy group
was lower and performance more variable when compared
to the control subjects, the difference between groups
was not significant. There was considerable overlap
of individual scores; on the AX task, for example, only
4 of the 12 patients in the lobotomy group scored below
the range of performance established by the control
group. The bracketed values in Table 4 indicate the
scores achieved by the lobotomy group when the most deviant case (completely unable to perform one version of
the task) was removed from the group statistics. In
any case, the deficit in CPT performance characterizing
the lobotomy group is difficult to interpret since the
schizophrenia prompting the surgery would also be expected to be associated with some instances of impaired
performance (50).

It is worth keeping in mind, however, that although
the data of Table 4 do not support the notion that the
frontal lobes are essential in the type of attentive
behavior measured by the CPT, during the substantial
period of time intervening between surgery and testing,
some recovery of function or compensatory behavior could
have occurred. Larger deficits among frontally damaged
patients might have been observed earlier in the post-
surgical period.

SOME SPECULATIONS CONCERNING ETIOLOGY

If it is true that pathology of the mesopontine regions of the brainstem plays a critical role in producing the kinds of attention defects that have been
described in this chapter, then it is appropriate to
ask how such pathology may arise. Probable causes
would seen to fall into three categories: Genetic, toxic, and congenital. By *genetic* is meant that some
structural and/or biochemical fault of this critical
area of the brain exists as an inherited trait, and is
transmitted along with other physical characteristics.
The work of Metrakos and Metrakos (33) provides some
evidence that this is the case with petit mal epilepsy; Rosenthal and Kety (55) have gathered in an edited
volume some of the evidence for a genetic component in
schizophrenia.

Toxic and *congenital* factors refer to: (a) the pres-

ence of some toxin or poison during the gestational
period which alters the normal development of critical
brain areas (candidates for such a role in prenatal
development include alcohol, tranquilizer drugs, anti-
convulsants, and other central nervous system depres-
sants); (b) physical damage to brain structures due
to such traumata as stretching, tearing, and compression that often accompany a difficult labor and/or delivery; (c) toxins which may be present only during
postnatal life such as nitrogenous wastes which are not
excreted by the impaired kidney in uremia and excess
phenylalanine in phenylketonuria.

With regard to congenital factors, Towbin (68, 69)
has called attention to the importance of pre- and
perinatal events in generating cerebral and spinal
pathology. He has remarked (69) that the most dangerous journey we ever take in our life is the one down
the birth canal and has provided evidence of structural
damage to brainstem regions, in particular, which can
accompany an arduous forceps delivery (68). Toxic substances may exert damaging effects, either pre- or
postnatally, by depriving certain brain tissues of oxygen. The work of Windle (75, 76) and Myers (45, 46)
has emphasized that experimental asphyxia in monkeys
may produce damage to brainstem structures whether as
a result of acute umbilical cord clamp at term or of
prolonged cord clamp in midpregnancy.

ATTENTION AND NEUROPEPTIDES

Consideration of attentional problems has always
formed a part, at least informally, of the usual clinical assessment of pyschopathologically or neurologi-
cally disturbed patients. However, formal measurement
of sustained attentive capacity is rarely done, even
with testing approaches that rely upon a standard battery of tests. The studies described here appear to
lend encouragement to the use of tasks such as the
CPT, since it has been useful in studies of epileptic,
psychotic, and metabolic disorders, and in the study
of disturbances such as hyperkinesis. Animal studies
can complement the human studies; they aid in specify-
ing the functions which are impaired, in appreciating
the nature of the brain alterations which underlie
these functional changes, and their possible etiology.
Hopefully, they will aid in guiding the eventual development of new therapeutic approaches. The balance
of this chapter will consider the evidence provided
from the neuropeptide attention research, and consider
whether sufficient data are at hand to warrant the assertion that a new approach to attention and, in particular, a new therapeutic approach is now possible.

The chapters presented in this volume as well as
other published studies (35, 59) have provided evidence
which suggests that administration of certain neuropeptides can produce increments in performance of rats and
human subjects on various tasks. Although these
changes in behavior have been discussed in terms of enhanced learning or memory capacity, the prevailing belief appears to be that the fundamental, core change is
in visual attention and that the other behavioral alterations are secondary to this. What are the behavioral alterations that have led to the inference that
attention is enhanced? There are three studies in rats
(4, 6, 10) which are said to provide evidence of attentional change. It seems fair to say however, that the
work described by Endröczi (10) bears only indirectly
on this issue, since the primary contribution of that
work is to show that better performance on maze and
avoidance type tasks, and enhanced exploratory behavior are associated with greater catecholamine turnover.
The interpretation of these changes is not unambiguous,
however, and motivational or cognitive factors could
be involved as well as modification in attentive capacity. Alternative explanations could also be applied
to the findings of Champney et al. (6). The modest effect these workers found on avoidance and reversal
tasks with administration of ACTH 4-9 was seen in males
only, and required a fair degree of excavation of the
data to become manifest. The study by Beckwith et al.
(4) provided an explicit test of attentive functioning
with the dimensional model as first proposed by Sutherland and Mackintosh (4). Unfortunately, since no
statistically significant results were found in that
study, the work can best be described as suggestive or
preliminary, only.
    There is somewhat greater consistency in the results
of studies that have employed human subjects. Miller
et al. (34), Miller et al. (35), Sandman et al. (59),
and Sandman et al. (60) have all reported a small but
reliable enhancement of scores in the Benton Visual Retention Test, usually with the ACTH 4-10/MSH fragment.
The work by Sandman et al. (60) reported in this volume
indicates that this effect is seen in mentally retarded
as well as normal subjects, a particularly significant
contribution and one to which we will return later.
The two studies by Sandman and colleagues have reported
changes or enhancements in performance from measures of
dimensional or extra dimensional shift during complex
visual discrimination learning tasks. However, one of
these studies (59) involved a long infusion of ACTH/MSH
over a period of several hours. The complex changes
which are interpreted as reflecting altered attention
have to be viewed against the "baseline" depression

produced by the compound, and are at least somewhat
ambiguous. This criticism does not apply to the study
by the authors presented here, and the result is rather
less ambiguous. In addition to these findings, positive results from a number of investigations have contributed some bits and pieces of data: some improvement
in the CPT, the Digit Symbol Substitution Task, and in
MQ (34); and some enhancement in parts of the Halstead-
Reitan neuropsychological battery (60). On the other
hand, Miller et al. (35) were unable to find improvement in disjunctive reaction time with ACTH 4-10. Miller et al., (34) have also described some alterations
in late components of visual evoked potentials following neuropeptide administration in man. However, it is
not certain how much of this VEP effect may be due to
effects on baseline EEGs which have been previously
described by this group [i.e., decreased 3 to 7 Hz activity; increased 7 to 12 Hz and 12+ activity (35)].

A reasonable summary of the behavioral data, is that
there are a few suggestive findings of improvement, following administration of ACTH fragments, on tasks measuring some aspect of visual-attentive-mnemonic functioning. Enhancement, when it occurs, tends to be
small; there have been no studies (to our knowledge)
with very large, resounding effects. The belief that
something beneficial happens to attention seems to be
the result, for the most part, of accumulation of 0.05
level findings, and the most consistent effects have
been seen with the Benton task (four studies) and in
dimensional shifts (one clear effect, one less clear
effect).

This is not an overwhelming array of findings, and
there are several possible interpretations that can be
discussed at this point.

1. The changes may have nothing to do with attention
and may be discussed more fruitfully in some other
terms. More effort should be directed toward separa-
ting motivational from attentional effects. In particular, since many of the animal studies have used avoidance tasks, psychophysical investigations should be
carried out, analagous to the one by Panksepp and his
colleagues (51) regarding positive reinforcers, to determine whether the aversiveness of noxious stimuli is
altered by the administration of neuropeptides.

2. The test model is wrong, i.e., the changes may reflect attentional processes, but since normal well-
rested young subjects are very good at attentional
tasks, one needs to start from a different baseline.
That is, to avoid ceiling effects, the proper subjects
to study are those who are fatigued, bored, or pathologically weakened in attention.

Various possibilities suggest themselves:

(a) Study normal persons who are fatigued or deprived
of sleep for varying periods of time. In a research
program somewhat similar to the present neuropeptide
effort, Kornetsky et al. (30) found improvement in
CPT performance with *d*-amphetamine only when the
subjects were deprived of sleep for up to 68 hours.
An essential part of this experiment was that sleep
deprivation produced profound impairment in the CPT;
in a prior study we were unable to show significant
improvement in normal, rested subjects (70). It is
possible that some of the neuropeptide effects described in man in this volume and in prior studies
might also represent an anti-fatigue or anti-bore-
dom effect. This would be in accord with the results of the numerous studies with amphetamine.
Weiss and Laties (74) concluded in their exhaustive
review that there was no convincing evidence that
this drug did anything beyond restoring depressed
function to normal levels. Some support for extending this interpretation to the effect of neuropeptides is provided in the present volume, albeit in
a slightly different context and model. Strand and
co-workers (63) report that ACTH fragments act to
delay fatigue in muscle, both in experimental animals and in patients with muscle disease.

A corollary recommendation here would be to use
amphetamine controls in future work, since the effects of this drug are well known and could provide
useful baseline or comparative information.

(b) Study persons in whom pathologically deficient attention is a prominent symptom. Table 3 summarizes
the results of CPT investigations with various clinical populations including those with psycho- and
neuropathology, hyperkinetic disorders, and various
metabolic deficiencies. It is conceivable that
neuropeptide administration may have dramatic effects in some of these populations. It should be
added that the work by Sandman and associates (60)
presented here is a promising step in that direction.

The thrust of these suggestions is that the concept of super- or hypernormal attention may not be a
fruitful one and that experimental efforts to demonstrate it are misdirected.

3. The test instruments that have been employed are
not optimally sensitive to attentional changes. More
use should be made of CPT-like tasks. Henry Appleton
and Paul Miller of our laboratory have recently developed, following the suggestion of Dr. Phillip Rennick
of the Lafayette Clinic, a version of the CPT which
might be of use in testing neuropeptide effects. The

task automatically becomes progressively more difficult, in terms of stimulus parameters, when the subject
makes correct responses, and easier when he makes errors. The subject is free to achieve the maximum performance level of which he is capable. Miller et al.
(34) apparently used a procedure similar to this, but
the very high scores obtained by their subjects suggests that the task parameters did not vary over a sufficient range.

Another advantage of the CPT is its adaptability for
the study of attention in animal subjects such as the
rat (27) and the monkey. Monkeys, in particular, present great potential advantages as experimental subjects in this work, as we have tried to demonstrate
earlier in this chapter. Of particular interest is our
finding that there is an area of the monkey brainstem
that is critical for the maintenance of sustained visual attention. Conceivably this might be a focus for
future ACTH-attention-oriented research since Gispen et
al. (15) have pointed out that some behavioral effects
of ACTH fragments are paralleled by their effects on
brainstem protein metabolism.

In addition to the measures of dimensional attention
employed by Sandman and his colleagues (58, 59, 60),
greater use should be made of the habituation-orienta-
tion paradigm for several reasons:

The operational procedures resulting in specific behavioral changes observable in man and a wide range of
subhuman species are well known.

Habituation and orientation are less tied to motivational variables than are measures of attention which
depend on positive and negative reinforcement and on
learned behavior.

The electrophysiological correlates and the neural
analogues already demonstrated within the framework
of habituation and orientation would provide a context
for understanding neuropeptide central nervous system
effects. In this regard, the putative role of the
hippocampus in mediating neuropeptide effects (6, 34,
58) might be more directly established by studying habituation and orientation-behaviors for which the hippocampus is probably especially important (72).

Neuropeptide effects on other aspects of attentive
behavior could be tested as well. The focusing or re-
striction of attention as studied by Callaway (5) using
the Stroop Test, might be related to dimensional attention and thus subject to alteration by neuropeptides.

A final comment or two: It is not clear at this
point whether it is useful to begin to analyze neuropeptide effects on attention in terms of stimulus re-
ception-central processing-motor output as we have attempted to do for our models of the petit mal absence.

The neuropeptide effect still appears somewhat evane-
scent and ephemeral with respect to attention enhancement. Consequently it might be argued that more experimental effort should be devoted to providing a solid,
unambiguous, and convincing attention effect before
proceeding to a more molecular analysis. The data so
far gathered are suggestive and seductive, but more
time, data (and maturing) are needed.

ACKNOWLEDGMENTS

    Support for much of the work described here was pro-
vided by grants from the National Institutes of Health,
United States Public Health Service: MH-10324, MH-12568,
NIDA CDA 00257, and NS 12201. Dr. Mirsky is supported
by a Research Scientist Award K5-MH-14915. During her
dissertation study, parts of which are described here,
Dr. Orren was supported by a Predoctoral Fellowship
MH-40360.
    A special procedure used to extract evoked poten-
tials from the high amplitude spike-wave activity is
described by Orren (1974).

REFERENCES

1. Ajmone Marsan, C. (1969): Pathophysiology of the EEG pattern
   characteristic of petit mal epilepsy, a critical review of
   some of the experimental data. In: *The Physiopathogenesis of
   the Epilepsies,* edited by H. Gastaut, H. Jasper, J. Bancaud,
   and A. Waltregny, pp. 237-248. Charles C. Thomas, Illinois.
2. Anderson, V. E., Siegel, F. S., Fisch, R. O., and Wirt, R. D.
   (1969): Responses of phenylketonuric children on a continuous
   performance test. *J. Abnorm. Psychol.,* 74:358-362.
3. Bakay Pragay, E., Mirsky, A. F., Fullerton, B. C., Oshima, H.,
   and Arnold, S. W. (1975): Effect of electrical stimulation
   of the brain on visually controlled (attentive) behavior in
   Macaca mulatta. *Exp. Neurol.,* 49:203-220.
4. Beckwith, B. E., Sandman, C. A., and Kastin, A. J. (1976):
   The influence of three short-chain peptides (MSH, MSH/ACTH 4-
   10, MIF-1) on dimensional attention. *Pharmacol. Biochem.
   Behav. (Suppl.),* 5:11-16.
5. Callaway, E. III. (1959): The influence of amobarbital (amy-
   lobarbitone and methamphetamine on the focus of attention. *J.
   Ment. Sci.,* 105:382-392.
6. Champney, T. F., Sahley, T. L., and Sandman, C. A. (1976):
   Effects of neonatal cerebral ventricular injection of ACTH 4-
   9 and subsequent adult injections on learning in male and female albino rats. *Pharmacol. Biochem. Behav. (Suppl.),* 5:3-
   10.
7. Cohen, B. and Feldman, M. (1968): Relationship of electrical
   activity in pontine reticular formation and lateral geniculate
   body to rapid eye movements. *J. Neurophysiol.,* 31:806-817.

8. Cohen, B. and Feldman, M. (1971): Potential changes associated with rapid eye movement in the calcarine cortex. *Exp. Neurol.,* 31:100-113.

9. Crosby, K. G. (1968): Attention and distractibility in mentally retarded and average children. Unpublished doctoral dissertation. Boston University, Boston, Massachusetts.

10. Endröczi, E. (1976): Brain mechanisms involved in ACTH-induced changes of exploratory activity and conditioned avoidance behavior. *(This volume.)*

11. Fedio, P. and Mirsky, A. F. (1969): Selective intellectual deficits in children with temporal lobe or centrencephalic epilepsy. *Neuropsychologia,* 7:286-300.

12. Feldman, M. and Cohen, B. (1968): Electrical activity in the lateral geniculate body of the alert monkey associated with eye movements. *J. Neurophysiol.,* 31:1481-1483.

13. Gastaut, H., Rohmer, F., Cossette, A., and Kurtz, D. (1969): Introduction to the study of functional generalized epilepsies. In: *The Physiopathogenesis of the Epilepsies,* edited by H. Gastaut, H. Jasper, J. Bancaud, and A. Waltregny, pp. 5-25. Charles C. Thomas, Illinois.

14. Geller, M. and Geller, A. (1970): Brief amnestic effects of spike-wave discharges. *Neurology* (Minneap.), 20:1089-1095.

15. Gispen, W. H., Reith, M. E. A., Schotman, P., Wiegant, V. M., Zwiers, H., and de Wied, D. (1976): The CNS and ACTH-like peptides: Neurochemical response and interaction with opiates. *(This volume.)*

16. Glosser, G., Butters, N., and Orzack, M. (1974): Unpublished data. Personal communication.

17. Goldman, P. S., Crawford, H. T., Stokes, L. P., Galkin, T. W., and Rosvold, H. E. (1974): Sex-dependent behavioral effects of cerebral cortical lesions in the developing rhesus monkey. *Science,* 186:540-542.

18. Grunebaum, H., Weiss, J. L., Gallant, D., and Cohler, B. J. (1974): Attention in young children of psychotic mothers. *Am. J. Psychiatry,* 131:887-891.

19. Herman, J., Mirsky, A. F., Ricks, N. and Gallant, D. (1977): Behavioral and electrographic measures of attention in children at risk for schizophrenia. *J. Abnorm. Psychol.,* 86(1):27-33.

20. Jacob, J. C., Gloor, P., Elwan, O. H., Dossetor, J. B. and Pateras, V. R. (1965): Electroencephalographic changes in chronic renal failure. *Neurology,* 15:419-429.

21. Jasper, H. H. and Droogleever-Fortuyn, J. (1947): Experimental studies on the functional anatomy of petit mal epilepsy. *Res. Publ. Assoc. Res. Nerv. Ment. Dis.,* 26:272-298.

22. Jasper, H. H., Ward, A. A., and Pope, A. (1969): *Basic Mechanisms of the Epilepsies,* edited by H. H. Jasper, A. A. Ward, and A. Pope, p. 835. Little, Brown and Co., Boston.

23. Kasper, J. C., Millicap, J. C., Backus, R., Child, D., and Shulman, J. L. (1971): A study of the relationship between neurological evidence of brain damage in children and activity and distractibility. *J. Consult. Clin. Psychol.,* 36:329-337.

24. Kopeloff, L. M., Barrera, S. E., and Kopeloff, N. (1942): Recurrent convulsive seizures in animals produced by immuno- logic and chemical means. *Am. J. Psychiatry,* 89:881-902.
25. Kopeloff, L. M., Chusid, J. C., and Kopeloff, N. (1954): Chronic experimental epilepsy in *Macaca mulatta. Neurology,* 4:218-227.
26. Kopeloff, L. M., Chusid, J. C., and Kopeloff, N. (1955): Epilepsy in *Macaca mulatta* after cortical or intracerebral alumina. *A.M.A. Arch. Neurol. Psychiatry,* 74:523-526.
27. Kornetsky, C. and Eliasson, M. (1969): Reticular stimula- tion and chlorpromazine: An animal model for schizophrenic overarousal. *Science,* 165:1273-1274.
28. Kornetsky, C. and Humphries, O. (1953): Psychological ef- fects of centrally acting drugs in man. Effects of chlorpro- mazine and secobarbital on visual and motor behavior. *J. Ment. Sci.,* 104:1093-1099.
29. Kornetsky, C. and Mirsky, A. F. (1966): On certain psycho- pharmacological and physiological differences between schizo- phrenic and normal persons. *Psychopharmacologia,* 8:309-318.
30. Kornetsky, C., Mirsky, A. F., Kessler, E. K., and Dorff, J. E. (1959): The effects of dextroamphetamine on behavioral deficits produced by sleep loss in humans. *J. Pharmacol. Exp. Ther.,* 127:46-50.
31. Lansdell, H. and Mirsky, A. F. (1964): Attention in focal and centrencephalic epilepsy. *Exp. Neurol.,* 9:463-469.
32. Luria, A. F. (1973): The frontal lobes and the regulation of behavior. In: *Psychophysiology of the Frontal Lobes,* edi- ted by K. H. Pribram and A. R. Luria, pp. 3-26. Academic Press, New York.
33. Metrakos, K. and Metrakos, J. (1961): Genetics of convulsive disorders: II. Genetic and electroencephalographic studies in centrencephalic epilepsy. *Neurology,* 11:474-483.
34. Miller, L. H., Harris, L. C., Kastin, A. J., and Van Riezen, H. (1976): A neuropeptide influence on attention and memory in man. *Pharmacol. Biochem. Behav. (Suppl.),* 5:17-22.
35. Miller, L. H., Kastin, A. J., Sandman, C. A., Fink, M., and VanVeen, W. J. (1974): Polypeptide influences on attention, memory and anxiety in man. *Pharmacol. Biochem. Behav.,* 2:663- 668.
36. Mirsky, A. F. (1969): Neuropsychological bases of schizo- phrenia. *Ann. Rev. Psychol.,* 20:321-348.
36a.Mirsky, A. F., Bakay Pragay, E., and Harris, S. (1977): Evoked potential correlates of stimulation-induced impairment of attention in *macaca mulatta. Exp. Neurol. (In press.)*
37. Mirsky, A. F. and Bloch, S. (1967): Effects of chlorproma- zine, secobarbital and sleep deprivation on attention in mon- keys. *Psychopharmacologia,* 10:388-399.
38. Mirsky, A. F. and Kornetsky, C. (1964): On the dissimilar effects of drugs on the digit symbol substitution and continu- ous performance test. *Psychopharmacologia,* 5:161-177.
39. Mirsky, A. F. and Orzack, M. H. (1976): Psychosurgery Pilot

Study. Proceedings of the National Commission for the Protection of Human Subjects in Biomedical and Behavioral Research.

40. Mirsky, A. F. and Oshima, H. (1973): Effects of subcortical aluminum cream lesions on attentive behavior and electroencephalogram in monkeys. *Exp. Neurol.*, 39:1-18.

41. Mirsky, A. F., Primac, D. W., Ajmone Marsan, C., Rosvold, H. E., and Stevens, J. R. (1960): A comparison of the psychological test performance of patients with focal and nonfocal epilepsy. *Exp. Neurol.*, 2:75-89.

42. Mirsky, A. F. and Tecce, J. J. (1968): The analysis of visual evoked potentials during spike and wave EEG activity. *Epilepsia*, 9:211-220.

43. Mirsky, A. F. and Van Buren, J. M. (1965): On the nature of the "absence" in centrencephalic epilepsy: A study of some behavioral, electroencephalographic and autonomic factors. *EEG Clin. Neurophysiol.*, 18:334-348.

44. Murawski, B. J. (1970): The continuous performance test: A measure of sustained attention in human uremics. In: *Proceedings of the Workshop on Behavioral Bioassays in Uremia*. DHEW Publication No. (NIH) 72-37, edited by R. B. Coletti and K. K. Krueger, pp. 54-61. U.S. Government Printing Office, Washington.

45. Myers, R. E. (1969): The clinical and pathological effects of asphyxiation in the fetal rhesus monkey. In: *Diagnosis and Treatment of Fetal Disorders*, edited by K. Adamson, pp. 226-249. Springer-Verlag, New York.

46. Myers, R. E. (1971): Brain damage induced by umbilical cord compression at different gestational ages. In: *Second Conference on Experimental Medicine and Surgery in Primates*, edited by E. I. Goldsmith and J. Moor-Jankowski, pp. 394-425. S. Karger, New York.

47. Olsen, S. (1961): The brain in uremia. *Acta Psychiol. Scand.*, 36: (Suppl. 156) 129.

48. Orren, M. (1974): Visuomotor behavior and visual evoked potentials during petit mal seizures. Unpublished doctoral dissertation. Boston University, Boston, Massachusetts.

49. Orzack, M. H. and Kornetsky, C. (1966): Attention dysfunction in chronic schizophrenia. *Arch. Gen. Psychiatry*, 14:323-326.

50. Orzack, M. H. and Kornetsky, C. (1971): Environmental and familial predictors of attention behavior in chronic schizophrenics. *J. Psychiatr. Res.*, 9:21-29.

51. Panksepp, J., Reilly, P., Bishop, P., Meeker, R. B., Vilberg, T. R., and Kastin, A. J. (1976): Effects of α-MSH on motivation, vigilance and brain respiration. *Pharmacol. Biochem. Behav. (Suppl.)*, 5:59-64.

52. Penfield, W. and Jasper, H. (1954): *Epilepsy and the Functional Anatomy of the Human Brain*, p. 895. Little Brown & Co., Boston.

53. Purpura, D. P., Penry, J. K., Tower, D. M., Woodbury, D. M., and Walter, R. (Eds.) (1972): *Experimental Models of Epilepsy:*

A Manual for the Laboratory Worker, p. 615. Raven Press, New York.

54. Ricks, N. L. (1974): Sustained attention and the effects of distraction in underachieving second grade children. Unpublished doctoral dissertation, Boston University, Boston, Massachusetts.

55. Rosenthal, D. and Kety, S. S. (Eds.) (1968): *The Transmission of Schizophrenia,* p. 345. Pergamon Press, New York.

56. Rosvold, H. E. and Mirsky, A. F. (1955): Five-year follow up of Yale lobotomy series. Unpublished data.

57. Rosvold, H. E., Mirsky, A. F., Sarason, I., Bransome, E. D. Jr., and Beck, L. H. (1956): A continuous performance test of brain damage. *J. Consult. Psychol.,* 20:343-350.

58. Sandman, C. A., Denman, P. M., Miller, L. H., Knott, J. R., Kastin, A. J., and Schally, A. V. (1971): Electroencephalographic measures of melanocyte stimulating hormone activity. *J. Comp. Physiol. Psychol.,* 76:103-109.

59. Sandman, C. A., George, J. M., Nolan, J. D., Van Riezen, H., and Kastin, A. J. (1975): Enhancement of attention in man with ACTH/MSH 4-10. *Physiol. Behav.,* 15:427-431.

60. Sandman, C. A., George, J., Walker, B., Nolan, J. D. and Kastin, A. J. (1976): Neuropeptide MSH/ACTH 4-10 enhances attention in the mentally retarded. *Pharmacol. Biochem. Behav. (Suppl.),* 5:23-28.

61. Schreiner, G. E. (1959): Mental and personality changes in the uremic syndrome. *Med. Ann. D. C.,* 28:316-323.

62. Stammeyer, E. C. (1961): The effects of distraction on performance in schizophrenic, psychoneurotic and normal individuals. The Catholic University of America Press, Washington, D.C., Ph.D. dissertation.

63. Strand, F. L., Cayer, A., Gonzalez, E., and Stoboy, H. (1976): Peptide enhancement of neuromuscular function: Animal and clinical studies. *Pharmacol. Biochem. Behav. (Suppl.),* 5:179-188.

64. Sutherland, N. S. and Macintosh, N. J. (1971): *Mechanisms of Animal Discrimination Learning,* Academic Press, New York.

65. Sykes, D. H., Douglas, V. I., and Morgenstern, G. (1973): Sustained attention in hyperactive children. *J. Child Psychol. Psychiatry,* 14:213-220.

66. Sykes, D. H., Douglas, V. I., Weiss, G. and Minde, K. K. (1971): Attention in hyperactive children and the effect of methylphenidate (Ritalin). *J. Child Psychol. Psychiatry,* 12: 129-139.

67. Teschan, P. E. (1970): The effect of uremia on behavior: The concept of behavioral bioassays in the pursuit of uremic toxins. In: *Proceedings of the Workshop on Behavioral Bioassays in Uremia,* edited by R. B. Colletti and K. K. Drueger, pp. 5-17. U.S. Government Printing Office, Washington, D. C.

68. Towbin, A. (1969a): Latent spinal cord and brain stem injury in newborn infants. *Dev. Med. Child Neurol.,* 11:54-68.

69. Towbin, A. (1969b): Mental retardation due to germinal matrix infarction. *Science,* 164:156-161.

70. Townsend, A. and Mirsky, A. F. (1960): A comparison of the effects of meprobamate, phenobarbital and d-amphetamine on two psychological tests. *J. Nerv. Ment. Dis.*, 130:212-216.
71. Victor, M., Adams, R. D., and Collins, G. H. (1971): *The Wernicke-Korsakoff Syndrome*. F. A. Davis, Philadelphia, Pennsylvania, p. 206.
72. Vinogradova, O. S. (1970): Registration of information and the limbic system. In: *Short-Term Changes in Neural Activity and Behavior*, edited by G. Horn and R. A. Hinde, pp. 95-140. University Press, Cambridge, England.
73. Weir, B. (1964): Spike-wave from stimulation of the reticular core. *Arch. Neurol.*, 11:209-218.
74. Weiss, B. and Laties, V. G. (1962): Enhancement of human performance by caffeine and the amphetamines. *Pharmacol. Rev.*, 14:1-36.
75. Windle, W. F. (1968): Brain damage at birth: Functional and structural modification with time. *J. Am. Med. Assoc.*, 206: 1967-1972.
76. Windle, W. F. (1969): Brain damage by asphyxia at birth. *Sci. Am.*, 221:76-84.
77. Wohlberg, G. W. and Kornetsky, C. (1973): Sustained attention in remitted schizophrenics. *Arch. Gen. Psychiatry*, 28: 533-537.

Neuropeptide Influences on the Brain and Behavior, edited by L.H. Miller, C.A. Sandman, and A.J. Kastin. Raven Press, New York © 1977.

Some Implications of Current Neuropeptide Studies for Clinical Psychophysiology of the Future

Sanford I. Cohen

Division of Psychiatry, Boston University Medical Center, Boston, Massachusetts 02118

INTRODUCTION

As one reviews the many outstanding papers in the growing peptide literature, it is interesting to note the absence of several areas of inquiry:

(1) The importance of environmental stress in the release of peptides or the effects of peptides in modulating the response to stress as viewed from a multilevel, integrative point of view has been virtually ignored.

(2) The relative absence of any serious commitment to the study of individual differences, especially those concerned with personality, perception, cognition, emotion, behavior is disturbing. Passing reference has been made by some, and a few investigators such as Miller (34) have undertaken studies where these variables have been more seriously considered.

Investigators and clinicians who in the past have been concerned with integrative CNS functions, especially those who have been interested in the relationship of biochemical and neurophysiological functions to normal and abnormal psychological functions, may have a *déjà vu* experience as they became aware of these lacks. It seems that each time a new biochemical-behavioral correlate is identified, the precision with which environmental contingencies, personality variables, and behavioral analysis is carried out diminishes. It is almost as if we all get caught up in the "magic bullet wish," i.e., a wish that one molecule (or fragment) will explain complex behavior and that modification of an "abnormal" molecule will change abnormal complex psychological functions. This chapter will examine the broader effect peptides may have on the organization and activation of brain

functions in greater depth than generally discussed in
the literature. It may be that the most parsimonious
explanation of the correlations obtained, i.e., the effect of ACTH 4-10/MSH on selective attentional variables, is too narrow an hypothesis and could lead to
too much "pebble polishing" by constantly refining
ways to prove the same observation. One goal of this
chapter is to suggest a synthetic framework by which
one can view the peptide data and develop strategies
for new studies.

We will summarize a few points related to the effects of neuropeptides on CNS functions, especially
some of the relationships and correlations which have
been demonstrated between learning and peptide substances, as well as some of the effects of some hormones on specific brain areas (10). The purpose will
be to develop a base for hypothesizing about some of
the processes which may mediate the effects of environmental stress on psychophysiological responses.
Further, an effort will be made to address some issues
related to the role of peptides such as ACTH in the release of stress induced emergency responses and the
role of peptides in the learning of new behavior.

Certain hormones like ACTH originally have "first
messenger" type functions, or perhaps it would be better to identify these as activating functions. This
function is concerned with triggering-off patterns of
body responses which are already programmed in the organism. The material presented here will attempt to
discuss the question, can hormonal substances with
these activating functions be fragmented or modified so
that a portion of the original hormonal molecule becomes responsible for an organizing function—like a
"second messenger." The new CNS functions which would
be organized under the influence of this hormone substance would involve a pattern including (1) selective
attending to external stimuli which were not previously
considered significant, and (2) mobilizing and expres-
sing a variety of new outputs (behavior) which are not
directly concerned with survival.

One of the most impressive points in the literature
is the profound effect that very small quantities of
the peptides have, as well as the difficulty, in obtaining the substance. Guillemin (18, 19) had described
the successful isolation of purified TRF. This required the development of highly sophisticated separation methods, as well as a hypothalamic tissue collection system involving hundreds of trained dissectors,
large numbers of sheep, and 50 tons of hypothalamic
starting material. He points out that final success
resulted from obtaining 1 mg of material from 300,000
sheep hypothalami.

It is startling to appreciate that a tripeptide can exert such powerful hormonal controls. It is not surprising that there are a large number of investigators attempting to solve the riddle of the mechanism of TRF synthesis, and the location of the cells which release the tripeptide. Since the amount of material in the hypothalamus is very small, the localization of TRF cells will not be easy, yet this step is essential to demonstrate the neuronal circuits involved in the regulation. It seems likely that, at best, a small number of hypothalamic cells can control a whole range of feedback and feed-forward steps by which the thyroid gland regulates cellular metabolism throughout the body.

Another important factor highlighted in the literature is the possibility that central neurons might utilize peptides as intercellular messengers. Many of these peptides are synthesized in the CNS and are known to possess a high degree of specific biological activity on peripheral target organs.

The evidence which exists regarding neurons producing and responding to polypeptides is available primarily in relation to the hypothalamus. But, this brain region also mediates a large number of responses to the environment. The interaction of neurons and peptides may be more widespread, however, and not exclusive to the hypothalamus. For example, the action of angiotensin in the setting off of drinking behavior requires that large chains of motorneurons be activated once the initial signal to drink has been registered in the hypothalamus (48).

If hormones that act on neurons utilize information transfer systems (42), then small amounts could produce significant cellular changes. The efferent limb of the TRF-TSH-thyroxine reflex has a molecular magnification of nearly six orders of magnitude, and it is possible that 2 to 3 µg of hypothalamic neurons with hormone responsiveness could be the basis of a variety of complex behavioral patterns and controls.

One important basic assumption which is made is that the possible importance of polypeptides in relation to psychophysiological responses to environmental stress is probably based on the activities of the hypothalamus and limbic system. Although the hypothalamus comprises less than 5% of the brain's weight, it is credited with an enormous number of vital functions (56). It is felt that its integrative role is possible because it receives an abundant input of information from neural and endocrine sources, and helps regulate the endocrine and autonomic nervous systems while also modulating the activity of other brain areas. Further, hormones which are mainly peptides produced either in the hypothalamus

or pituitary may act on the brain to influence complex
neural functions such as behavior.

The behaviors which peptide hormones may control
could include innate as well as learned patterns. The
role of peptides in innate behavior could be viewed as
merely an extension of the known hormonal functions of
these substances. There may be nothing surprising in
the possibility that hormonal peptides can control such
elementary behavioral patterns as feeding, sleep, re-
production, territorial defense, aggressive behavior-
all intimately linked to survival.

Consideration of the possible role in the acquisition and preservation of new patterns of behavior implies they may have something to do with the mechanisms
of conditioning, learning and memory. It has also been
suggested that peptides which influence behavior and
learning may act on brain protein metabolism by modulating the presence of certain proteins which could be
specific for certain brain functions. The capacity for
ACTH to influence avoidance behavior seems to parallel
its effectiveness in influencing brainstem protein synthesis (1). Further, ACTH may affect noradrenergic
mechanisms by increasing the turnover of NA (16).

The influence of ACTH-like peptides on CNS cells
which may be relevant to learning can be conceptualized
as follows:

ACTH-like——Interact on surface of——Induced conforma-
Peptides   plasma membrane of   tional change and
              effector cell.   stimulates in-
              (There may be specific   creased production
              peptidergic receptors   of cAMP (2nd mes-
              in various brain areas)   senger).
                                                ↓
                                        Mediates the in-
                                        formation on pep-
                                        tide-cell membrane
                                        binding.
                                                ↓
                                        Triggers biochemi-
                                        cal events under-
                                        lying the func-
                                        tional response of
                                        the effector cell.
                                                ↓
                        Change in AMP-dependent protein ki-
                        nase activity, which may cause change
                        in membrane phosphorylation and in
                        macromolecule metabolism.   ↓

May be basis of modulatory influence of neuropeptides on neurotransmission.

Learning a new behavior is often associated with release of pituitary hormones, e.g., ACTH——> increased
availability of hormones. This may provide biochemical
mediators by which protein metabolism is activated and
plasticity in the nervous system is facilitated—necessary to form and maintain new behavior (15, 39, 40, 57).

NEUROPEPTIDES AND THE PSYCHOPHYSIOLOGY OF STRESS

Let us now turn to some studies of stress and related neuroendocrine mechanisms. We will attempt to
relate some of the comments in this section to some of
the more basic mechanisms mentioned previously. Some
ideas will be presented on individual differences in
stress responsivity and individual differences in the
acquisition and retention of C.R. especially as this
may be taken to reflect the development of internal
models of external reality formed in the brain which
may be influenced by peptide hormones.
The response to external stimuli, stressful or not,
can be viewed in at least two ways:
(1) Pre-programmed responses, e.g., to danger. The
organism may need to learn a multiplicity of signals
which indicate threat or danger but recognition sets
off pre-programmed responses, such as fight or flight;
(2) Learned adaptive responses requiring new percep-
tions, cognitions, and complex behaviors in which future consequences of the event or behavior are considered. This requires determining the characteristics
and significance of an event, then selecting an appropriate new behavioral response which has to be learned.

Research involving the effects of stress on CNS activity, behavior, emotions and adaptation to life situations was very vigorously pursued in the 1950s and
60s. The neuroendocrine mechanisms considered involved
(1) hypothalamo-adrenomedullary mechanisms, and (2) hy-
pophyseal-adrenocortical axes, with increased secretion
of (a) epinephrine, (b) noradrenaline, (c) corticosteroids, and (d) thyroxine. Although it was felt there
were probably many other mechanisms, those were considered to be the most relevant.
Since those initial studies based largely on formu-
lations developed by Cannon on fight/flight mechanisms
(5) and by Selye (47) in his general adaptation theory,
two major thrusts have advanced our understanding.
Firstly, the neurophysiological and endocrine mechanism

involved has been more precisely defined. Secondly,
considerable efforts have been undertaken to understand
the psychological response to life stress. Mason (32)
emphasized the need for not only a research strategy
which involved multihormonal measures but a strategy
which adequately recognized the importance of psycho-
socially induced emotional stimuli and the need to
avoid too much emphasis on nonspecificity of stress re-
sponsibility or too much reliance on neurobiological
mechanisms to fully understand the response in man to
stressful events.

Mason (32) has pointed out that one general principle that has emerged in endocrinology is that most if
not all hormones respond to multiple stimuli, especially those considered stressful. This includes cortisol,
epinephrine, norepinephrine, thyroxine, growth hormone,
testosterone, etc. The multihormonal patterns seem to
be organized in a rather specific or selective manner,
probably dependent on complex interdependencies in hormonal actions at metabolic levels.

He also urged investigators to keep individual differences in mind, including differences in how situations are perceived, differences in behavioral responses, and differences in CNS response characteristics. Rose (43) suggests that research in psychoneuroendocrinology, possibly more than in any other field,
has demonstrated that environmental stimuli significantly affect physiological functioning. In classical
endocrinology, the control of individual endocrine
glands was believed to be by a closed negative feedback
loop. Increased secretion from the glands served to
inhibit secretion of the specific tropic hormone from
the pituitary. This autoregulatory concept was inade-
quate to explain a few different phenomena. It could
not account for the circadian or diurnal rhythm observed in various circulating hormones, e.g., cortisol
and testosterone. Furthermore, it could not account
for the increases observed following exposure to stress.
It did not explain the independent activity of releasing hormones on the brain in addition to its effect on
pituitary and other endocrine glands. In fact, a
closed feedback loop would tend to inhibit the increased levels often observed.

ACTH has, of course, been shown to parallel levels
of cortisol confirming the fact that a simple negative
feedback system is not sufficient to explain alterations in cortisol secretion.

The essentials of the systems operating in response
to stress are currently described as follows: information concerning stress coming either from external
sources, such as change in body temperature, is received and integrated by the central nervous system

(CNS) and is presumably delivered to the hypothalamus and the basal area of the brain. The hypothalamus secretes a substance called corticocotropin (CRF) and other releasing factors, that stimulate the pituitary to secrete the hormone ACTH. This is turn stimulates the cortex of the adrenal gland to increase its synthesis and secretion of hormones; however, in addition, both CRF and ACTH, which are both polypeptides, seem to have direct effects on the brain. If the adrenal gland is removed, the pituitary secretes abnormally high amounts of ACTH, presumably because the absence of the adrenal hormone allows unrestricted secretion. This is the portion of the ACTH molecule that is directly concerned with the stimulation of the adrenal cortex.

Having referred to Mason's (32) notions that an integrative CNS multihormonal framework is necessary to study the response to stress, it is interesting to note that Corson (9) emphasizes similar points but in addition emphasizes the importance of differentiating acute and chronic stress and stressful situations which are avoidable and not avoidable. Further, he highlights the importance of individual differences. Kimble (24) suggests that the study of unavoidable shock and in general the utilization of a learned helplessness paradigm was an important experimental strategy to be undertaken.

Corson describes studies in dogs in which he attempted to correlate and integrate behavioral responses in conditioned reflex experiments with neuroendocrine and neurophysiological responses. It would appear to be more profitable not to single out a particular neural or endocrine response to psychologic stress but to simultaneously study as many behavioral, physiologic, and endocrine responses as possible taking into account the existence of individual differences. His work involved chronic experiments dealing with conditioned and unconditioned responses to nociceptive stimuli. He demonstrated the involvement of vasopressin in the response of dogs to psychologic stress. He found reproducible individual differences with some dogs exhibiting a marked and persistent release of vasopressin in response to repeated stress while other dogs failed to show such responses to the same stimuli.

The question arose, what is the function of vasopressin in adaptive responses to stress? One may conceive of vasopressin release in response to a "fight or flight" situation as serving the function of fluid conservation, an adaptation that could serve a useful purpose in the case of hemorrhage. Vasopressin release to symbols of danger may represent an anticipatory adaptive response in preparation for combat.

Quite apart from its water conservation properties,

vasopressin may have other important functions, e.g.,
it can exert profound vasoconstrictive influences including the coronaries (45). Further, it has been implicated as a link between CNS and the release of ACTH.
A number of authors have also reviewed evidence suggesting links between the neurohypophyses and adenohy-
pophyses (25). In this connection it is of course pertinent that a basic peptide with ACTH releasing properties has been described as the corticotropic releasing
factor (46).

In studies reported in the literature it has been
noted that in addition to the effect of vasopressin on
blood pressure and water regulation, it also appears
to increase consolidation of long-term memory during
learning (60). It is of interest that vasopressin,
like MSH and ACTH, increases the resistance of active
and passive avoidance responses to extinction (10, 11).
An absence of vasopressin has been reported to lead to
a deficit in avoidance learning (12, 36). It has also
been noted that lesions in the hippocampus seem to prevent vasopressin and ACTH from exerting their ability
to preserve avoidance response but the lesions themselves may not modify the rate of extinction. However,
lesions in the hippocampus may retard the rate of acquisition of the avoidance response (62).

In another type of study the mechanism of action of
the peptides in stressful situations has been looked at
in terms of their possible interaction with brain transmitter substances. Endröczi (14) in his studies had
noted that brain norepinephrine levels seemed sensitive
to various stressors and that animals who showed good
retention of avoidance responses showed a greater decrease in brain norepinephrine (greater turnover) than
poor retainers. He also demonostrated a relation of
norepinephrine turnover to performance. Further, it
has been suggested that brain biogenic amine responses
to stress may be hormonally mediated.

Briefly, then, the findings suggest that some of the
peptide hormones released during the learning of adaptive behavior in relation to stressful stimuli may be
important in modulating the storage, and later retention of specific information provided by the experience.
It is not clear however whether we are talking about an
organizing or activating effect.

Finally, Mason and Corson (9, 32) and others, have
suggested that differences in individual patterns of
hormonal responsivity to similar stresses requires attention.

INDIVIDUAL DIFFERENCES IN STRESS RESPONSIVITY

This section will consider individual differences in

stress responsivity and the possible role peptide hormones may have in the development of these differences
or, the differences in hormone activity that are an expression of individual difference.

Reference will be made to perceptual mode characteristics—field independence (FI) and field dependence
(FD). However, there is no intention to imply this is
the key personality or perceptive variable to be considered. It is utilized to illustrate some points
which can be made about individual differences in autonomic responsivity, cognition, and behavior which may
be related to differences in the organization of CNS
areas affected by neuropeptides.

A series of studies utilizing FI and FD subjects led
to the speculation that differences in perceptual mode
characteristics were a reflection of some differences
in CNS organization, i.e., a difference in the way in
which CNS handles internal and external signals or a
difference in the way the world gets organized in a
person's head so that predictions can be made about how
signals are related to one another. Many of the first
studies by Witkin (63) involving FI and FD were concerned with the relation of this perceptual dimension
to differences in styles of cognition, articulated or
global, and differences in personality, e.g., outer vs
inner directed. Witkin's work (63, 64) suggested that
this difference in perceptual mode seemed to have its
roots in different early mother-child relations with
the FD coming from situations where independent exploration of the world was not encouraged.

During the 1960s a large number of studies indicated
that FI and FD subjects responded differently to a variety of experimental situations, e.g., low sensory input, drugs, insulin hypoglycemia (6, 52). Differences
were reported in the way these subjects perceived and
reacted psychologically, and differences were noted in
a variety of physiological dimensions, e.g., GSR, EEG,
heart rate, free fatty acid mobilization (17, 33, 38,
51). In addition, differences in integrative neuropsychological functions began to emerge with the FD individual consistently showing difficulties in a variety
of spatial perceptual, sensory-motor and complex sensory tasks, especially those requiring the identification of stimuli embedded within some larger field or
tests involving stimuli in which stimuli presented se-
quentially had to be related to one another (6, 49, 50).

The differences which began to emerge in neuropsychological functions and in autonomic response suggested that differences in integrative CNS functions might
be in part responsible for the perceptual mode differences or be a correlate of it.

In an attempt to further delineate CNS reactivity in

FI and FD subjects especially in relation to the effect of external sensory signals on autonomic responses, a series of conditional reflex (CR) studies were
conducted. Only the conclusions of those studies will
be presented in this chapter. These findings suggested
that in this experimental situation the field-independent subjects showed evidence of more sympathetic neurogenic activity when stimulated (7, 20). This was
suggested by the cardio-acceleration and the greater
and more prolonged galvanic skin response (GSR) responsivity to specific stimuli and a higher frequency of
nonspecific skin resistance fluctuation. Field-independent subjects also showed a more pronounced differentiation of GSR responses to reinforced from nonreinforced CS during the extinction period. The experiment
suggested that there was some sort of a parallel between the psychologic differentiation described by Witkin in field-independent individuals and discriminated
conditional reflex reactivity of the balanced excitatory type. Further, field-independent subjects resembled Lacey's cardiac "labile" subjects (27, 28), a
group who displayed evidence of active sympathetic neurogenic cardiac activity.
    More recent work by Dronsejko suggests the relation
between perceptual mode differences and discriminated
autonomic nervous system (ANS) response characteristics
(13). In her studies she utilized a delayed conditioning paradigm and demonstrated that with a sufficiently
long CS-US interval a biphasic acceleration-decelera-
tion heart rate conditioned or anticipatory response
could be demonstrated. Instructional sets did not significantly alter cardiac activity but did influence responses in interaction with individual differences in
perceptual mode. One question she asked of the data
was, did FI subjects show an adaptive pattern of cardiac responding? The data included that FI subjects in a
situation where they were expecting the very first UC
reacted with cardiac deceleration rather than acceleration in FD. She felt this was indicative of attentive
observation and searching of the environment rather
than an anxious-arousal response.
    Other experiments in which specific preparatory in-
structions were given revealed that FI subjects showed
clearer cardiac deceleration which she felt was suggestive of looking for specific elements in the environment. The first CR experiments to which reference
was made indicated that FI showed discriminated cardiac
acceleration of greater magnitude and larger duration
than FD subjects, but in the work of Dronsejko the FI
subjects showed a much clearer cardiodecelerative CR.
    The major point is that in a wide variety of studies
(to which I have not done justice) persons who score FI

on a perceptual test and who show an articulated cognitive style showed more selective and seemingly appropriate autonomic response patterns. Most important is that discriminated responses persisted into the extinction period for longer periods of time in both types of experiments. FD subjects seemed to respond to reinforced CS's only when they were being reinforced. The longer period of time that the FI continued to respond to the previously reinforced CS during the extinction period suggested the possibility that they may have acquired a more stable internal model of the external signal relationships.

This then leads us to consider some notions about internal models of external reality. According to Sokolov (53, 54), incoming stimuli leave some traces in the nervous system. He called these traces the neuronal model. The function of this model is to preserve information about direction and intensity of stimuli. Subsequent inputs are then compared with the model and if they do not match an orienting response occurs. If they do match, the orienting response is blocked. So-called FD persons may merely be persons who have a less stable internal norm or neuronal model. One would expect an FD would show an orienting response for a longer period than FI persons. This is what has been reported. It seems like FI persons manifest more appropriate and selective arousal. It is possible that the FD person is more anxiously vigilant and scans the environment more frequently because it takes longer for new stimuli, even a familiar one, to be matched with previous input, or it may be that slight changes in the characteristics of input stimuli lead to orienting responses.

Witkin found that children are initially field-dependent and become more field-independent as they mature (63, 64). This suggests that field dependency may be associated with a more primitive, less mature, less integrated, or less organized perceptual apparatus or CNS, especially as it concerns the integration of external and internal signals and the formation of a stable internal norm. It is also interesting that in other types of studies, the learning of motor avoidance behavior has been reported to be accompanied by evidence of sympathetic neurogenic activity in response to anticipatory signals (8). In a conditioned avoidance experiment, FI subjects learned a motor avoidance response more readily and showed more sympathetic activity. This may reflect the activation of brain areas concerned with motor activity which also leads to cardiovascular changes necessary to supply muscular areas activated by the motor efferents. On the other hand, the internal interoceptive cues associated with sympa-

thetic discharges or alterations in brain functions associated with adrenergic stimulation may be changes
that are necessary for avoidance learning to occur.
This might involve excitation of brain areas concerned
with a motivational state appropriate for learning de-
fensive avoidance reactions and a level of responsiveness to external cues in which discrimination is enhanced and appropriate motor activity is facilitated.

The studies of Brown and Heninger (3) were concerned
with correlating stress induced growth hormone release
and perceptual mode. This work further suggested the
possibility that differences in CNS organization might
be related to individual variations in stress hormone
responsivity and perceptual, cognitive, and coping
styles. These studies were based on the observation
that even though growth hormone has been shown to increase in humans undergoing stressful procedures, these
changes occur in only a percentage of persons studied.
Their study demonstrated that one-third of their subjects showed a growth hormone increase during a presumably stressful situation.

Their findings suggested that this presumably
stress-induced growth hormone response was not related
to any measurable or obvious degree of subjective distress or state variable at the time of catheterization
but rather to the perceptual style of the subject,
i.e., FI vs FD. In the absence of definitive evidence
for a relationship between a "state" variable such as
anxiety and GH release, they felt their findings indicate that stable individual differences in the propen-
sity to release GH during stress may account for differential GH as much if not more so than changes in
subjective state.

Another group (55) has investigated the relationship
between field dependence and one parameter of thyroid
activity. More specifically, they tested the hypothesis that extremely field dependent individuals would
differ from FI in RA iodine uptake levels.

The ingestion of triiodothyronine by normal subjects
may produce perceptual distortion, and intensification
of after images (59). More recently, Kopell (26) has
shown that while the ability to attend to a significant
stimulus was not affected by T3 ingestion, attention to
nonsignificant information was enhanced. One conclusion was that in experimentally induced hyperthyroidism
the individual becomes limited in his ability to screen
out extraneous stimuli. This is an essential function
in disembedding an item from its context in tests of
FD.

Of great interest is the correlation found in a control group of euthyroid subjects. The longer the duration of visual negative after images, the lower the RA

iodine uptake. After image phenomena are thought to be related to the persistence or fading of neural excitation evoked by visual stimuli (64), further, differences in diffusion and the strength of neural trace have been invoked by some to explain FI and FD modes of perceiving (21).

The results of perceptual mode thyroid studies indicated that greater field dependence is associated with higher RA iodine uptake. However, there was no way to determine whether this was primarily due to differences in function in the thyroid, pituitary, or hypothalamus.

In a number of papers a relationship has been postulated between attentional parameters and peptides. As indicated previously, differences in attentional characteristics have been hypothesized in FI and FD subjects. Therefore, it would seem important to carefully study neuropeptide differences found in FI and FD and other specific personality and perceptual dimensions. It should be noted that Miller has already begun some studies in this area (35). One intriguing point Miller reported was that in spite of the "ceiling effect" which obscured differences in the FI subjects he tested who received ACTH and saline, differences were found in FI given ACTH as opposed to controls (saline) at the point where they had to change expectancies. This might mean a point at which the rapid development of a new internal model of external reality occurs. It would be interesting to see if FD with ACTH would have done as well as the FI.

The question to raise at this point is whether the administration of ACTH facilitated the CNS functions necessary to subserve the learning of new relationships between stimuli and between external stimuli and an organism's response.

Since heart rate has been mentioned in relation to FI and FD subjects, it may be useful to be reminded of one of the few papers in which this autonomic variable has been reported. Sandman (44) reported that mentally retarded subjects improved after the administration of peptide hormones in some tests, e.g., tests of intra-dimensional shifts. They also noticed a significant heart rate deceleration to the test signal. This relation was interpreted in line with Lacey's notions that a decreased heart rate can be a part of a pattern where more attention is paid to environmental stimuli and the intake of stimuli is facilitated (27-30).

Mentally retarded persons are FD or stimulus bound as are all brain damaged patients, children and aged persons. However, these different groups may differ in the reason that they are field dependent, e.g., in some there may be a problem in attending to stimuli or too

much responding to irrelevant stimuli; in others the
internal noise may be an impediment or some problem may
exist in the storage of signals, or the integration of
new and old signals. Whatever the explanation, the
mentally retarded subjects after being given peptides
displayed a heart rate pattern which accompanies or facilitates increased intake of external signals and
showed an increased ability to perform certain tests.

One further point about peptides, learning, and
heart rate. In a number of papers, e.g., Kastin (23),
it has been postulated that some peptides facilitate
learning of conditioned avoidance response (CAR) by increasing the ability to pay attention (either to the
stimuli or the task). It has been noted by a number of
psychophysiologists that a slow heart rate often accompanies attention to environmental stimuli. Further, it
has been noted that fast heart rate learners are slow
conditioned avoidance learners.

One speculation from this data is that some organisms (or organisms under the influence of specific
substances) have the capacity to organize sensory perceptual experiences and goal directed motor responses.
This capacity may include a pattern of ANS responses
which is specifically facilitative and not merely a
nonspecific response.

Some of the data is beginning to suggest that ACTH
4-10, MSH, and possibly other peptide substances are
concerned with the organization in the CNS of a pattern
which includes the capacity to identify and discriminate complex signals together with the learning of appropriate new behavioral responses and ANS changes
which facilitate perception and learning, i.e., an organizing function.

The other portion of the ACTH molecule may be more
related to the more classic activating function of ACTH,
i.e., its involvement in the release of peripheral adrenal cortical hormones concerned with the organism's
response to environmental stress. This response may be
expressed by pre-programmed adaptive fight/flight type
activity. The question being begged is whether ACTH 4-
10 has more to do with nongenetic, newly learned adaptive responses, and whether it facilitates the development of a new neuronal model which allows the organism
to respond appropriately and consistently to new environmental signals with nongenetically programmed behaviors.

In Rigter's opinion (41), the view that ACTH-like
peptides improve (selective) attention may also explain
the improvement of retrieval by ACTH 4-10. He points
out behavior consists of a chain of learned or genetically determined motor patterns (programs). The individual links (programs) are selected on the basis of an

evaluation of perceptive input and memory of previous
experiences and coupled to each other to produce the
smoothly running process of controlled behavior. The
control depends mainly on two brain functions. One is
the capacity of the brain to retrieve and activate
these programs. The second is the process of selecting
the correct program. Some of the research suggests
that both the selection capacity and the retrievability
of programs are under motivational control and that
this control mechanism is located in the nonspecific
reticulothalamic system (22). He proposes that ACTH
(fragments) activate this mechanism. Lesion studies
(2), implantation studies (62), and electrophysiological work (58) suggest that the locus of action of ACTH-
like peptides is in the nonspecific reticulothalamic
system.

The two functions of retrieval and selection capacity decline in aging subjects. It is also of interest
that FI diminishes with age. It might be argued that
the cause of this decline is a deficiency of the hormonal control of these functions.

There is also some evidence that MSH may be released
when an organism is exposed to psychological or physical stress. Panksepp (37) felt that the role of MSH in
the response to stress may be a function of the fact
that the target of this hormone may be the pigmented
cells of the ANS. MSH may possibly lead to direct effects on the locus ceruleus. It is felt by some that
the l. ceruleus may participate in organizing stress
related responses and states of vigilance.

Part of Panksepp's hypothesis is that a main function of MSH is to modulate central autonomic tone. He
feels from such autonomic action one might assume that
the behavior of animals in many situations would be
stabilized (this could be taken to imply a more stable
internal model) rather than shifted. Therefore, MSH
might tend to reduce the variability of behavior.

The speculations in the previous section suggest
that it would be useful to study whether the neuropeptides can have organizing effects in the infant and
adult organism. Levine's work (31) is extremely important to consider since it provides us with a model of
how hormones can affect CNS organization and behavior.

The details of Levine's studies are important but
unfortunately cannot be included in this chapter. A
few conclusions from his work which have relevance to
this chapter will be presented. In one group of studies he showed that infant animals who had been handled,
stimulated, and stressed while young when they were
tested as adults learned adaptive avoidance responses
in conditioning experiments better than animals not
handled or stressed when young. There may be some

vague parallel between optimally stressed infant rats who are better learners of avoidance response to adult stress and FI persons who in their development have been allowed by their mother to actively explore the world and within limits to suffer the consequences of their acts. These FI persons are better avoidance learners than FD.

Does this mean that the brain peptides which facilitate the learning of or the retention of avoidance responses are influenced by this early interaction? Levine's most recent hypothesis postulates that one of the major consequences of early stimulation may be to endow the organism with capacities to make finer discriminations concerning the relevant aspects in the environment. The animal is then able to make responses more appropriate to the demands of the environment. Perhaps this is the real meaning of adaptiveness, that is, the ability to make appropriate discriminations in a particular situation and respond according to the demands of the situation.

One model for the influence of hormonal substances on brain function and specific behavior patterns can be examined in relation to sexual behavior. It has been suggested (31) that gonadal hormones act on the central nervous system in different ways at two different stages of development. First, during fetal or neonatal life, sex hormones organize the sexually undifferentiated brain with regard to patterns of gonadotropin secretion. Specifically, this hypothesis states that androgens acting on the CNS during critical periods of development are responsible for the programming of male patterns of gonadotropin secretion and sex behavior in much the same way they determine the development of anatomical sexual characteristics. Second, during adult life gonadal hormones activate the sexually differentiated brain and elicit responses which were programmed earlier. Third, one of the components of the process of sexual differentiation is to render the tissues that are responsive to gonadal hormone differentially sensitive in the male and female.

These experiments were concerned mainly with sexual behavior and rather clearly indicate the importance of hormones in organizing various areas of the CNS. In addition, these hormones appear to influence the sensitivity of certain areas of the brain to certain external signals and to the release of certain motor patterns in adult life.

The emphasis in Levine's work is based on the assumption that the function of gonadal hormones in infancy is to organize the CNS with regard to neuroendocrine function and patterns of behavior. The focus in this work by Levine is on reproductive behavior, but there are numerous reports that have indicated that there are sex differences in nonsexual behavior. There are numerous reports about sex difference in other behaviors, e.g., aggressive behavior. Virtually all these reports suggest aggressive behavioral patterns are more easily elicited in males.

A point of interest in relation to some of the previous comments made about perceptual mode is that males appear to be more FI than females. However, it is quite unclear whether this perceptual difference is due to biological sensory perceptual differences, or is explicable on the basis of socially induced differences during development. One characteristic difference between FI and FD persons is that the FI is more comfortable with and more able to express or display agressive behavior.

It is generally agreed that because of the observed sexual difference in aggressive behavior we need to more precisely delineate the organizational role of testosterone on brain functions. Further, the role of different peptides in the organization of the developing brain especially in relation to complex programs of behavior should be an item of high priority in future investigations.

A point which needs to be emphasized is that there seem to be permanent irreversible effects of androgens that occur early in development which have been called organizing effects of hormones on the brain, and these stand in contrast to transient reversible activating effects of the same hormones secreted in adulthood.

There is a need to determine what interactions occur between the so-called organizing and activating effects the peptides have on the developing mature organism. Further, there is a need to distinguish the effects of hormonal substance on (a) pre-programmed behavior, (b) perception, motivation, and behavior organized during early life when mother-infant reactions are significant factors, (c) adult behavioral responses to new, novel stimuli, and (d) learned adaptive behavioral patterns. It is important not to merely talk of peptide-behavior correlations but to distinguish the type of behavioral pattern.

CONCLUSION

It is possible that one may be born with the capacity to react to certain threats, i.e., traces may be genetically pre-programmed which involve recognition of specific danger signals and the release of adaptive behaviors. Society has become more organized and complex and the signals to which we react are less obvious dangers. In addition, the behaviors are no longer purely

biological adaptive responses. As the signals to which
we react become more symbolic, it seems logical to assume that it was necessary to develop a capacity to react to these second or symbolic signals with behavior
appropriate to the cultural and societal meaning of the
signal, and to react with consideration to future consequences of our behavior as well as on the basis of
immediate needs or impulses.

Further, it has become necessary to develop a capacity to relate two or more signals, i.e., to be able to
predict the relation of environmental events which are
coupled. This implies that in addition to the model of
the world which is built in or pre-programmed, the capacity to adapt in society requires learning a new series of related signals or the need to develop addi-
tions to the internal model of the world which may be
provided at birth.

It is possible that hormones which are the so-called
first messengers have the function of triggering off
pre-programmed responses, e.g., ACTH. It is generally
felt that first messengers do not develop, initiate, or
set in motion the construction of new input-output patterns but that they are mainly concerned with setting
off reactions which are already organized. The usual
functions of these first messengers—activating hormones—may not have been adequate to subserve the need
to learn signals and to develop new patterns of responding, i.e., they were not adequate to subsume functions related to learning that became required as human
society changed. The "way out" question obviously being begged is whether in the course of evolution fragments of some of these activating type hormones took on
a new "organizing" function or whether some organisms
through mutations developed new CNS sensitivities to
portions of hormonal molecules. These mutants would
then have hormonal substances which had new functions,
namely, to subserve attentional and learning mechanisms
enabling them to organize a broader model of reality
and a greater range of adaptive techniques and perceptual capabilities.

It is possible that the effects already described
for a substance like ACTH could be integrated into the
hypothesis being developed. There is a considerable
body of evidence which suggests that fear is a signal
which is genetically pre-programmed in man, as well as
the rest of mammalia. Stimuli which are stressful,
especially those that produce fear, may then be related
to the release of ACTH. The ACTH would be part of an
emergency response system which helps to trigger off
pre-programmed responses to danger. This would represent the emergence of recorded engram, in this instance
one which was wired into the system.

This emotional signal indicating that one is confronted with danger was, and in many instances still
is, absolutely necessary for survival. To lack a fear
response could prevent flight from dangerous situations.
This fear response probably consists of perceptual recognition of danger, affective signal, motor behavioral
impulse, and physiological changes to support motor activity. It is possible that the release of this pre-
programmed complex CNS pattern might be adaptive when
confronted with some new, novel, unknown, uncertain
situations. This was especially true when man lived a
more primitive existence. However, the automatic perception of a new, novel environmental event as dangerous and subsequent release of a "fear reaction" could
prevent more careful attention to the components of
this new stimulus and could prevent efforts to explore
new behaviors in relation to the signal. The epineph-
rine-ACTH-corticosterone relations involved in carrying
out activation type functions might set off these
"fear" patterns. It has also been noted that after the
injection of ACTH 4-10, an animal might perceive a big
footshock (fear inducing) as if it were a small shock.
This would imply that the fear response of the animal
would be less and reduce the likelihood that innate,
unlearned, pre-programmed fear reactions were released.

In human subjects it has been reported that ACTH 4-
10 decreases anxiety, increases attention, improves
visual memory, etc. (34). In general ACTH 4-10 may
create conditions more conducive for the learning of
new relations between environmental stimuli and the
learning of new adaptive or appetitive responses.

What has been suggested may seen overly optimistic
in respect to our ability to understand complex behavior as it relates to molecules and molecular fragments.
However, our guidelines were the words of Don Santiago
Ramon y Cajal (4):

> The individual who in the presence of an arduous
> problem does not feel his enthusiasm grow and not
> feel his soul flooded by the anticipatory emotion
> of pleasure, should abandon scientific research,
> for Nature does not grant her favors to those of a
> cold disposition, coldness often being an unmis-
> takable sign of impotence.

REFERENCES

1. Barondes, S. (1975): Neurochemistry and behavior. In: *Comprehensive Textbook of Psychiatry, Vol. 2*, edited by A. Freed-
   man, H. Kaplan and B. Sadock, pp. 128-132. Williams and Wilkins, Baltimore.
2. Bohus, B. and de Wied, D. (1967): Avoidance and escape be-

havior following medial thalamic lesions in rats. *J. Comp. Physiol. Psychol.*, 64:26-30.

3. Brown, W., and Heninger, G. (1976): Stress induced hormone release: Psychologic and physiologic correlates. *Psychosom. Med.*, 38:145-147.

4. Cajal, Don Santiago Ramon y (1893): *Precepts and Counsels on Scientific Investigation,* quoted in: *Brain Research Institute Tenth Anniversary Symposium,* UCLA, 1972, BRI Publications, Los Angeles, p. 6.

5. Cannon, W. B. (1929): *Bodily Changes in Pain, Hunger, Fear and Rage.* Appleton-Century-Crofts, New York.

6. Cohen, S. I. (1967): Central nervous system functioning in altered sensory environments. In: *Psychological Stress,* edited by M. Appley and R. Trumbull, pp. 77-122. Appleton-Century-Crofts, New York.

7. Cohen, S. I. (1964): Neurobiological considerations for behavior therapy. In: *Behavior Therapy: Appraisal and Status,* edited by C. Franks, pp. 589-605. McGraw-Hill, New York.

8. Cohen, S. I., Shmavonian, B., Hein, P., and Graham, L. (1966): Cardiovascular responsivity in classical and instrumental conditioning. In: *Proceedings XVIII International Congress of Psychology,* pp. 94-103. Moscow

9. Corson, S. (1966): Neuroendocrine and behavioral response patterns to psychological stress. *Ann. N. Y. Acad. Sci.*, 125:890-918.

10. de Wied, D. (1969): Effects of peptide hormones on behavior. In: *Frontiers in Neuroendocrinology,* edited by W. F. Ganong and L. Martini, pp. 97-140. Oxford University Press, New York.

11. de Wied, D. (1973): Pituitary-adrenal system hormones and behavior. In: *The Neurosciences, Third Study Program,* edited by F. O. Schmitt and F. G. Wordon, pp. 653-666. M.I.T. Press, Cambridge.

12. de Wied, D., Bohus, B., and van Wimersma Greidanus, TjB. (1975): Memory deficit in rats with hereditary diabetes insipidus. *Brain Res.*, 85:152-156.

13. Dronsejko, K. (1972): Effects of CS duration and instructional set on cardiac anticipatory responses to stress in field dependent and independent subjects. *Psychophysiology,* 9:1-113.

14. Endröczi, E. (1977): Brain mechanisms involved in ACTH-induced changes of exploratory activity and conditioned avoidance behavior. *(This volume.)*

15. Gispen, W. H., Reith, M., Schotman, P., Wiegant, V., Zwiers, H. and de Wied, D. (1977): The CNS and ACTH-like peptides: Neurochemical responses and interaction with opiates. *(This volume.)*

16. Gold, P. and McGaugh, J. L. (1977): Hormones and memory. *(This volume.)*

17. Goldstein, H. S., Pardes, H., Small, A., and Steinberg, M. (1970): Psychological differentiation and specificity of response. *J. Nerv. Ment. Dis.* 151:97-103.

18. Guillemin, R. (1972): Characteristics and identification of pituitary releasing factors from the hypothalamus. *Neurosci. Res. Progr. Bull.*, 10:193.

19. Guillemin, R., and Burgus, R. (1972): The hormones of the hypothalamus. *Sci. Am.*, 227:24-33.

20. Hein, P., Cohen, S., and Shmavonian, B. (1966): Perceptual mode and cardiac conditioning. *Psychophysiology*, 3:101-107.

21. Immergluck, L. (1968): Individual differences in figural after effect potency. *Psychosom. Sci.*, 10:203-204.

22. Kalsbeek, J. (1925): Le concept de la capacite reduite et la charge mentale. In: *Age et Contraintes de Travail*, edited by A. Laville, C. Teiger and A. Wisner. N.E.B. Editions Scientifiques, Paris.

23. Kastin, R. J., Miller, L., Nockton, R., Sandman, C. D., Schally, A. V., and Stratton, L. O. (1973): Behavioral aspects of melanocyte-stimulating hormone. *Prog. Brain Res.*, 39:461-470.

24. Kimble, G. A. (1977): Is learning involved in neuropeptide effects on behavior? *(This volume.)*

25. Kleeman, C. R., and Cutler, R. E. (1963): The neurohypophysis. *Ann. Rev. Physiol.*, 25:385-432.

26. Kopell, B., Wittner, W., Lunde, D., Warrick, G., and Edwards, D. (1970): Influence of tri-iodothyronine on selective attention in man as measured by visual average evoked potential. *Psychosom. Med.*, 32:495-502.

27. Lacey, J., and Lacey, B. (1958): The relationship of resting autonomic activity to motor impulsivity. *Res. Pub. Assoc. Nerv. Ment. Dis.*, 36:144.

28. Lacey, J. (1963): The visceral level: Situational autonomic response patterns. In: *Expression of Emotions in Man*, edited by P. K. Knapp, pp. 161-196. International University Press, New York.

29. Lacey, J. (1967): Somatic response patterning and stress. In: *Psychological Stress*, edited by M. Appley and R. Trumbull, pp. 14-36. Appleton-Century-Crofts, New York.

30. Lacey, J. (1974): Studies of heart rate and other bodily processes in sensorimotor behavior. In: *Cardiovascular Psychophysiology*, edited by Obrist, Black, Brenner, and DiCara, pp. 538-564. Aldine Publishers, Chicago.

31. Levine, S. (1974): Developmental psychobiology. In: *American Handbook of Psychiatry, Vol. 6*, edited by S. Arietti, A. Hamburg, and H. K. Brodie, pp. 335-351. Basic Books, New York.

32. Mason, J. W. (1975): A historical view of the stress field. *J. Hum. Stress*, 1:22-36.

33. McGaugh, W., Silverman, A., and Bogdonoff, M. (1968): Patterns of fat mobilization in field dependent and independent subjects. *Psychosom. Med.*, 27:245-256.

34. Miller, L. H., Harris, L. C., Van Riezen, H., and Kastin, A. J. (1976): A neuropeptide influence on attention and memory in man. *Pharmacol. Biochem. Behav. (Suppl.)*, 5:17-21.

35. Miller, L., Kastin, A., Sandman, C., Fink, M., and VanVeen, W.

(1974): Polypeptide influences on attention, memory and anxiety in man. In: *Pharmacology, Biochemistry and Behavior,
Vol. 2*, pp. 663-668. Ankho International, Inc., Phoenix.

36. Miller, M., Barranda, E., Dean, M., and Brush, R. (1976):
Does the rat with hereditary diabetes insipidus have impaired
avoidance learning and/or performance. *Pharmacol. Biochem.
Behav. (Suppl.)*, 5:35-40.

37. Panksepp, J., Reilly, P., Bishop, P., Meeker, R., Vilberg, T.,
and Kastin, A. (1976): Effects of alpha-MSH on motivation,
vigilance and brain respiration. *Pharmacol. Biochem. Behav.
(Suppl.)*, 5:59-64.

38. Pillsbury, J., Meyerowitz, S., Salzman, L. F., and Satran, R.
(1967): EEG correlates of perceptual style. *Psychosom. Med.*,
29:441-449.

39. Rall, T. W. (1972): Role of adenosine 3',5' monophosphate
(cyclic AMP) in actions of catecholamines. *Pharmacol. Rev.*,
24:399-409.

40. Renaud, L. P., Martin, J. B., and Brazeau, P. (1977): Hypothalamic releasing factors: Physiological evidence for a regulatory action on central neurons and pathways for their distribution in brain. *(This volume.)*

41. Rigter, H., Janssens-Elbertse, R., and van Riezen, H. (1977):
Reversal of amnesia by an orally active ACTH 4-10 analog.
(This volume.)

42. Rodbell, M. (1972): Polypeptide receptor mechanisms in amino
acids and polypeptides in neuronal function. *Neurosci. Res.
Prog. Bull.*, 10:183-185.

43. Rose, R. M. (1976): Statement included in *Report of the
President's Biomedical Research Panel*, April 30, 1976, Department of Health, Education and Welfare Publication No. (OS)76-
500.

44. Sandman, C., George, J., Walker, B., Nolan, J. and Kastin, A.
(1976): The heptapeptide MSH/ACTH 4-10 enhances attention in
the mentally retarded. *Pharmacol. Biochem. Behav. (Suppl.)*,
5:23-28.

45. Sawyer, W., Munsick, R. and van Dyke, H. (1960): Antidiuretic hormone. *Circulation*, 21:1027-1037.

46. Schally, A. and Guillemin, R. (1963): Isolation and chemical characterization of a beta-CRF from pig posterior pituitary glands. *Proc. Soc. Exp. Biol. Med.*, 112:1014-1017.

47. Selye, H. (1963): *The Wisdom of the Body*. W. W. Norton and
Company, New York.

48. Severs, W. and Daniels-Severs, R. (1973): Effects of angio-
tensin on the central nervous system. In: *Pharmacological
Reveiws*, Vol. 25 #3, pp. 415-448. Williams and Wilkins,
Baltimore.

49. Silverman, A. J. (1971): Perception, personality and brain
lateralization. In: *Proceedings Vth World Congress of Psychiatry*, Mexico City.

50. Silverman, A. J., Adevai, G., and McGaugh, W. (1966): Some
relationships between handedness and perception. *J. Psychosom. Res.*, 10:151-158.

51. Silverman, A. J., and McGaugh, W. (1971): Personality, stress and venous flow rates. *J. Psychosom. Res.*, 15:315-322.
52. Silverman, A. J., McGaugh, W., and Bogdonoff, M. (1967): Perceptual correlates of the physiological response to insulin. *Psychosom. Med.*, 29:252-264.
53. Sokolov, E. (1960): Neuronal models and the orienting reflex. In: *Central Nervous System and Behavior: Transactions of 3d Conference*, edited by M. Brazier, Josiah Macey Jr. Foundation, New York.
54. Sokolov, E. (1963): *Perception and the Conditioned Reflex*. Pergamon Press, New York.
55. Sousa-Poza, J., Rohrberg, R., Bellabarba, D., and Ruest, P. (1976): Physiological concomitants (I^{131} uptake) of field dependence. *Psychosom. Med.*, 38:19-26.
56. Strand, F. L. (1975): The influence of hormones on the nervous system. *Bioscience*, 25:568-577.
57. Ungar, G. (1975): Peptides and behavior. *Int. Rev. Neurobiol.*, 17:37-60.
58. Urban, I., Lopes da Silva, F. H., Storm Van Leeuwen, W., and de Wied, D. (1974): A frequency shift in the hippocampal theta activity: An electrical correlate of central action of ACTH analogues in the dog. *Brain Res.*, 69:361-365.
59. Wilson, W., Johnson, J., and Feist, F. (1964): Thyroid hormone and brain function. *Electroencephalogr. Clin. Neurophysiol.*, 16:329-331.
60. van Wimersma Greidanus, TjB., Bohus, B., and de Wied, D.: The role of vasopressin in memory processes. In: *Hormones, Homeostasis of the Brain; Progress in Brain Research, Vol. 42*, edited by W. H. Gispen, TjB. van Wimersma Greidanus, B. Bohus and D. de Wied, pp. 135-141. Elsevier, New York.
61. van Wimersma Greidanus, TjB. and de Wied, D. (1976): The dorsal hippocampus as a site of action of neuropeptides on avoidance behavior. *Pharmacol. Biochem. Behav.(Suppl.)*, 5: 29-34.
62. van Wimersma Greidanus, Tjb. and de Wied, D. (1971): Effects of systemic and intracerebral administration of two opposite acting ACTH-related peptides on extinction of conditioned avoidance behavior. *Neuroendocrinology*, 7:291-301.
63. Witkin, H. (1962): *Psychological Differentiation*. Wiley, New York.
64. Witkin, H. and Altman, P. (1967): Cognitive style. *Int. J. Neurol.*, 6:119-137.

Subject Index